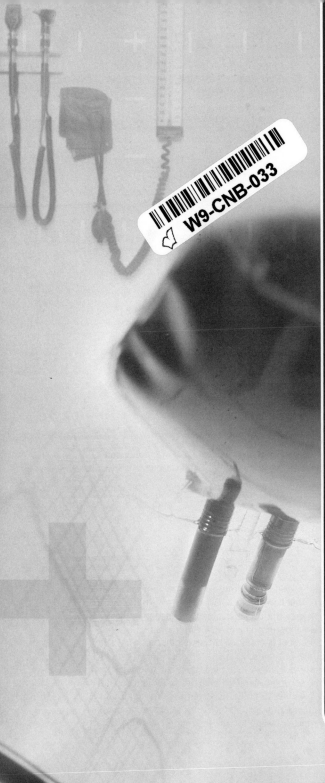

AMERICAN
ASSOCIATION
of CRITICAL-CARE
NURSES

AACN
Protocols for Practice

Care of
Mechanically
Ventilated Patients

Second Edition

Edited by
Suzanne M. Burns
RN, MSN, RRT, ACNP, CCRN,
FAAN, FCCM, FAANP
University of Virginia Health System
Charlottesville, Virginia

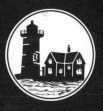

JONES AND BARTLETT PUBLISHERS

Sudbury, Massachusetts

BOSTON   TORONTO   LONDON   SINGAPORE

World Headquarters

Jones and Bartlett Publishers
40 Tall Pine Drive
Sudbury, MA 01776
978-443-5000
info@jbpub.com
www.jbpub.com

Jones and Bartlett Publishers Canada
6339 Ormindale Way
Mississauga, Ontario L5V 1J2
CANADA

Jones and Bartlett Publishers International
Barb House, Barb Mews
London W6 7PA
UK

Jones and Bartlett's books and products are available through most bookstores and online booksellers. To contact Jones and Bartlett Publishers directly, call 800-832-0034, fax 978-443-8000, or visit our website, www.jbpub.com.

Substantial discounts on bulk quantities of Jones and Bartlett's publications are available to corporations, professional associations, and other qualified organizations. For details and specific discount information, contact the special sales department at Jones and Bartlett via the above contact information or send an email to specialsales@jbpub.com.

Library of Congress Cataloging-in-Publication Data
AACN protocols for practice. Care of mechanically ventilated patients
/ [edited by] Suzanne Burns.
 p. ; cm.
Includes bibliographical references.
ISBN-13: 978-0-7637-4080-1
ISBN-10: 0-7637-4080-2
1. Respiratory intensive care. 2. Respiratory therapy. 3. Respiration, Artificial. 4. Respirators (Medical equipment)
5. Critical care nursing. I. Burns, Suzanne M. II. American Association of Critical-Care Nurses. III. Title: American Association of Critical-Care Nurses protocols for practice. IV. Title: Protocols for practice. V. Title: Care of mechanically ventilated patients.
[DNLM: 1. Respiration, Artificial--nursing. 2. Clinical Protocols. 3. Nursing Care--methods. 4. Respiration, Artificial-methods. WY 163 A111 2006]
RC735.R48A33 2006
616.2'0046--dc22
                    2006006211
6048

The authors, editor, and publisher have made every effort to provide accurate information. However, they are not responsible for errors, omissions, or for any outcomes related to the use of the contents of this book and take no responsibility for the use of the products described. Treatments and side effects described in this book may not be applicable to all patients; likewise, some patients may require a dose or experience a side effect that is not described herein. The reader should confer with his or her own physician regarding specific treatments and side effects. Drugs and medical devices are discussed that may have limited availability controlled by the Food and Drug Administration (FDA) for use only in a research study or clinical trial. The drug information presented has been derived from reference sources, recently published data, and pharmaceutical research data. Research, clinical practice, and government regulations often change the accepted standard in this field. When consideration is being given to use of any drug in the clinical setting, the health care provider or reader is responsible for determining FDA status of the drug, reading the package insert, reviewing prescribing information for the most up-to-date recommendations on dose, precautions, and contraindications, and determining the appropriate usage for the product. This is especially important in the case of drugs that are new or seldom used.

Production Credits
Acquisitions Editor: Kevin Sullivan
Associate Editor: Amy Sibley
Production Director: Amy Rose
Associate Production Editor: Daniel Stone
Marketing Managers: Emily Ekle and Sophie Fleck
Manufacturing and Inventory Coordinator: Amy Bacus
Composition: Jason Miranda, Spoke & Wheel
Cover Design: Timothy Dziewit
Cover Image: © Photos.com
Printing and Binding: Courier-Stoughton
Cover Printing: Courier-Stoughton

Printed in the United States of America
10 09 08 07 06   10 9 8 7 6 5 4 3 2 1

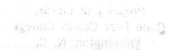

Contents

Chapter 5   Nutritional Support for Mechanically Ventilated Patients   191

Carol Ress Parrish

Joe Krenitsky

Kate Willcutts

Chapter 6   Sedation and Neuromuscular Blockade in Mechanically Ventilated Patients   253

Jill Luer

About the Protocols

Recognizing that clinical practice must continually evolve to keep up with current science, busy bedside clinicians and advanced practice nurses asked the American Association of Critical-Care Nurses for help in using available research to change acute and critical care practice. They asked for studies to be translated into a format in which findings were demystified and their strength evaluated. They would use this tool to advocate for necessary changes in practice because such changes were based on the latest evidence and because they carried the weight of the association's credibility and influence.

In 1994 the American Association of Critical-Care Nurses began developing research-based practice protocols as one of several responses to this request. AACN's *Protocols for Practice* are designed to provide clinicians at the point of care with the latest patient care research findings in a format that is easy to understand and integrate into clinical practice. The protocols outline the latest thinking on how to best provide care when using technology and in specific patient care situations. Experts in each topic area develop a concise list of recommendations that are appropriate to incorporate into practice routines for patients with a particular situation or device. Recommendations are based on a comprehensive review of the science related to the situation or technology and include only those that are based on research and/or expert consensus positions.

PROTOCOL STRUCTURE

Clinical recommendations represent the core of each protocol. Recommendations are organized in a logical order, usually chronologically, starting with the time before a device is used or an occurrence begins and continuing until after the device is discontinued or the occurrence ends. Recommendations address the following:

Selection of Patients: including indications, contraindications, and special considerations for use, such as age, physiologic status, and intermittent or continuous monitoring. Depending on the device or procedure, a clinical decision-making algorithm may be provided.

Application of Device and Initial Use: where appropriate, important considerations during device or procedure application, such as patient preparation, preapplication calibration, and preparation of application site.

Ongoing Monitoring: important considerations for maintaining the patient during the procedure or for monitoring the device, such as monitoring frequency and clinical factors influencing accuracy and positioning.

Prevention of Complications: key strategies for prevention or early identification of complications, such as infection, skin breakdown, pain, or discomfort.

Quality Control: requirements to maintain accuracy of the device under circumstances of normal use.

Recommendation Level: each recommendation is rated according to the level of information available to support the statement. A scale ranging from I to VI represents progressively stronger levels of scientific basis for the recommendation. Ratings are defined as:

I Manufacturer's recommendation only.
II Theory-based. No research data to support recommendations. Recommendations from expert consensus groups may exist.
III Laboratory data only. No clinical data to support recommendations.
IV Limited clinical studies to support recommendations.
V Clinical studies in more than 1 or 2 different populations and situations to support recommendations.
VI Clinical studies in a variety of patient populations and situations to support recommendations.

Along with clinical recommendations, each protocol includes these elements:

- **Case Study:** One or more brief case studies describing a common patient care situation related to the protocol topic.
- **General Description:** general description of the device or patient care situation addressed by the protocol.

- **Accuracy:** for medical devices, a general description of the accuracy of the device, including precision and bias, with range of accuracy given when variation exists between models and/or manufacturers.
- **Competency:** specific skill or knowledge verification that is important in determining a nurse's competency.
- **Ethical Considerations:** ethical implications or considerations related to the device or patient care situation.
- **Occupational Hazards:** hazards that may be associated with a device or patient care situation, such as electrical safety or exposure to blood-borne pathogens.
- **Future Research:** suggested areas of future research needed to strengthen the research basis of practice related to the protocol content. This may include key points of research methodology important for clinical studies in this category, such as dependent variables to be measured or confounding variables to be considered.
- **Annotated Bibliography:** summary of important aspects of key studies on the topic.
- **Suggested Readings:** resources for additional information on the protocol topic.

USING THE PROTOCOLS

The protocols are designed to guide care in a variety of acute and critical care settings, including intensive care, progressive care, and medical-surgical units. Selected topics may also be appropriate for long-term and home care. Clinicians should select those elements that apply to their practice setting.

The protocols are not intended to be used as a step-by-step procedure or comprehensive education resource alone. For this reason, each protocol includes additional information sources. Where available and appropriate, protocols include other essential information such as details about the proper application of devices or patient management algo-

rithms. Clinicians may consider first using a protocol to assess the topic's current status in their practice. From this baseline assessment, they can evaluate the merits of changing current practice drawing from the protocol's evaluation of evidence that would support a change in practice.

Protocols will be valuable adjuncts in nursing education because they succinctly summarize the state of the science on a specific topic and identify areas for future research. Nursing students are often exposed to wide variation in practice in equally varied clinical settings. Protocols help to identify whether a variation is based on science.

Experienced researchers will find the protocols useful in identifying areas of inquiry. The evidence supporting each action in a protocol is rated according to its level of scientific information. Lower level ratings indicate there is insufficient research to support a strong scientific base. Users with limited expertise in research methods will find that the protocols accurately summarize the research base using a user-friendly, concise approach with minimal jargon. They have been reviewed for scientific merit, readability, and clinical usefulness as of the time of publication.

AACN PRACTICE ALERTS

Recognizing that clinical practice is ever evolving, the American Association of Critical-Care Nurses issues practice alerts as a real-time complement to the protocols. Practice alerts are succinct dynamic directives supported by authoritative evidence to ensure excellence in practice and a safe and humane work environment. The alerts address nursing and multidisciplinary activities of importance to acutely and critically ill patients and environments in order to close the gap between research and practice, provide guidance in changing practice, standardize practice, and identify and inform about advances and new trends in the science. Practice alerts are posted at www.aacn.org.

Acknowledgments

Thanks to the scientific and clinical reviewers who assisted in developing the second edition of these protocols:

- Airway Management—Jill Malen, Robert Virag, John J. Gallagher
- Invasive and Noninvasive Modes and Methods of Mechanical Ventilation—Kathleen M. Stacy, Kathryn Von Rueden
- Weaning from Mechanical Ventilation—Wes Ely, Franklin McGuire, Rose Lewis, Charles Fisher
- Beyond the ICU: Home Care Management of Patients Receiving Mechanical Ventilation—Zara Brenner, Diane M. Salipante, Maureen A. Seckel
- Nutritional Support for Mechanically Ventilated Patients—Charles Mueller, Norma Metheny
- Sedation and Neuromuscular Blockade—Rebecca Haynes Hockman, Richard Arbour

Thanks to Le Banh, MS, RD, CNSD; Theresa Fessler, MS, RD, CNSD; Emily Gasser, RD, CNSD; Amy Radigan, RD, CNSD; Sherrie Walker, RD; and Nicole Waldron, RD, for their contributions to Chapter 5, Nutritional Support.

Thanks to the AACN national office staff, whose assistance was invaluable to many aspects of the project: Marilyn Herigstad, Justine Medina, and Teresa Wavra.

Special appreciation to Marianne Chulay, who developed and implemented the practice protocols initiative for the American Association of Critical-Care Nurses, and to Barbara Gill MacArthur, executive editor for this series.

Contributors

Suzanne M. Burns, RN, MSN, RRT, ACNP, CCRN, FAAN, FCCM, FAANP
Professor of Nursing, Acute and Specialty Care
School of Nursing
Advanced Practice Nurse 2, MICU
University of Virginia Health System
Charlottesville, Virginia

Margaret M. Ecklund, RN, MS, CCRN, APRN-BC
Clinician VI—Pulmonary Medicine
Rochester General Hospital
Rochester, New York

Robert E. St. John, RN, MSN, RRT
Director Clinical Research
Nellcor, a unit of Mallinckrodt/Tyco Healthcare
Adjunct Clinical Instructor of Nursing
St. Louis University School of Nursing
St. Louis, Missouri

Joe Krenitsky, MS, RD
Nutrition Support Specialist
University of Virginia Health System
Charlottesville, Virginia

Jill Luer, PharmD
Senior Medical Director
Helix Medical Communications
San Mateo, California

Carol Rees Parrish, MS, RD
Nutrition Support Specialist
University of Virginia Health System
Digestive Health Center of Excellence
Charlottesville, Virginia

Lynelle N. B. Pierce, RN, MS, CCRN
Critical Care Clinical Nurse Specialist
University of Kansas Hospital
Kansas City, Kansas

Maureen A. Seckel, RN, MSN, APRN-BC, CCRN
Clinical Nurse Specialist, Medical Critical Care/Pulmonary
Christiana Care Health Services
Newark, Delaware

Kate Willcutts, MS RD, CNSD
Assistant Clinical Manager/Nutrition Support Specialist
University of Virginia Hospital
Instructor, School of Nursing
Charlottesville, Virginia

Airway Management

Robert E. St. John, RN, MSN, RRT

Maureen A. Seckel, RN, MSN, APRN-BC, CCRN

Airway Management

CASE STUDY

The family of Mrs Smith, a 72-year-old woman, called 911 after noting she was unable to be aroused. Upon arrival, the paramedics intubated her orally with an 8-mm inner-diameter endotracheal (ET) tube. She had a 3-day history of fever, lethargy, and complaints of a cough. Her medical history included smoking 50 packs of cigarettes a year, chronic obstructive pulmonary disease (COPD), congestive heart failure (CHF), and chronic atrial fibrillation. Upon arrival at the medical center, she was volume resuscitated in the emergency department, treatment was initiated for severe sepsis and pneumonia, and she was transferred to the medical ICU on mechanical ventilation. Over the next 3 days, Mrs Smith improved and she was able to be weaned off her vasopressors. Her neurological status was also improving, and she was now alert and oriented and able to communicate through gestures to the medical staff and her family. She was receiving intravenous fentanyl 25 µg every 2 hours as needed for pain and was on a continuous infusion of propofol at 35 µg/kg per minute for sedation.

Mrs Smith required periodic suctioning, which yielded moderate amounts of white to yellow secretions. Although the need for suctioning was assessed every hour, she only required suctioning (via a closed in-line suction catheter) every 2 to 3 hours during the day. Mrs Smith was oxygenated with 100% oxygen via the ventilator's 100% button before, during, and after suctioning.

On day 4 of Mrs Smith's admission, the plan of care dictated a weaning readiness assessment during her holiday from sedation and the possibility of extubation. The nurse explained to Mrs Smith what the plan was and also communicated with the respiratory therapist to coordinate a time. The propofol was turned off, and Mrs Smith continued to be alert and oriented. Prior to performing a weaning assess-

ment, Mrs Smith asked for the bedpan. As the nurse and her colleague were removing the bedpan, they noted she was also incontinent and quickly worked to clean her by lowering the head of bed and turning her side-to-side to remove the linens. Mrs Smith quickly became increasingly agitated and started pulling at her ET tube.

The nurse raised the head of the bed and explained to Mrs Smith the importance of not pulling on the ET tube. Mrs Smith continued to be agitated and twisted and turned in the bed. The nurse restrained Mrs Smith after explaining the importance of not pulling on the ET tube and continued to assess and attempt to calm her. Mrs Smith became increasingly tachypneic and tachycardic, and her oxygen saturation level, as estimated by pulse oximetry (SpO_2), dropped to 85% from a baseline of 94%.

The nurse quickly preoxygenated and suctioned Mrs. Smith who was coughing and gagging. The first suction pass removed a large, thick, green mucus plug. The respiratory therapist came in the room and began to assist. Because Mrs Smith's SpO_2 level was still 85% to 88%, the therapist decided to hyperventilate the patient with a hand-held resuscitation bag with a positive end-expiratory pressure (PEEP) valve and 100% oxygen prior to resuming suction attempts. The nurse suctioned with a 14-Fr catheter, while the therapist "bagged" the patient. Both continually reassured the patient. After several minutes Mrs Smith appeared more relaxed, and her heart rate, respiratory rate, and oxygen saturation returned to her normal baseline levels. The nurse notified the physician, and Mrs Smith received an additional respiratory treatment, was restarted on her propofol, and the plan was revised to rest for a few hours and reassess for weaning readiness and possible extubation later that day.

The significant respiratory compromise illustrated in this case demonstrates the importance of airway management in the critically ill patient. Mrs Smith had a history of COPD and excessive mucus production. Plus the presence of a cuffed ET tube decreased the patient's ability to clear secretions effectively. These factors contributed to her inability to tolerate changes in airway resistance caused by the secretions and the resultant increased work of breathing.

The first response to agitation in any critically ill patient is to assess for a possible physiologic cause such as hypoxemia. The use of restraints and/or sedatives is an adjunct to providing safe airway management and should not supersede assessment skills for the cause of agitation and respiratory distress.

Thorough airway assessment and management are critical to any acutely ill patient. The practitioners in this case communicated and worked together to rapidly assess, treat, and formulate a plan to provide care and maintain patient safety.

GENERAL DESCRIPTION

Airway management is a priority for any critically ill patient. Many critically ill patients require insertion of an artificial airway, such as an ET or a tracheostomy tube. These artificial airways are typically used to provide a patent airway when the patient is unable to manage his or her own secretions and/or to provide positive pressure mechanical ventilation. Artificial airways are used for both short- and long-term airway management. Endotracheal tubes are the most common type of short-term artificial airway used in critical care. These tubes can be placed either nasally or orally by skilled personnel.

Tracheostomy tubes, which are generally used for longer-term airway management, may also be necessary when upper airway obstruction or trauma prohibits the use of an ET tube. Recent information also suggests that early tracheostomy in patients who may require prolonged mechanical ventilation (longer than 10 days) may improve outcomes. Both ET and tracheostomy tubes are available in a variety of sizes and materials. Special features are commonly available. The choice of tube is based on individual patient requirements. Appendices 1A, 1B, and 1C provide more information on tube selection.

PERFORMANCE CHARACTERISTICS: TECHNICAL STANDARDS FOR TRACHEAL TUBES

Manufacturers of ET and tracheostomy tubes conform to a variety of regulations governing production standards. The American Society for Testing and Materials International, (ASTM) a nonprofit organization, provides a forum for producers, physicians, and allied health care providers to develop standards for artificial airway devices and other anesthesia and respiratory equipment. Decisions are reached by group consensus; producers' compliance with these standards is voluntary. The committee on anesthesia and respiratory equipment standards, known as F29, addresses 5 aspects of ET tube construction: general requirements for materials used in the manufacturing of tracheal tubes, cuff and tubing characteristics, permissible dimensions of tracheal tubes and connectors, required markings, and product packaging and labeling.

The ASTM F29 committee has been delegated by the American National Standards Institute (ANSI) to represent the United States in the development and harmonization of international standards by the International Standards Organization (ISO) technical committee 121. Many ISO standards, such as the ET tube and tracheostomy tube standards, have been adopted as American National Standards, replacing older ASTM standards in this process.

The US Food and Drug Administration (FDA) Center for Devices and Radiological Health encourages compliance by recognizing certain standards in the review of premarket device submissions. The FDA believes that conformance with recognized consensus standards can provide a reasonable assurance of safety and effectiveness for many applicable aspects of medical devices and may help establish the substantial equivalence of a new device to a legally marketed predicate device.

The FDA-recognized standard for ET tubes and connectors is ISO 5361. Two recognized standards for tracheostomy tubes are ISO 5366-1 for adult tracheostomy tubes and connectors and ISO 5366-3 for pediatric tracheostomy tubes and connectors.

Materials

Any material intended for insertion into a patient must be biocompatible and nontoxic to human tissue. Different levels of biocompatibility testing are required for each type of device depending on the area and duration of tissue contact. ISO 10993 standard regarding biological evaluation of medical devices identifies a testing matrix for 3 levels of device categories consisting of 8 levels of body contact, further categorized as long- or short-contact duration with the body. These device categories are then aligned with a checklist of 12 levels of biological effect testing, including cytotoxicity, sensitization, irritation, hemocompatibility, and reproductive or developmental changes.

One well-accepted test method determines cytotoxicity of a material. This technique can be performed in vitro by exposing cells grown in glass flasks filled with nutrient fluids that were exposed to the materials. After several days the cells are examined microscopically for cellular damage. Another well-accepted method for assessing material toxicity is via rabbit implantation: a technique that involves implanting strips of the tube material in question into the muscle of a rabbit. After several days, depending on the duration that the material is intended for use, the tissue surrounding the center portion of each implant is examined for hemorrhage, film, or encapsulation. If there is no significant tissue reaction, then the material is deemed safe.

The FDA recognizes certain sections of the ISO 10993 standard but also provides further guidance on these requirements in their own guidance document known as the Bluebook Memo G95-1.

Surface Characteristics

The external surface of the ET tube should generally be smooth. Sharp points or rough edges should not be found, particularly on the patient end. The internal surface of the tube should likewise be generally smooth. These characteristics are important, and minimize the risk of mucosal damage during insertion or with long-term use of the tube.

Rigidity

Endotracheal tubes must be stiff enough to be easily inserted but must soften sufficiently at body temperature to conform to the patient's airway anatomy. The degree of softness should not allow the tube to kink. Certain specialty tubes and those composed of materials (eg, silicone) that can kink easily may be reinforced with metal wire for greater stability. This is also important to know in certain clinical situations—for example, an ET or tracheostomy tube that contains magnetically permeable metal components should not be used during MRI (magnetid resonance imaging) studies. Most cuffed tubes contain stainless steel springs with low magnetic permeability. Clinicians should always follow the manufacturer's directions for use for specific indications when using such tubes.

Lumen Integrity

Endotracheal tubes must be flexible yet resilient enough to prevent kinking or collapsing that might be caused by an inflated cuff (a rare complication). This complication is clinically recognized by a sudden increase in airway resistance coincident with cuff inflation. Single-use ET tubes with low-pressure cuffs are unlikely to cause this type of problem.

Balloon Cuffs

The balloon cuff is typically designed in such a way that it has low-pressure, high-volume characteristics as well as a cross-sectional diameter larger than its tracheal diameter. The reason that a low sealing pressure design feature is desirable is because high-pressure cuffs have been associated with serious tracheal complications (eg, tracheoesophageal fistula, tracheal stenosis, tracheal-innominate artery fistula). In addition, the low-pressure, high-volume cuffs have also proved to be more effective than the high-pressure, low-volume cuffs in preventing aspiration. Lastly, balloon cuffs should inflate symmetrically and not leak. Ideally, manufacturers should perform a leak test on every ET and tracheostomy tube before final packaging. The cuff should also be checked by the clinician prior to inserting the tube in the patient.

Required Product Markings

Each tracheal tube should be marked with the inner diameter (ID), outer diameter (OD), and designation of whether the tube is intended for oral, nasal, or either insertion. The marking materials used should be nontoxic, and the markings should remain clearly legible during use. The length of the tube from the patient end is usually marked on the tube in centimeters. The manufacturer always includes its name or trademark on the tube, and a radiopaque marker is usually placed at the patient end of the tube or along the entire tube length.

For tracheostomy tubes, the inner and outer diameters, product size and style designation, and name manufacturer are clearly marked on the tube neck flange or plate. The tracheostomy tube must have radiopaque qualities; this is accomplished by using radiopaque materials (eg, metal, polyvinyl chloride [PVC]) to manufacture the tracheostomy tube or by placing some type of radiopaque marker at the patient end of the tube or along the entire length of the outer cannula.

Packaging and Labeling

The manufacturer should provide appropriate warnings for standard uses of the product. For example, a common warning with cuffed ET tubes might include a statement about the effects of anesthetic gases on cuff volume and pressure and about the injurious effects of high temperature, ultraviolet light, and fluorescent lighting on stored tubes. Examples of other package information are cleaning instructions (if applicable), maximum length of use before replacement is needed, certain clinical limitations, and other precautions.

Package information should also state the method of sterility or, if nonsterile, appropriate directions for sterilization. Disposable tubes should be clearly marked for single use only; reusable tubes should include the necessary information for cleaning and sterilization. The product's outer package or carton should be clearly labeled with size and style. Other important data frequently seen on packaging materials are manufacturer name, date, lot number, and expiration date. The expiration date is particularly important as the manufacturer cannot guarantee proper and safe performance of the tube beyond this time.

COMPETENCY

Airway management is a collaborative function shared by nurses, respiratory therapists, and physicians. Along with familiarity of the facility or agency policies and procedures, basic competencies required by all disciplines include these abilities:

- Assist with the insertion or repositioning of artificial airways in emergency and nonemergency situations, including securing the tubes properly, and monitoring untoward events during and after the procedure.

- Determine adequacy of airway patency, airway positioning, and ventilation while on the unit, during patient position changes, and during patient transport.
- Maintain airway patency using common interventions (eg, ET suctioning, humidification, medication administration, inner cannula care, or securing tubes).
- Identify and prevent complications associated with artificial airways (eg, infection, skin breakdown, unplanned extubation, or decannulation).
- Facilitate communication in short-term or long-term airway patients.

ETHICAL CONSIDERATIONS

As the technology of critical care has increased, so have the ethical considerations.

Ethical issues related to airway management generally focus on several ethical principles. These include beneficence (doing good), nonmalfeasance (doing no harm), patient autonomy, and moral conflict. Patient autonomy, or the right to determine what will be done for one's self, also implies decisional capacity. Decisional capacity is the ability to comprehend information and to evaluate risks and consequences and to be able to communicate wishes, desires, and understanding of risks and benefits. This may be difficult to determine in a critical care environment because of many factors: language, cultural, and communication barriers; emotional distress; and decreased sensorium and delirium due to critical illness and medications. Surrogates may be chosen by the patient and often include family members or friends to assist in decision making. It may also be necessary for the court system to appoint a legal guardian is some cases. Surrogates serve as advocates to reflect the patient's wishes. Moral conflict can result from differing values, positions, and conflicts between the medical team and the patient and or surrogate. For example, the health care team may struggle with providing care they feel is not beneficial to the patient. The hospital's ethics consultation service is helpful in these cases and should be contacted when ethical conflicts occur.

Physical restraint use is not required for all intubated patients or those with an artificial airway. However, restraints in the ICU are at times necessary to avoid the consequences of abrupt self-extubation or to prevent injury of the staff, as in the case of a combative patient. Some moral conflict is inevitable when patient autonomy is overruled by the caregivers for patient and/or caregiver safety.

The decision of the patient (or surrogate) to permit placement of an artificial airway such as an ET tube or tracheostomy for the purpose of airway protection or mechanical ventilatory support is often difficult, particularly in long-term or chronically, critically ill patients. Issues of withholding treatment often surround decisions related to tracheostomy placement, intubation, extubation, and/or reintubation (eg, when a gravely ill patient fails extubation).

Often the issues result in conflict between caregivers, patients, and families. In many instances, patients have an advance directive that provides some guidance to the health care team about desired treatments and procedures should the patient become seriously ill and be unable to communicate. However, most advance directives are framed to address patient wishes only in a terminal condition or permanent vegetative state. The potential for moral conflict and distress increases when an advance directive, durable power of attorney for health care, or prior discussion of the patient's wishes are not available. Sometimes, when the medical outcome is ambiguous (ie, not terminal but very poor prognosis), the patient and/or surrogate may desire all aggressive measures despite recommendations of the health care team. Additional conflict may occur when the surrogate opposes the patient's wishes or the health care team disagrees about withdrawing care. The institution's ethics consultation service should be used as a resource in circumstances of unresolved moral conflict; it can also provide support to the patients, surrogates, and the health care team.

OCCUPATIONAL HAZARDS

Staff working with artificial airways are at high risk for exposure to organisms that are airborne or spread by contact, for example, tuberculosis, bacteria including antibiotic-resistant organisms, hepatitis, herpes, and so on. However, these hazards can be minimized by effective hand washing before and after patient contact, gloving before contact with any respiratory equipment, and wearing masks and protective eye wear per institution protocol. Additionally, the use of closed in-line suction catheters, closed ventilator circuits with water traps, heated wires to decrease moisture in ventilator tubing, and other hospital policies can help to decrease exposure.

FUTURE RESEARCH

Although numerous studies have been done to determine the risk factors associated with ventilator-associated pneumonia (VAP), prospective, randomized controlled trials (RCT) are necessary to resolve outstanding issues. (See Annotated Bibliography: 4, 5, 7, 8). The impact of oral care on the psychological well-being of the patient is known and theorized to help prevent VAP. However, research is needed to define what constitutes adequate oral hygiene and whether the risk of VAP is decreased if the measures are employed. Studies have demonstrated a decreased risk of VAP with the prophylactic use of chlorhexidine in select populations, but more studies using controls are needed before the results can be generalized.

Other variables that affect VAP are airway placement and tube type. The use of oral ET tubes instead of nasal has been demonstrated to prevent both hospital-acquired sinusitis and VAP. Continuous airway subglottic suctioning (CASS) tubes have been shown to delay or prevent early onset of VAP in patients who require ETs for more than 72 hours. But, CASS tubes do not appear to similarly affect late-onset VAP. Further, the use of the tubes has not been associated with positive outcomes such as decreased mortality, length of hospital and ICU stay, or duration of mechanical ventilation. Tracheostomy CASS tubes are also now available. Further research is needed to determine what, if any, impact these tubes will have on late-onset VAP. Additional airway enhancements such as antiseptic-impregnated ET tubes are also available and need to be studied.

Although suctioning is a basic tenet of airway management, research is still needed to substantiate the efficacy of traditional techniques. (See Annotated Bibliography: 1, 3, 6). Studies are needed to explore deep suctioning versus shallow technique and whether directional catheters designed for either right or left bronchus placement are effective and affect patient outcomes. The use of closed in-line suctioning has not demonstrated a decreased risk of VAP but does prevent loss of lung volume and PEEP along with reducing risk of caregiver exposure. Hyperoxygenation with 100% F_{IO_2} is a routine practice, yet it remains unclear whether this practice is warranted in patients with normal cardiopulmonary function (eg, postoperative patients). Physiologic data is available that demonstrates that saline instillation before suctioning decreases oxygen saturation, causes patient distress, and increases coughing. However, there is only anecdotal evidence suggesting that saline *thins* secretions despite widespread belief that it really does. It is also unclear whether the use of saline results in an increased risk of VAP. Randomized controlled trials are needed to definitively answer many of these questions.

Interventions to prevent unplanned extubation are important to determine. It is known that the use of physical restraints does not prevent all self-extubations. Alternatives to restraints such as ICU environmental options that decrease stimuli, the use of diversionary activities such as music and guided imagery, increased family access, and creative patient communication devices are important to test to determine their usefulness in the intubated patient.

Additionally, research has demonstrated that delirium is an often unrecognized complication of critical illness and can be a contributing factor in self-extubation. Continued work is needed on the prevention, assessment, and treatment of delirium. Recent consensus statements and research have shown that sedation holidays reduce the complications of critical illness from pharmacological interventions, reduce ventilator days, and do not increase the self-extubation rate. Further research is needed to determine strategies that balance appropriate care with patient safety and reduce the risk of complications.

Many aspects of tracheostomy care and stomal care require further study with large groups of patients. The optimal time for transitioning from ET to tracheostomy tube is unknown. Studies suggest early tracheostomy may offer benefits over delayed tracheostomy in patients for whom mechanical ventilation for longer than 10 to 14 days is predicted. Unfortunately, what determines *early* has not been consistently defined in the research, and additional work is needed.

Numerous materials are used to make tracheostomy tubes (metal, silicone, PVC, and so on). To date no RCTs have been accomplished comparing these materials in terms of patient comfort, complications, and ease of use. Additional studies need to be done challenging or supporting the practice of routine changing or replacing of inner cannulas. It is theorized that changing the inner cannula prevents occlusion and bacterial colonization, yet only one study has tested this hypothesis to date and found it lacking. Several tracheostomy manufacturers currently produce tubes without inner cannulas, making the point moot.

Lastly, research is needed on how best to care for the tracheostomy stoma. (See Annotated Bibliography: 2). There is little research supporting current practices of stoma care, including routine tracheostomy tube changes. In addition, the tradition of "downsizing" tracheostomy tubes is just that, tradition. To date, no data exist that clarify the necessity and/or timing of the practice.

SUGGESTED READINGS

American Association of Critical-Care Nurses. Ventilator-associated pneumonia [AACN practice alert]. Available at: http://www.aacn.org/AACN/practiceAlert.nsf/Files/VAP/$file/VAP.pdf. Accessed November 16, 2005.

ASTM International. Available at: http://www.astm.org. Accessed November 16, 2005.

ASTM International. Committee F29 on Anesthestic and Respiratory Equipment. Available at: http:// www.astm .org/cgi-bin/SoftCart.exe/COMMIT/COMMITTEE /F29.htm?L+mystore+fmit1039+1132203609. Accessed November 16, 2005.

Lynn-McHale Wiegand DJ, Carlson KK, eds. *AACN Procedure Manual for Critical Care.* 5th ed. Philadelphia, Pa: Elsevier; 2005:1–86.

Dezfulian C, Shohania K, Collard HR, Kim HM, Matthay MA, Saint S. Subglottic secretion drainage for preventing ventilator-associated pneumonia: a meta-analysis. *Am J Med.* 2005;118:11–18.

US Food and Drug Administration. *Required Biocompatibility Training and Toxicology Profiles for Evaluation of Medical Devices.* May 1, 1995, (G95-1). Available at: http://www.fda.gov/cdrh/g951.html. Accessed November 16, 2005.

Fenstermacher D, Hong D. Mechanical ventilation—what have we learned? *Crit Care Nurs Q.* 2004;27:258–294.

Grap MJ, Munro C, Ashtiani B, Bryant S. Oral care interventions in critical care: frequency and documentation. *Am J Crit Care.* 2003;12:113–119.

Happ MB. Communicating with mechanically ventilated patients: state of the science. *AACN Clin Issues.* 2001;12:247–258.

ASTM International. ANS/ISO 5361-99 *Anaesthetic and Respiratory Equipment—Tracheal Tubes and Connectors Approved as an American National Standard by ASTM International.* Available at: http://www.astm.org/cgi-bin/SoftCart.exe/STORE/filtrexx40.cgi?U+mystore+djmh1197+L+ISO5361+/usr6/htdocs/astm.org/DATABASE.CART/REDLINE_PAGES/ANSISO5361.htm. Accessed November 16, 2005.

ASTM International. ANS/ISO5366.1-00E *Anaesthetic and Respiratory Equipment-Tracheostomy Tubes—Part 1: Tubes and Connectors for Use in Adults Approved as an American National Standard by ASTM International.* Available at: http://www.astm.org/cgi-bin/SoftCart.exe/STORE/filtrexx40.cgi?U+mystore+djmh1197+L+TRACHEOSTOMY+/usr6/htdocs/astm.org/DATABASE.CART/REDLINE_PAGES/ANSISO53661.htm. Accessed November 16, 2005.

ASTM International. ISO 5366.3-03 *Anaesthetic and Respiratory Equipment-Tracheostomy Tubes—Part 3: Paediatric Tracheostomy Tubes.* Available at: http://www.astm.org/cgibin/SoftCart.exe/STORE/filtrexx40.cgi?U+mystore+djmh1197+L+ANAESTHETIC:RESPIRATORY:TRACHEOSTOMY:PART:3+/usr6/htdocs/astm.org/DATABASE.CART/REDLINE_PAGES/ISO53663.htm. Accessed November 16, 2005.

International Organization for Standardization. *Biological Evaluation of Medical Devices:* Parts 1 through 12. Available at: http://www.iso.org/iso/en/StandardsQueryFormHandler.StandardsQueryFormHandler?scope=CATALOGUE&sortOrder=ISO&committee=ALL&isoDocType=ALL&title=true&keyword=10993. Accessed November 17, 2005.

Jacobi J, Fraser GL, Coursin DB, et al. Clinical practice guidelines for the sustained use of sedatives and analgesics in the critically ill adult. *Crit Care Med.* 2002;30:119–141.

Kollef MH. Prevention of hospital-associated pneumonia and ventilator-associated pneumonia. *Crit Care Med.* 2004;32:1396–1405.

Maccioli GA, Dorman T, Brown BR, et al. Clinical practice guidelines for the maintenance of patient physical safety in the intensive care unit: Use of restraining therapies-American College of Critical Care Medicine Task Force 2001-2002. *Crit Care Med.* 2003;31:2665–2676.

Metheny NA, Scallom ME, Edwards SJ. Effect of gastrointestinal motility and feeding tube site on aspiration risk in critically ill patients: a review. *Issues in Pulm Nurs.* 2004:33:131–145.

Oh H, Seo W. A meta-analysis of the effects of various interventions in preventing endotracheal suction-induced hypoxemia. *J Clin Nurs.* 2003;12:912-924.

St. John RE, Malen JF. Contemporary issues in adult tracheostomy management. *Crit Care Nurs Clin N Am.* 2004;16:413-430.

US Department of Health and Human Services, Food and Drug Administration, Center for Devices and Radiological Health, Office of Science and Technology and Office of Device Evaluation. *Recognition and Use of Consensus Standards: Final Guidance for Industry and FDA Staff.* June 20, 2001. Available at: http://www.fda.gov/cdrh/ost/guidance/321.html. Accessed November 17, 2005.

Van Hooser DT. *Airway clearance with closed-system suctioning.* American Association of Critical-Care Nurses Web site. Available at: http://www.aacn.org/pdfLibra.NSF/Files/Airwayweb/$file/Airwayweb.pdf. Accessed November 17, 2005.

CLINICAL RECOMMENDATIONS

The rating scales for the Level of Recommendation range from I to IV, with levels indicated as follows: I, manufactuer's recommendations only; II, theory based, no research data to support recommendations; recommendations from expert consensus group may exist; III, laboratory data only, no clinical data to support recommendations; IV, limited clinical studies to support recommendations; V, clinical studies in more than 1 or 2 different populations and situations to support recommendations; VI, clinical studies in a variety of patient populations and situations to support recommendations.

Period of Use	Recommendation	Rationale for Recommendation	Level of Recommendation	Supporting References	Comments
Selection of Patients	Indications for artificial airways: • Upper airway obstruction (eg, secondary to swelling, trauma, tumor, bleeding) • Apnea • Ineffective clearance of secretions • High risk of aspiration (ie, unable to protect the airway) • Respiratory distress • Two major types of artificial airways are commonly used in the critical care setting: • Endotracheal tubes (ET) • Tracheostomy tubes		II: Theory based, no research data to support recommendations; recommendations from expert consensus group may exist	See Other References: 2, 11, 13, 76, 96, 109, 141, 147, 175, 183, 203	Signs of partially obstructed upper airway: ineffective efforts to ventilate, paradoxical respiration, stridor, use of accessory muscles, and choking gestures Signs of complete airway obstruction: respiratory efforts with no breath sounds or suggestion of airflow movement
	ETs are appropriate for short-term airway protection or mechanical ventilation.	Patients with ETs are at risk of developing complications (eg, ulceration of the nasal and oral mucosa, sinusitis, laryngeal damage).	II: Theory based, no research data to support recommendations; recommendations from expert consensus group may exist	See Other References: 2, 4, 7, 11, 22, 45, 58, 61, 73, 76, 80, 97, 101, 118, 119, 127, 129, 141, 146, 157, 163, 167, 174, 175, 182, 183, 184, 185, 186, 200	
	Surgically or percutaneously inserted airways such as tracheostomy tubes are used for longer-term airway protection or mechanical ventilation (eg, patients with persistent absence of protective reflexes, home care), when endotracheal intubation is not possible (eg, facial trauma, upper airway obstruction), or for improved patient comfort (unable to tolerate noninvasive mechanical ventilation).	Transitioning from an ET to a tracheostomy tube helps prevent some of these complications but places the patient at risk for complications of tracheostomy (eg, stomal infections, pneumothorax, subcutaneous emphysema, hemorrhage, tracheal stenosis, tracheomalacia, and granulation tissue).	IV: Limited clinical studies to support recommendations	See Other References: 7, 32, 52, 54, 60, 70, 80, 88, 89, 95, 101, 114, 133, 141, 148, 149, 163, 173, 177, 181, 182, 183, 184, 190, 203, 204, 208	The optimal time for transitioning from ET to tracheostomy tube is unknown. Recent studies favor the use of early tracheostomy (ie, 2 days after intubation) in terms of favorable outcomes. Early tracheotomy may have advantages over delayed tracheostomy in critically ill medical patients in whom mechanical ventilation longer than 10 to 14 days is predicted. The definition of early tracheostomy varies in the literature

Period of Use	Recommendation	Rationale for Recommendation	Level of Recommendation	Supporting References	Comments
Selection of Patients *(cont.)*					from 48 hours to 10 days. It has previously been suggested that early tracheostomy may be indicated when prolonged artificial airway support is anticipated or to enhance patient comfort. See "Preventing Complications"
	Two less commonly used temporizing airways are the Combitube and the laryngeal airway mask.	Both may be used to provide an emergency airway while resuscitating a profoundly unconscious patient who requires invasive artificial ventilation and when endotracheal intubation is not readily available or has failed to establish an airway.	II: Theory based, no research data to support recommendations; recommendations from expert consensus group may exist	See Other References: 11, 13, 22, 76, 133, 141, 186	See Appendix 1B
Application of Device and Initial Use	Endotracheal or tracheostomy tubes must be of an appropriate size (Appendix 1A).				
	Endotracheal Tubes The size of an ET is based on bodyweight. Sizes range from an internal diameter (ID) of 2.0 mm for a neonate to 9.0 mm for a large adult (for an average sized woman, 7.5–8.0 mm; for an average sized man, 8.0–9.0 mm. Pediatric tube sizes can be estimated two ways: • Based on size of child's little finger (equal to tube's outer diameter) when age is unknown or when calculation not possible • (Age in years + 16) / 4 = x mm ID		II: Theory based, no research data to support recommendations; recommendations from expert consensus group may exist	See Other References: 11, 113, 141, 186	The inner and outer diameters of ETs vary depending on the manufacturer. See tube package insert for details of inner- and outer-diameter tube sizes. See pediatric-specific guidelines for more information on sizing.
	The tube with the largest clinically acceptable ID should be used to minimize resistance to airflow.	Resistance to flow is inversely related to the fourth power of the radius of the tube (ie, the larger the ID, the lower the resistance to airflow).	V: Clinical studies in more than one or two different patient populations and situations to support recommendations	See Other References: 19, 20, 55, 60, 72, 102, 174, 175, 176	See Appendix 1B for a comparison of the various tube types

Period of Use	Recommendation	Rationale for Recommendation	Level of Recommendation	Supporting References	Comments
Application of Device and Initial Use *(cont.)*		A small ID increases the resistance of airflow through the tube and has the potential to increase the patient's work of breathing.			The ID of an artificial airway has a more significant effect than the length of the airway device on resistance to airflow.
	Oral vs. Nasal Endotracheal Tubes Base selection of type of tube on factors such as:	Nasal intubation requires smaller diameter tubes to allow passage through the nares.	II: Theory based, no research data to support recommendations; recommendations from expert consensus group may exist	See Other References: 13, 45, 71, 186	Decisions regarding oral vs nasal tubes depend on the skill of the person intubating the patient as well as the clinical condition of the patient.
	• Future need for bronchoscopy	Small ID ETs make passing a bronchoscope more difficult.			
	• Risk of sinusitis and ventilator associated pneumonia (especially important if long-term ventilation is likely)	Orally placed ETs have been shown to be associated with less sinusitis than nasotracheal tubes.	V: Clinical studies in more than one or two different populations and situations to support recommendations	See Other References: 14, 15, 38, 42, 46, 58, 94, 112, 118, 119, 122, 141, 146, 152, 157, 168, 179, 207	Also consider use of an orogastric tube rather than nasogastric tubes to reduce risk of nosocomial sinusitis. Staff education and hand washing continues to be an effective intervention in preventing VAP, along with changing gloves prior to touching respiratory equipment.
	Choose ET and tracheostomy tubes of appropriate size and with desirable features. Ideally, any cuffed ET or tracheostomy tube should have high-volume/low-pressure characteristics. Low cuff inflation pressures are important to minimize the amount of pressure exerted against the lateral wall of the trachea. (See "Preventing Complications" below.)	High-volume/low-pressure cuffs conform more readily to the trachea, providing an adequate seal with lower tracheal wall pressures and less chance of reduced tracheal blood flow or ischemia and subsequent tracheal damage (eg, tracheal stenosis, malacia).	IV: Limited clinical studies to support recommendations	See Other References: 11, 22, 50, 61, 88, 89, 114, 127, 129, 140, 141, 163, 182, 190, 199, 200, 204, 206	
	If feasible, use an ET or continuous aspiration subglottic suction (CASS) tube with a dorsal lumen above the endotracheal cuff to allow subglottic suctioning. CASS tubes may be indicated for the prevention of ventilator-associated pneumonia in patients who require mechanical ventilation greater than 72 hours.	Subglottic secretion drainage is accomplished by a separate dorsal lumen that opens directly above the cuff of an ET tube. Secretions pool above the cuff allowing for leakage of these secretions into the lower airways and is thought to increase the risk of pneumonia. Recent meta-analysis on CASS tubes suggests that use of the tubes may prevent or delay early-onset VAP.	V: Clinical studies in more than one or two different patient populations and situations to support recommendations	See Annotated Bibliography: 1, 4 See Other References: 10, 25, 36, 57, 59, 86, 104, 119, 122, 133, 141 173, 179, 191, 195	One recent study (Other References: 24) has demonstrated mucosal damage secondary to the use of these tubes in animal models. Additionally, research is needed with CASS tubes to clarify whether reduction in VAP is associated with decreased mortality, decreased length of stay, and duration of mechanical ventilation.

Period of Use	Recommendation	Rationale for Recommendation	Level of Recommendation	Supporting References	Comments
Application of Device and Initial Use *(cont.)*	*Tracheostomy Tubes* Select a tracheostomy tube appropriate for the patient's need.	Tracheostomy tubes are available in a variety of sizes and styles and with special features.	II: Theory based, no research data to support recommendations; recommendations from expert consensus group may exist	See Other References: 7, 76, 78, 95, 102, 141, 149, 173, 181, 199, 203, 205, 208	See Appendix 1C for a discussion of various types of tracheostomy tubes
	Assisting with Intubation Procedure Ensure equipment and medications for emergency management of the airway (eg, laryngoscope battery/bulb) are readily accessible and functioning properly.	Airway management is a priority for critically ill patients. Equipment must be available for emergency intubation and reintubation.	II: Theory based, no research data to support recommendations; recommendations from expert consensus group may exist	See Other References: 2, 11, 12, 13, 22, 71, 76, 107, 130, 141, 178, 181, 186	
	Explain the intubation procedure to patients and families. Include what they will feel, see, and hear during and following the intubation procedure. Include information about the inability to speak, the ventilator, restraints, and so on, as appropriate. Repeated explanations are likely to be necessary.	With nonemergency intubation (eg, following elective surgery), the patient may exhibit anxiety preoperatively and need to be given information in a straightforward but reassuring manner. Patients may not remember what they have been told so information may need to be repeated following intubation.	II: Theory based, no research data to support recommendations; recommendations from expert consensus group may exist	See Other References: 2, 4, 11, 13, 105, 131, 141, 159	Recognize that ET intubation is often performed as an emergency procedure and, therefore, only limited explanations may be possible. During this time it is critical to explain details to the family or significant others.
	Postintubation Care Verify correct tube placement by clinical assessment and appropriate monitoring. The following steps are important in assessing tube placement:				
	• Evaluate end-tidal CO_2 ($ETCO_2$) using capnography to verify tracheal placement.	$ETCO_2$ monitoring allows immediate evaluation of tube placement (trachea vs. esophagus). $ETCO_2$ is a highly reliable method of confirming tracheal (vs. esophageal) intubation. $ETCO_2$ monitors measure and display the amount of exhaled CO_2 from the lungs. If the ET tube has been inadvertently placed into	VI: Clinical studies in a variety of patient populations and situations to support recommendations	See Other References: 2, 4, 8, 12, 13, 22, 56, 76, 87, 97, 141, 181, 186	$ETCO_2$ may also be useful to assess inadvertent gastric tube insertion into an airway (Other References: 33, 34). Having end-tidal technology available does not replace the need for clinician physical assessment. The ability for $ETCO_2$ monitors to detect exhaled carbon dioxide depends on adequate pulmonary blood flow to the

Period of Use	Recommendation	Rationale for Recommendation	Level of Recommendation	Supporting References	Comments
Application of Device and Initial Use *(cont.)*	*Postintubation Care (cont.)*	the esophagus, no CO_2 is exhaled, and a CO_2 waveform or color change (if using a colormetric device) will not appear (See below).			lung. In the absence of blood flow (ie, massive pulmonary emboli, cardiac arrest), $ETCO_2$ may be less useful for tube placement detection since there may be no CO_2 exchange at the alveolar capillary level.
		Simple handheld semi-quantitative CO_2 detectors that change color when exposed to CO_2 gas called *colormetric CO_2 devices* are available for use.			Colorimetric devices have the advantages of being portable and disposable.
	• Auscultate breath sounds to verify tracheal vs. esophagus intubation. Auscultate over the abdomen as well as the chest.	Clinical assessment of tube location can be misleading. Case reports have demonstrated that chest auscultation alone may fail to identify esophageal intubation.	II: Theory based, no research data to support recommendations; recommendations from expert consensus group may exist	See Other References: 2, 4, 11, 12, 13, 97, 130, 141, 175, 183	Air movement or gurgling sounds over the epigastrium may indicate possible esophageal intubation.
		Breath sounds should be auscultated bilaterally. ETs are frequently inadvertently advanced into the right mainstem bronchus. A right mainstem intubation will result in asymmetrical chest expansion and diminished left-sided breath sounds.			Observe the chest wall for adequate and equal chest expansion.
	• Assess oxygen saturation by noninvasive pulse oximetry, if available.	Oxygen saturation will fall if the esophagus has been inadvertently intubated. Saturation levels may or may not significantly decrease with right mainstem intubation.	II: Theory based, no research data to support recommendations; recommendations from expert consensus group may exist	See Other References: 2, 4, 11, 13, 76, 130, 141, 183, 186	Pulse oximetry, like capnography, should be used as an adjunct, not replacement, for direct physical assessment.
	• Obtain a chest X-ray. (Because the X-ray is not immediately available, it should not be used as the primary method of tube assessment.)	A postprocedure X-ray is necessary to assess correct placement (ie, distance from the carina).	V: Clinical studies in more than one or two different patient populations and situations to support recommendations	See Other References: 2, 4, 11, 71, 76, 87, 133, 141	Proper tube placement in the trachea can be confirmed without a chest X-ray by using a fiberoptic laryngoscope.
	The tip of the endotracheal tube should be 3–4 cm above the carina.	Endotracheal tubes have radiopaque lines that allow their position to be easily visualized on chest X-ray.	II: Theory based, no research data to support recommendations; recommendations from expert consensus group may exist	See Other References: 2, 4, 11, 45, 41	

Period of Use	Recommendation	Rationale for Recommendation	Level of Recommendation	Supporting References	Comments
Application of Device and Initial Use *(cont.)*	*Postintubation Care (cont.)* • Head position will affect ET tube placement as visualized by X-ray (if patient's head is tilted back, the tube is pulled up; if the head is down, the tube will be pushed down).		II: Theory based, no research data to support recommendations; recommendations from expert consensus group may exist	See Other References: 48, 192	
	• Tubes placed bronchoscopically may not require a postprocedure chest X-ray. (Follow institution policy.)	Allow for clinicians to assess and maintain proper tube position.			
	• Document the position of the endotracheal tube at the teeth or lip. (Levels are printed in cm along body of tube.)	Proper centimeter level will vary depending on patient anatomy, tube movement, method of securing tube, and repositioning.	II: Theory based, no research data to support recommendations; recommendations from expert consensus group may exist	See Other References: 2, 4, 76, 109, 133, 141, 183	It is unusual to see right mainstem intubation with nasotracheal intubation.
	Stabilizing the ET • Secure the tube to prevent movement, occlusion, and skin breakdown. Select method based on patient needs.	Many products are available to secure the ET, although costs and in-service time vary. Studies to date have not shown any method to be superior to any other.	II: Theory based, no research data to support recommendations; recommendations from expert consensus group may exist	See Other References: 2, 21, 45, 96, 110, 126, 131, 198	See Figure 1-1 for an example of securing methods using adhesive tape. Do not secure the tube until you have assessed placement by using one or more of the methods described above.

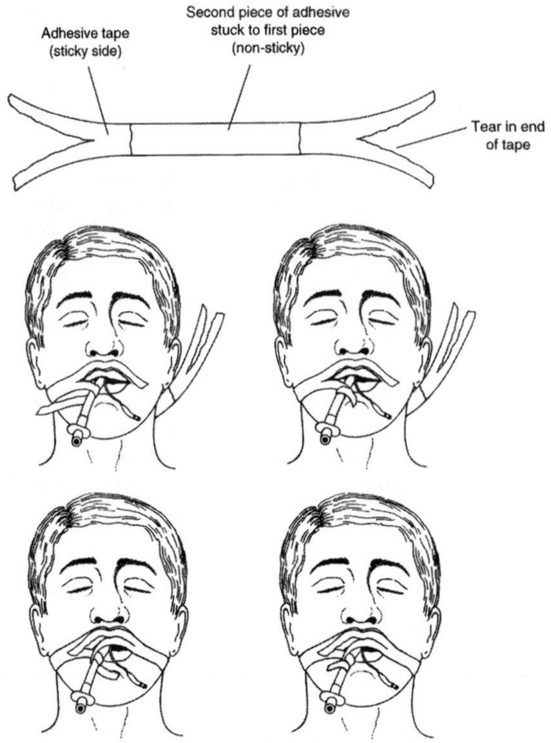

FIGURE 1-1: Methods for securing adhesive tape. Example of protocol for securing endotracheal tube using adhesive tape:

1. Clean the patient's skin with mild soap and water.
2. Remove oil from the skin with alcohol and allow to dry.
3. Apply a skin adhesive product to enhance tape adherence. (When the tape is removed, an adhesive remover will be necessary.)
4. Place a hydrocolloid membrane over the cheeks to protect friable skin.
5. Secure tube with adhesive tape as shown here.

Period of Use	Recommendation	Rationale for Recommendation	Level of Recommendation	Supporting References	Comments
Application of Device and Initial Use *(cont.)*	*Postintubation Care (cont.)* • A hydrocolloid membrane (eg, thin Duoderm) may be used over the cheek to protect friable skin, and the adhesive tape then secured to it.	Hydrocolloid membranes protect the skin as some patients have allergic reactions to the tape, and others develop skin tears as a result of repeated removal and reapplication of tape.	II: Theory based, no research data to support recommendations; recommendations from expert consensus group may exist	See Other References: 96	
	Stabilizing the Tracheostomy Tube Secure the tracheostomy tube to prevent dislocation. (A variety of products is available.)		II: Theory based, no research data to support recommendations; recommendations from expert consensus group may exist	See Other References: 45, 76, 78, 95, 141, 149, 173, 182, 199, 203	
	Tie cotton twill tape (trach ties), if used, with a knot rather than bows. Check to verify that ties are neither excessively tight nor loose.	Twill tape loosens when wet and may allow tube movement, leading to increased risk of tube displacement. Excessively tight tracheostomy ties may cause skin breakdown and pressure ulcers or increased carotid artery pressure.			Tube ties should be secure enough to prevent movement of tube but allow for 1 finger width of play to decrease risk of skin necrosis.
	Commercially available tracheotomy holders are available with foam backing and Velcro ties to permit adjusting the device to maintain patient comfort. Assess these tracheostomy tube holders for proper placement, following manufacturer instructions.	Tracheostomy tube holders will also stretch when wet and when in use over time. Some clinicians prefer twill tape to secure tube until the stoma track has been fully established (5–7 days).			Recheck securement for loosening. Most tracheostomy tube holders are composed of latex-free materials. Always check with manufacturer before applying.
Ongoing Monitoring	*Endotracheal Tube* Assess tube position via chest X-ray whenever it is suspected that the tube position has changed.	Changes in patient position may result in inadvertent ET tube malposition. Inappropriate or incomplete securing of the tube may also cause displacement and require a reevaluation of tube position. ET misplacement can result in serious complications (eg, pneumothorax, hypercapnia, hypoxemia).	II: Theory based, no research data to support recommendations; recommendations from expert consensus group may exist	See Other References: 87, 141	

Period of Use	Recommendation	Rationale for Recommendation	Level of Recommendation	Supporting References	Comments
Ongoing Monitoring *(cont.)*	*Ventilator Alarms* • Follow facility or agency guidelines/policy for monitoring and responding to ventilator alarms.	Depending on geography of unit or location of ventilator patient, ventilator alarms may be transmitted via pager, central station, or remain localized to the ventilator itself to promote maximum patient safety.		See Other References: 8	Also included in Joint Commission on Accreditation of Health Care Organizations (JCAHO), Sentinel Event Alert 25: "Preventing Ventilator-Related Deaths and or Injuries"
	Retaping the ET • For safety, two people should perform retaping.	Having two people for the procedure decreases the chance of an accidental extubation.	II: Theory based, no research data to support recommendations; recommendations from expert consensus group may exist	See Other References: 97, 141	
	• Move the ET from one side of the mouth to the other when retaping. • Retape and move the ET from side to side periodically based on patient need. (There is no universally accepted time frame.) • Assess the position of the tube after retaping to determine if it has moved.	Moving the tube position helps prevent ulceration of the lips and tongue.	II: Theory based, no research data to support recommendations; recommendations from expert consensus group may exist	See Other References: 96, 182	Providing meticulous oral care is critical in preventing the development of candidiasis or other infections of the mouth related to poor oral hygiene.
	Tracheostomy Tubes • Resecure the tracheostomy tube, or change the tube holder any time the holder becomes excessively loosened or wet.	Secretions promote maceration of tissue. Avoiding free tube movement minimizes patient discomfort and prevents tube displacement.	II: Theory based, no research data to support recommendations; recommendations from expert consensus group may exist	See Other References: 141, 182	
	Monitoring Cuff Pressures Cuff pressures are measured periodically (eg, every shift); however, the "correct" frequency is not known. Maximum cuff pressures should not exceed 24–30 cm H_2O or 20–25 mm Hg. Adequate cuff inflation (> 20 cm H_2O) helps to prevent large volume aspiration, decreases the risk of inadvertent	Cuff pressures that are too high can reduce tracheal mucosal perfusion pressure and cause ischemia, ulceration, necrosis, and possible exposure of the cartilage.	IV: Limited clinical studies to support recommendations	See Other References: 2, 14, 25, 45, 53, 88, 89, 90, 107, 141	Perfusion pressure of the trachea ranges from 30 mm Hg at the arterial side to 18 mm Hg at the venous side. When high airway pressures are present, neither cuff measurement nor the minimal leak technique may be accurate.

Period of Use	Recommendation	Rationale for Recommendation	Level of Recommendation	Supporting References	Comments
Ongoing Monitoring *(cont.)*	*Monitoring Cuff Pressures (cont.)* extubation, provides a patent airway for ventilation and suctioning, and decreases the risk of VAP. Two alternative cuff inflation techniques are used:				
	• The minimal leak technique (MLT) is defined as air inflation of the tube cuff until any leak stops, then a small amount of air is slowly removed until a slight leak is observed at peak inflation pressure.	Some clinicians suggest that cuff pressures do not need monitoring if MLT is used. However, it is reasonable to measure and record pressures at routine intervals, regardless of the inflation method used.	II: Theory based, no research data to support recommendations; recommendations from expert consensus group may exist	See Other References: 25, 45, 53, 56, 90, 109, 129, 146, 166, 182	Air leaks are commonly heard when high peak airway pressures are generated with or without PEEP or if the tube being used is too small relative to the diameter of the patient's trachea.
	• The minimal occlusive volume (MOV) technique is defined as air inflation of the tube cuff until the air flow heard escaping around the cuff during a positive pressure breath ceases. It is not necessary to periodically deflate the cuffs of low-pressure tubes (as long as cuff pressures are routinely monitored). See Appendix 1C (Types of Tracheostomy Tubes) for information regarding alternative cuffs, including foam cuffs and tight-to-shaft cuffs.				
	If high peak airway pressures are required to obtain a clinically acceptable seal, it may be necessary to replace the tube.	Increasing pressures necessary to seal the airway adequately indicate tracheal dilation or tracheomalacia. Repositioning of the tube and changing to a larger or longer tube may be needed.	II: Theory based, no research data to support recommendations; recommendations from expert consensus group may exist	See Other References: 45, 53, 182	Hemostats should not be routinely used on the cuff inflation line as this may damage the integrity of the tubing. Hemostats may be necessary as a temporizing measure if the balloon is damaged prior to changing the tube.

Period of Use	Recommendation	Rationale for Recommendation	Level of Recommendation	Supporting References	Comments
Ongoing Monitoring *(cont.)*	*Head of the Bed Elevation* All patients receiving mechanical ventilation should have the head of the bed (HOB) elevated at a minimum of 30° to 45° unless medically contraindicated.	Supine positioning has shown to be a risk factor for developing VAP. VAP is the leading cause of morbidity and mortality in the ICU.	VI: Clinical studies in a variety of patient populations and situations to support recommendations	See Other References: 10, 14, 38, 42, 46, 73, 86, 94, 107, 118, 119, 122, 141, 157, 166, 168, 197, 207	Also included in Joint Commission on Accreditation of Health Care Organizations (JCAHO), ICU Core Measures. Patients with tube feedings and artificial airway should also have the head of the bed at 30° to 45°.
	Oral Care Assess oral cavity for presence of plaque, dried or coated secretions, signs of infection, skin breakdown from oral airways, loose teeth, removable appliances, and bleeding. Brush teeth twice a day with soft toothbrush, and swab mouth every 2–4 hours with foam swabs. Rinse mouth with water or normal saline (per institution policy). Moisturize oral cavity and lips with water-based moisturizer.	Brushing the teeth assists in preventing plaque formation and periodontal disease and may help prevent ventilator-associated pneumonia. Additional orders/treatment may be needed for thrush, herpes, trauma, etc. Teeth and removable appliances can be aspirated or impede the airway.	II: Theory based, no research data to support recommendations; recommendations from expert consensus group may exist	See Annotated Bibliography: 1, 4 See Other References: 36, 65, 83, 84, 100, 117, 133, 170, 171	Limited research has shown a decrease in VAP with the use of chlorhexadine rinses in cardiac surgery patients only.
	Tracheostomy Care Keep the area around the stoma as clean and dry as possible. Follow institutional policy for method and frequency of stoma site care.	Moisture promotes maceration of the site. If dressing is needed, use precut gauze dressings only. Precut gauze has sealed edges with decreased potential for aspiration of fibers.	II: Theory based, no research data to support recommendations; recommendations from expert consensus group may exist	See Annotated Bibliography: 2 See Other References: 141, 148, 182, 203	A small preliminary pilot study recently demonstrated that an antimicrobial drain sponge dressing decreases the prevalance of four pathogens in the long-term trach population. However, until outcomes of additional studies with larger samples are accomplished, the practice cannot be encouraged. (Annotated Bibliography: 2)

Period of Use	Recommendation	Rationale for Recommendation	Level of Recommendation	Supporting References	Comments
Ongoing Monitoring (*cont.*)	Periodic cleaning of the reusable inner cannula or changing of the disposable inner cannula may be necessary to identify narrowing of the inner diameter from encrusted sections or tenacious secretions. Controversy exists on the required frequency.	Changing or cleaning the inner cannula keeps the airway patent. However, not all tracheostomy products have inner cannulas.	II: Theory based, no research data to support recommendations; recommendations from expert consensus group may exist	See Other References: 35, 141, 182	Most institutions change/clean inner cannulas every 8–12 hours. However, a preliminary study suggests that routine changing (ie, every 24 hours) versus every 3 days, does not increase the incidence of occlusion or colonization. (Other References: 35) However, this finding may not be generalized to patients with tracheostomy tubes cared for outside of the critical care unit because the level of nursing vigilance may not be similar to the conditions of the study patients. Routine inspection or changing and cleaning of the inner cannula according to institutional policy may still be warranted until additional studies are accomplished. However, with the increased use of tracheostomies without inner cannulas, this may be less of an issue.
	Changing the tracheostomy tube may be necessary secondary to patient needs (upsize, downsize, new cuff, cuffless, etc) and for routine assessment and care.	The first tracheostomy tube change should not be performed until the stoma tissue tract is established (7–14 days), and it should be done by trained providers. Follow manufacturer recommendations for tracheostomy tube life and replacement recommendation frequency.	II: Theory based, no research data to support recommendations; recommendations from expert consensus group may exist	See Other References: 141, 182, 205	Regular tracheostomy tube changes may cause a decrease in granulation tissue formation. Most institutions and home care agencies perform regular tracheostomy tube changes that vary from 2 weeks, months, or greater for long-term trach patients.
	Promote effective patient-provider communication through techniques such as paper and pencil, letter/word boards, and one-way speaking valves (see Appendix 1E for more detail).	The type of communication technique used will depend on the patient's condition.	II: Theory based, no research data to support recommendations; recommendations from expert consensus group may exist	See Other References: 45, 47, 93, 137, 182, 201, 203	

Period of Use	Recommendation	Rationale for Recommendation	Level of Recommendation	Supporting References	Comments
Ongoing Monitoring *(cont.)*	One-way speaking valves, depending on design, may be used for patients with tracheostomy tubes who do not require ventilatory support and for in-line use with mechanical ventilators. Do not use in patients with poor lung compliance, high inspired oxygen requirements, diminished laryngeal muscular function, or vocal cord dysfunction. Patients with copious secretions may not tolerate the devices. Do not use speaking valves in patients with foam cuff tubes. All cuffed tubes must be completely deflated before using.	One-way speaking valves allow patients (who have functioning vocal cords) with tracheostomies (both on and off the ventilator) to speak. They are useful primarily in patients who can breathe around their tracheostomy tube. There must be a 15-mm connector on the end of the tracheostomy tube for valve attachment. Failure to completely deflate the tube cuff with a speaking valve attached will prevent the patient from being able to exhale, cause immediate acute respiratory distress, and possible death. If the patient is unable to exhale with the cuff completely deflated, consider placing a smaller tube and/or a cuffless tube if appropriate.		See Other References: 24, 47, 63, 78, 95, 102, 141, 149, 173, 177, 182, 203	Consider early involvement of a speech pathologist for formal speech evaluation. Monitor patient closely when first initiating the use of a one-way speaking valve. Speaking valves should not be worn during sleep. Consider the use of talking tracheostomy tubes for long-term ventilator patients if unable to tolerate a speaking valve. Consult with speech pathologist about the potential use of an electrolarynx device in those patients who do not tolerate a valve.
Extubation	Patients who no longer meet the criteria for an artificial airway are candidates for extubation. Indications for extubation include: • Underlying condition that originally led to the need for artificial airway is reversed or improved • Hemodynamically stable with no new reasons for continued artificial airway support • Able to clear pulmonary secretions based on assessment of respiratory mechanics (ie, able to generate a forceful cough) • Airway problems (ie, obstruction) have resolved. • Mechanical ventilatory support is no longer needed. (See Chapter 3, Weaning from Mechanical Ventilation.)		II: Theory based, no research data to support recommendations; recommendations from expert consensus group may exist	See Other References: 7, 16, 17, 45, 76, 182	

Period of Use	Recommendation	Rationale for Recommendation	Level of Recommendation	Supporting References	Comments
Extubation *(cont.)*	*Procedure for Extubation*				
	Prepare the patient and family for the process.		II: Theory based, no research data to support recommendations; recommendations from expert consensus group may exist		
	Assemble equipment needed for the procedure.	Decreases chance of desaturation during the extubation process.			May use 100% button on certain ventilators.
	Preoxygenate with 100% oxygen.				
	Place the patient in semi- or high-Fowler's position.	Decreases the risk of aspiration of secretions following cuff deflation.			
	Suction through the ET and then above the cuff via the oropharynx.				
	Remove the endotracheal tube as follows:				
	• Oxygenate the patient well after suctioning.	Oxygen prevents or limits hypoxemia as a result of suctioning.	III: Laboratory data only, no clinical data to support recommendations	See Other References: 3, 11, 45, 109	
	• Remove the tape or holding device securing the endotracheal tube.	Failure to completely deflate cuff before removal may result in vocal cord damage.			
	• Completely deflate the cuff and ask the patient to cough. May need to suction through ET again.				
	• Instruct the patient to take in a deep breath; remove the tube at peak inspiration.	Vocal cords are maximally abducted at peak inspiration.			
		Initial cough response expected immediately following extubation should be more forceful starting from a point of maximal inspiration vs. expiration.			
	Administer oxygen via face mask or nasal cannula if appropriate.	Prevent hypoxemia immediately postextubation.			
	Adjust inspired oxygen concentration if indicated based on arterial blood gases or pulse oximetry.				

Period of Use	Recommendation	Rationale for Recommendation	Level of Recommendation	Supporting References	Comments
Extubation *(cont.)*	Use cool mist if sore throat and hoarseness is a concern.	Thought to possibly decrease laryngeal edema.	II: Theory based, no research data to support recommendations; recommendations from expert consensus group may exist	See Other References: 141	Providing supplemental high-level humidity (bland aerosol of sterile water) using a large volume nebulizer via face mask or face tent is of questionable value. It also may be contraindicated in patients with increased airway resistance.
	Evaluate patient frequently for complications associated with extubation such as stridor, hoarseness, changes in vital signs, or SpO$_2$. Note: Postextubation glottic edema can develop within minutes or several hours following extubation. Routine physical assessment of the patient, including auscultation over the trachea, is critical.	Stridor or hoarseness may signify upper airway laryngospasm or glottic edema. If severe laryngospasm persists, reintubation may be required. Heart rate (HR) and blood pressure (BP) changes may be seen with vagal stimulation as well as hypoxemia. Oxygen saturation may decrease if patient is unable to maintain a patent airway.		See Other References: 2, 3, 13, 141, 183	Racemic epinephrine may be administered by aerosol inhalation if stridor develops and is thought to be related to glottic edema. Reintubation must be considered as the swelling can dramatically worsen.
	Assess patients at risk for postextubation stridor (eg, laryngotracheal injury, edema) before removing tube.	A low cuff leak volume (10%–12%) around the endotracheal tube prior to extubation may be useful for identifying patients at risk for stridor or reintubation.	IV: Limited clinical studies to support recommendations	See Other References: 3, 105, 138, 141, 169	As in some documented cases, there may be indications for the use of systemic steroids before attempting extubation. In certain cases, it may be appropriate for extubation to occur under bronchoscopic guidance to identify and document any upper airway abnormality.
	Decannulation (Tracheostomy) Once a tracheostomy tube is no longer required, decannulation may be accomplished. Indications for decannulation are the same as for ET tube extubation.	The process of downsizing allows patients to gradually become accustomed to breathing on their own while maintaining some degree of airway protection. Downsizing also permits improved air passage through the vocal cords and around the trach tube.	II: Theory based, no research data to support recommendations; recommendations from expert consensus group may exist	See Other References: 17, 30, 45, 182	After removal of the tube, the stoma will close on its own in a matter of days. Change dressing per institution protocol. Instruct patient to place finger over dressing while speaking for improved vocalization while stoma heals

Period of Use	Recommendation	Rationale for Recommendation	Level of Recommendation	Supporting References	Comments
Extubation (*cont.*)	There are several methods employed for decannulation (eg, decreasing tube size or downsizing); replacing with a fenestrated tube or with a tracheal stoma button). See Appendix 1C for advantages and disadvantages of fenestrated tubes and tracheostomy buttons.	No specific timing has been established for optimal decannulation or technique.			The decision to use a particular decannulation technique depends on patient requirements as well as the experience and preferences of the attending physician and nurses caring for the patient.
Maintaining Patency of the Artificial Airway	Provide humidified oxygen or air, with temperature of the inspired gas based on patient requirements. For example, humidification is typically delivered at room or body temperature (35°C–37°C) but may be warmed in special circumstances (eg, hypothermic patients). Cool humidification is typically reserved for patients immediately after extubation to decrease upper airway swelling.	Artificial airways bypass the nose and mouth, thus preventing normal warming, humidification, and filtering. A lack of humidification will result in the drying of secretions within the airway and make the removal of secretions difficult. Also, accumulated secretions that thicken can adhere to the inner lumen of the airway and effectively increase inspiratory and expiratory resistance to airflow.	II: Theory based, no research data to support recommendations; recommendations from expert consensus group may exist	See Other References: 14, 29, 81, 87, 141	Condensate should be carefully emptied from ventilator circuits and prevented from entering the endotracheal tube or nebulizer. Passive humidifiers or heat-moisture exchangers decrease condensation, but research has not demonstrated their effectiveness as a VAP prevention adjunct.
Endotracheal Suction	Suctioning should be performed when clinically indicated. Routine suctioning schedules solely based on ordered frequency alone (eg, every 2 hours) are not appropriate. Clinical indications for suctioning include: • Secretions in the ET tube • Frequent or sustained coughing • Adventitious breath sounds on auscultation (rhonchi) • Desaturation (low SpO_2) • Increased peak airway pressures • Sudden onset of respiratory distress whenever airway patency is questioned	Endotracheal suctioning can be associated with adverse complications such as hypoxemia, arrhythmias, increased mean arterial BP, and potential for tracheal damage.	II: Theory based, no research data to support recommendations; recommendations from expert consensus group may exist	See Annotated Bibliography: 2 See Other References: 1, 23, 28, 41, 43, 44, 45, 49, 81, 82, 133, 136, 150, 159, 172, 191	See Appendix 1F for terminology associated with various suctioning procedures. Patients have reported pain with routine ICU interventions such as repositioning and suctioning. Consider analgesia along with sedation as needed.

Period of Use	Recommendation	Rationale for Recommendation	Level of Recommendation	Supporting References	Comments
Endotracheal Suction *(cont.)*	• Hyperoxygenate the patient for at least 30 seconds before and after each pass of the suction catheter regardless of suction technique used (open or closed) or method of delivery (manual or ventilator).	Hyperoxygenation has been shown to decrease the occurrence of desaturation associated with suctioning. Hypoxemia can usually be avoided with both manual and ventilator methods of hyperoxygenation. In limited studies, PaO$_2$ or O$_2$ saturation increases are higher with ventilator than with manual delivery.	IV: Limited clinical studies to support recommendations	See Annotated Bibliography: 1, 6 See Other References: 1, 9, 74, 150	
	If the patient does not tolerate suctioning despite hyperoxygenation, try following steps:		II: Theory based, no research data to support recommendations; recommendations from expert consensus group may exist		Hyperventilation is difficult to accomplish with a handheld resuscitator. Most deliver only 600–800 mL even when two hands are used.
	• Assure that 100% oxygen is being delivered. • Maintain PEEP during suctioning. (A closed or in-line suction system may be helpful.) If manual ventilation with a handheld resuscitator is used for open-system suctioning, be sure it has a PEEP attachment with the appropriate setting. • Switch to another method of suctioning (eg, in-line). • Allow longer recovery intervals between suction passes.	Closed inline suction has not demonstrated a decrease in VAP; however, it can minimize the physiologic risks of suctioning by maintaining PEEP and avoiding lung derecruitment from loss of lung volume. Additionally it reduces risk of caregiver exposure to secretions.	IV: Limited clinical studies to support recommendations	See Other References: 74, 79, 39, 130, 194	
	Hyperventilation may be used in situations where the patient does not tolerate suctioning with hyperoxygenation alone. Hyperventilation may be delivered manually (with a handheld resuscitator) or via the ventilator.		II: Theory based, no research data to support recommendations; recommendations from expert consensus group may exist	See Other References: 82, 123, 188	

Period of Use	Recommendation	Rationale for Recommendation	Level of Recommendation	Supporting References	Comments
Endotracheal Suction *(cont.)*	The suction catheter should be passed into the ET or tracheostomy tube without suction being applied. Apply suction to the catheter as it is withdrawn from the tube.	Suction should be applied only as needed (to remove secretions) and for as short a time as possible to minimize the chance of desaturation.	II: Theory based, no research data to support recommendations; recommendations from expert consensus group may exist	See Other References: 1, 18, 116, 124, 125, 133, 141, 191	There have been studies in animal models suggesting that deep suctioning should be avoided. In select patients, it may be appropriate to use measured depth suctioning based on the length of the endotracheal tube. This is particularly important in neonates and pediatrics.
	Suction should be applied for no more than 10–15 seconds.	Both intermittent and continuous suction have similarly adverse effects on tracheal mucosa.		See Other References: 1, 41, 43, 44, 81, 82, 137, 141, 183, 191	
	The suction pressure level for an adult should be set at 100–120 mm Hg. If higher suction levels are necessary, consider precautions to prevent trauma such as the use of red rubber suction catheters. Follow manufacturer guidelines for suction pressure levels when using closed-suction catheter systems.	The amount of suction applied should only be high enough to effectively remove secretions.		See Other References: 1, 62, 123	Directional tip or coudé suction catheters are available for selective right or left mainstem bronchus placement. However, little data exist to support the hypothesis that the catheters can be placed preferentially.
	The number of suction passes required will be based on the amount of secretions and the patient's ability to tolerate the suctioning procedure.	Patients with large amount of secretions may require more frequent clinical assessment and may require multiple suction passes to effectively remove secretions.	II: Theory based, no research data to support recommendations; recommendations from expert consensus group may exist	See Other References: 1, 141, 150,	
	Monitor the patient during suctioning for complications including increased or decreased HR and BP, desaturation, increased intracranial pressure, and increased agitation.	Complications of ET suctioning include changes in HR, BP, and oxygen saturation. Anxiety during suctioning or hypoxia may contribute to increased agitation.	V: Clinical studies in more than one or two different patient populations and situations to support recommendations	See Other References: 23, 41, 76, 81, 82, 136, 141, 150, 183	
	Monitor patient for signs of suctioning effectiveness (eg, improved breath sounds, decreased work of breathing, improved oxygen saturation or blood gas values). If patient is on a volume-cycled ventilator, observe for reductions in both peak inspi-				

Period of Use	Recommendation	Rationale for Recommendation	Level of Recommendation	Supporting References	Comments
Endotracheal Suction *(cont.)*	ratory pressures and measured resistance. Patients receiving pressure-controlled ventilation should show improved tidal volume delivery.				
	Use of Saline Instillation During Suctioning				
	Saline should not be routinely instilled into ET or tracheostomy tubes before suctioning.	Oxygen saturation has been shown to decrease during suctioning when using saline instillation vs. no saline. Bolus saline is unable to liquefy or thin secretions due to lack of mucolytic activity.	IV: Limited clinical studies to support recommendations	See Selected Bibliography: 3 See Other References: 5, 6, 9, 27, 30, 79, 85, 88, 115, 141, 161, 165, 179, 183, 189, 191	Consider hydration or increasing humidity for thick secretions.
		Concerns related to potential lower airway contamination secondary to the instillation of saline raises concerns about the possibility of increased risk of nosocomial pneumonia.			
	Flush in-line catheters with saline after use.	Removes build-up of secretions in the suction line.	I: Manufacturers's recommendations only		
Preventing Complications	*Preventing Aspiration* Aspiration can be related to many factors in patients with artificial airways. Patients are at risk of aspiration and VAP from colonization of the stomach, upper airway, teeth, artificial airway, ventilator circuit and nasal sinuses. This section addresses potential strategies for preventing aspiration from enteral nutrition.			See Other References: 10, 38, 41, 101, 118	
	• Maintaining the ET or trach cuff pressure (See "Monitoring Cuff Pressures")	Even properly inflated and maintained cuffed tubes do not provide absolute protection from aspiration.	IV: Limited clinical studies to support recommendations	See Other References: 25, 45, 105, 114, 157	While a cuff may protect the patient from aspiration of large food particles, glucose-rich liquids can be aspirated around the sides or folds in the inflated cuff into the lung, thus increasing the risk of aspiration pneumonia.

Period of Use	Recommendation	Rationale for Recommendation	Level of Recommendation	Supporting References	Comments
Preventing Complications *(cont.)*	*Preventing Aspiration (cont.)*				
	• Placing the feeding tube distal to the stomach (small bowel) in critically ill patients	Small bowel feeding may be associated with decreased gastroesophageal regurgitation, an increase in nutrient delivery, a shorter time to achieve target nutrition, and lower rate of VAP. However, there have been no studies documenting improved outcomes and mortality of small bowel versus gastric feedings.	II, Theory based, no research data to support recommendations; recommendations from expert consensus group may exist	See Other References: 14, 98, 99, 103, 119, 135, 139, 145, 151	Enteral nutrition is preferred over parenteral to reduce risks of complications related to central catheters and to prevent atrophy of the intestinal mucosa that may increase risk of bacterial translocation. Refer to Protocol on Nutrition of the Mechanically Ventilated Patient.
	• Use of prokinetic agents	Prokinetic agents increase gastric motility. Consensus groups have recommended the use in patients who experience feeding intolerance.	II, Theory based, no research data to support recommendations; recommendations from expert consensus group may exist	See Other References: 42, 46, 63, 98, 99, 104, 139, 145	
	• Use of bedside methods to detect aspiration in tube-fed patients There are currently no recommended sensitive or specific bedside testing methods to detect aspiration.	Recent reports indicate that FD&C Blue dye No. 1 has the potential for harm and lacks sensitivity to detect small volume aspiration. Additionally, glucose oxidase reagent strips do not meet manufacturer recommendations for point-of-care testing.	IV: Limited clinical studies to support recommendations	See Annotated Bibliography: 5, 7 See Other References: 132, 139, 143, 144, 145, 180, 193	Testing for pepsin using a highly specific immunoassay has been researched in an exploratory study and may be a better test than previous methods for detecting pulmonary aspiration of gastric contents. Additional research is needed.
	Preventing Pressure and Shearing Injury Moving the tube from side to side and keeping the cuff pressure at the minimum pressure to seal the airway are measures to help prevent mucosal contact pressure injury. Adequate fixation of the tube will help to minimize movement of the tube in the airway. Another approach is to decrease pulling on the tube by using a 6-in piece of flexible corrugated tubing connected between the ET or tracheostomy tube and the Y connector of the ventilator tubing circuit. The use of a swivel	Pressure injury occurs from pressure of the endotracheal or tracheostomy tube against the posterior wall of the airway. Injury can also occur due to excessive tube cuff pressures. Shearing injury occurs with sharp movements of the head back and forth, up and down, and pulling on the ET and tracheostomy tube. Attempts to self-extubate also will lead to shearing.	II: Theory based, no research data to support recommendations; recommendations from expert consensus group may exist	See Other References: 126, 131, 142, 141, 145, 184, 185	Large-bore plastic naso/orogastric tubes placed in the esophagus can contribute to friction against the posterior wall of the trachea and lead to tissue breakdown, erosion, and subsequent development of tracheoesophageal fistula.

Period of Use	Recommendation	Rationale for Recommendation	Level of Recommendation	Supporting References	Comments
Preventing Complications *(cont.)*	*Preventing Pressure and Shearing Injury (cont.)* adapter on the tracheaostomy tube in conjunction with the corrugated tubing provides additional flexibility. It is important to keep the ventilator circuit stabilized and in proper position to decrease the amount of traction placed on the tube. Keeping the flex tube in line with the sternum aligns the trach tube in the center of the airway and prevents it from coming in contact with the airway wall.				
	Unplanned Extubations There are two types of unplanned extubations: self-extubation (patient removal) and accidental extubation (through movement or during procedures). Judicious use of restraints, sedation, and pain relief and frequent orientation and explanation of proceedings are used to improve patient compliance or tolerance. Care should be taken to observe and support the ventilator/oxygen circuit tubing during procedures and movement. The airway itself should always be adequately secured. Use of additional support measures to prevent pulling directly on the airway during movement and procedures is indicated.	Self-extubation is associated with agitation, confusion, restlessness, lack of restraints, and reintubation. Medical and trauma patients have a higher incidence of self-extubation with a higher rate of reintubation; surgical patients have a lower incidence of self-extubation and frequently do not need to be reintubated (probably a reflection that they are intubated longer than they need to be).	II: Theory based, no research data to support recommendations; recommendations from expert consensus group may exist	See Other References: 2, 21, 40, 51, 66, 67, 68, 69, 92, 96, 105, 110, 111, 134, 141, 142, 164, 183, 185, 186	See Appendix 1F
	Additional factors that may result in unplanned extubations include: • Improper length of the endotracheal tube • Improper support of respiratory tubing and/or airway during patient transfer or transport	Accidental extubations are associated with procedures, movement, and inadequate fixation of the tube.			

Period of Use	Recommendation	Rationale for Recommendation	Level of Recommendation	Supporting References	Comments
Preventing Complications (*cont.*)	*Unplanned Extubations* (*cont.*) • Inadequate securing method • Underinflation of the endotracheal cuff				
	Restraints Restraints are used to facilitate patient tolerance of invasive therapies and to avoid life-threatening consequences of abrupt cessation of these therapies. They must be used judiciously, not indiscriminately, to prevent premature removal of the endotracheal or tracheostomy tube. The type of restraint selected should be the least invasive option.	Patient and family/significant other teaching is important when restraints are used for patient safety. Reassessment for continued need of restraints should be done routinely. Most institutions have rigorous criteria outlining the use and ordering of restraints.	II: Theory based, no research data to support recommendations; recommendations from expert consensus group may exist	See Other References: 92, 105, 134, 164	Assess for skin breakdown from pulling against restraints and shearing on coccyx. Analgesics, sedatives, and neuroleptics should be considered and used to decrease the need for restraints and promote comfort. However, these drugs should not be overused as a chemical restraint.
	Preventing Delirium (*ICU Psychosis*) The most important step in delirium management is early recognition. Reorientation and other nonpharmacologic and pharmacologic strategies may be necessary.	Delirium occurs secondary to disease process, electrolyte imbalance, acid-base imbalance, sleep deprivation, and medications. It can also be a contributing factor in self-extubation. Delirium in the critically ill is associated with poor outcomes including longer hospital stay and increased mortality.	II: Theory based, no research data to support recommendations; recommendations from expert consensus group may exist	See Other References: 66, 67, 68, 69, 105, 128, 158	Consider use of a tool to assess delirium. For example, the Confusion Assessment Method (CAM-ICU) has been reported as a highly sensitive and specific tool in the evaluation of delirium in the critically ill.
	Maintaining Sleep Provide blocks of sleep (eg, 2–3 hours) whenever possible. Simulate room environment to incorporate day and night using window or room lighting.	Critically ill patients have increased awakenings and arousals than normal patients. They also experience decreased rapid eye movement (REM) and slow wave sleep. Lack of REM and levels 3 and 4 sleep predisposes to confusion and disorientation.	IV: Limited clinical studies to support recommendations	See Other References: 37, 77, 153, 154	

ANNOTATED BIBLIOGRAPHY

1. **Sole ML, Byers JF, Ludy JE, Zhang Y, Banta CM, Brummel K. A multisite survey of suctioning techniques and airway management practices.** *Am J Crit Care.* 2003;12:220–232.

Study Sample

The authors studied survey results from 1665 nurses and respiratory therapists at 27 sites throughout the United States on institutional policies and procedures related to closed-system suctioning and airway management of intubated patients.

Comparison Studied

In this descriptive, comparative, multisite study, nurses and respiratory therapists were surveyed to both describe institutional policies and procedures related to closed-system suctioning and airway management of intubated patients and to compare practices.

Study Procedures

Sites were recruited using network sampling through e-mail to colleagues and postings to the Society of Critical Care Medicine advanced practice nursing e-mail list. Sites were asked to participate if closed-system suctioning was used on more than 50% of intubated patients. Two surveys were used to collect data: the first survey covered suctioning techniques and airway management practices (STAMP) institutional policies and data, consisting of 45 multiple-choice and fill-in questions; and the second survey was a STAMP individual survey for nurses and respiratory therapists, with 32 multiple-choice questions and a single fill-in question. Test-retest reliability of 82% had been established from a previous pilot study.

Key Results

Less than 50% of sites had policies for oral care, oral and nasal suctioning, suctioning above the endotracheal cuff before repositioning, and changing bite blocks or oral airways. Instillation of normal saline was recommended at 74% of the sites. The closed-system catheters were changed every 24–48 hours at 63% of institutions surveys.

Study Strengths and Weaknesses

The strengths of this study included the instrument content validity and the multisite design. The major weakness is the survey design may inherently encourage bias in the sample. Regardless, the intent of the study was to describe current practices and serve as a preliminary step towards identifying areas for research.

Clinical Implications

The data suggests that current practice does not consistently reflect the most recent research related to changing closed-system tubing, use of normal saline, management of endotracheal cuff pressures, and oral care. Additionally, the study reinforced the importance of translating research-based evidence into clinical practice and institutional policies. Collaborative patient care between respiratory therapists and nurses along with the use of research is essential for optimal and consistent airway management.

2. **Motta GJ, Trigilia D. The effect of an antimicrobial drain sponge dressing on a specific bacterial isolates at tracheostomy sites.** *Ostomy Wound.* 2005;51:60–66.

Study Sample

The authors studied 10 patients over a period of 25 days in the neuroscience unit of a long-term rehabilitation hospital to compare the use of a nonwoven drain sponge dressing containing an antimicrobial to a nonimpregnated, nonwoven drain sponge on tracheostomy sites.

Comparison Studied

This prospective, descriptive, randomized, controlled study was designed to compare the use of a nonwoven drain sponge dressing containing an antimicrobial (polyhexamethylene biguanide) to a nonimpregnated, nonwoven drain sponge on tracheostomy sites.

Study Procedures

The study group received 5 daily consecutive dressing applications. Cultures were taken at enrollment and at days 1, 2, 3, and 4. Researchers also photographed the tracheostomy and surrounding skin along with clinical assessment parameters including pain, condition of the skin, color and odor of any drainage, and any other clinical findings.

Key Results

The treatment group (10 patients) and the control group (5 patients) completed the study. The treatment group had an absence of growth of 4 select pathogens (Methicillin-resistant *Staphylococcus aureus, Pseudomonas aeruginosa, Enterobacter cloacae,* and *Staphylococcus auereus*) for 11 days versus the control group of 6 days.

Study Strengths and Weaknesses

The small sample size and lack of outcome data makes it difficult to apply the findings to practice. Additionally, there was a clinically significant disparity between the tracheostomy duration of the control group (7.5 months) and the treatment group (14 months) despite random assignment.

Clinical Implications

The study suggests a role for additional research into whether using an impregnated tracheostomy drain sponge has a role in reducing healthcare-acquired pathogens. Wound infections of the tracheostomy site frequently occur despite routine care. Results suggest that antimicrobial drain sponge dressings may help control Methicillin-resistant *Staphylococcus aureus* and *Pseudomonas aeruginosa*.

3. Ridling DA, Martin LD, Bratton SL. Endotracheal suctioning with or without instillation of isotonic sodium chloride solutions in critically ill children. *Am J Crit Care*. 2003;12:212–219.

Study Sample

The authors used a convenience sample of 24 critically ill, endotracheally-intubated children in a 17-bed multispecialty pediatric intensive care unit.

Comparison Studied

A prospective, randomized study design was used. The purpose of the study was to compare the effects of endotracheal suctioning with or without instillation of isotonic sodium chloride on oxygen saturation as measured by pulse oximetry.

Study Procedures

Oxygen saturation was measured before suctioning and at 1, 2, and 10 minutes after each episode of suctioning for the duration of the patient's intubation. The subjects were randomized as follows: group 1—isotonic sodium chloride instilled before each suctioning episode, or group 2—subjects did not have any isotonic sodium chloride instilled. Additionally, the RNs and respiratory therapists received a review of the existing hospital policy on suctioning prior to initiation of the study. The procedure consisted of manual hyperoxygenation via anesthesia bag with 100% oxygen and same positive inspiratory pressure and positive end-expiratory pressure as ventilator settings before and after suctioning. Additionally per hospital procedure, the size of the catheter was approximately half the diameter of the endotracheal tube, and the catheter was inserted no more than 1 cm beyond the end of the tube. Suction was set at 80 mm Hg for infants up to 1 year and 100 mm Hg for all others.

Key Results

Of the 24 patients enrolled, 10 were in group 1 with 52 suctioning episodes, and 14 were in group 2 also with 52 suctioning episodes. Oxygen saturation was found to be significantly lower in subjects with the instillation of normal saline at 1 and 2 minutes, $P = .013$ and $P = .005$ respectively. No nosocomial pneumonias or tube occlusions were identified in either group.

Study Strengths and Weaknesses

Most of the children in this study, 23 out of 24 patients, had congenital cardiac disease and were recovering from cardiac surgery. Findings may not be generalizable to children with other critical care illnesses.

Clinical Implications

Instillation of normal saline had an adverse effect on oxygen saturation in children at 1 and 2 minutes after suctioning; however, oxygen saturation was not affected after 10 minutes. The adverse effects of normal saline instillation in children are similar to previous studies in adults. The study adds to the body of knowledge regarding the effects of normal saline instillation on physiological parameters.

4. Dezfulian C, Shohania K, Collard HR, Kim HM, Matthay MA, Saint S. Subglottic secretion drainage for preventing ventilator-associated pneumonia: a meta-analysis. *Am J Med*. 2005;118:11–18.

Study Sample

The authors retrieved 110 trials for the analysis. Five studies met the inclusion criteria of mechanically ventilated patients who were randomized to subglottic drainage versus no drainage and the incidence of pneumonia was reported. The 5 studies included a total of 896 patients.

Comparison Studied

This comprehensive, systematic meta-analysis of randomized controlled trials examined mechanically ventilated patients with endotracheal tubes who were assigned to standard endotracheal care versus subglottic suctioning.

Study Procedures

The authors searched databases for relevant studies from January 1966 to May 2003 using keywords: *glottis, suction, drainage, respiration, artificial, ventilation, mechanical, and pneumonia*. A second search was also done to identify any therapeutic or prevention strategies directed at ventilator-associated pneumonia. The authors of all included articles were contacted to ensure completeness of the search and to inquire regarding any unpublished research.

Key Results

The use of subglottic secretion drainage reduced the risk and incidence of ventilator-associated pneumonia by nearly half. Patients who received subglottic secretion drainage developed pneumonia 3.1 days later than patients who received standard endotracheal care and had a reduced risk of early-onset pneumonia based on bacterial etiology. Additionally, patients in the treatment group had 1.8 fewer days of mechanical ventilation and a 1.4 day shorter ICU stay. Hospital stay and mortality did not differ between the two groups. One of the 5 studies examined cardiac thoracic surgery patients who required short ventilator durations in contrast to the other 4 that all studied patients expected to remain ventilated longer than 72 hours. When removed from the analysis of the other 4 studies, the benefits of subglottic suctioning were even greater. This group had 2 fewer mechanical ventilator days and a 3-day shorter ICU stay. Pneumonia occured 6.8 days later and was less likely to be caused by organisms that typically characterize early onset of ventilator-associated pneumonia.

Study Strengths and Weaknesses

The clinical and statistical heterogeneity may have complicated the data analysis. Definitions for ventilator-associated pneumonia varied, all 5 studies required infiltrate on chest X-ray, while 2 used bronchoscopy for obtaining cultures, and 3 studies used nonbronchoscopic criteria. Additionally, methods varied in the use of subglottic drainage from continuous suction to manual aspiration.

Clinical Implications

Subglottic secretion suctioning reduces the risk of VAP nearly 50% with increased improvements in patients who were expected to be mechanically ventilated for longer than 72 hours. Drainage of subglottic secretions appears to be less effective in patients requiring mechanical ventilation longer than 72 hours. Subglottic secretion drainage appears to be an effective method to prevent ventilator-associated pneumonia and to decrease ventilator and ICU days in patients that are expected to require mechanical ventilation for more than 72 hours.

5. **Rabitsch W, Kostler WJ, Fiebiger W, Dielacher C, Losert H, Sherif C, Staudinger T, Seper E, Koller W, Daxbock F, Schuster E, Knobl P, Burgmann H, Frass M. Closed suctioning system reduces cross-contamination between bronchial system and gastric juices. *Anesth Analg*. 2004;99:886–892.**

Study Sample

The authors studied 24 intubated patients in a medical intensive care unit.

Comparison Studied

This prospective, randomized study was designed to evaluate whether a closed suctioning (CS) system influences crossover contamination between pulmonary system and gastric aspirates when compared with an open suctioning (OS) system.

Study Procedures

The study enrolled 24 consecutive patients who underwent mechanical ventilation. Inclusion criteria included expected length of ventilation greater than 72 hours and age greater than 18 years. Intubated patients were randomized into OS or CS groups. All patients were reintubated by using a tracheal tube exchanger no greater than 12 hours after initial intubation to the visualized endotracheal tube (VETT) system (Pulmonex). The VETT system consists of a PVC tube with fiber optics, a high-volume/low-pressure cuff, and a compact video camera allowing visualization of the lower

airways. Microbiological samples were obtained from tracheal secretions and gastric aspirates on day 1 and 3 and antibiograms were performed.

Key Results

The OS group had 5 cross-contaminations by antibiograms between tracheal and gastric secretions, and the CS group had none. Ventilator-associated pneumonia was also diagnosed in 5 of the OS group and in none of the CS group. Pulse oximetry did not differ between the 2 groups prior to suctioning but decreased immediately after suctioning in the OS group (statistically significant).

Study Strengths and Weaknesses

Limitations include the small sample size and the short length duration of study (ie, 1–3 days).

Clinical Implications

This is the first study to evaluate the use of CS versus OS with respect to the potential bacterial cross-contamination between gastric aspirates and the bronchial system. In this pilot study, CS appeared to prevent bacterial contamination and potential ventilator-associated pneumonia.

6. **Oh H, Seo W. A meta-analyis of the effects of various interventions in preventing endotracheal suction-induced hypoxemia. *J Clin Nurs*. 2003;12:912–924.**

Study Sample

The authors examined 30 studies that met criteria for inclusion.

Comparison Studied

The purpose of this meta-analysis was to clarify the effects of interventions that were applied to prevent endotracheal suction-induced hypoxia.

Study Procedures

The selection criteria for this meta-analysis included studies that investigated the effectiveness of interventions applied to prevent hypoxia post suctioning, studies published after 1970, human subject studies only, and included at least 1 intervention. Thirty studies were examined and included in the analysis; however, only 15 studies were included in the meta-analysis because detailed statistical data was not available for all studies.

Key Results

Results of the meta-analysis follow. Preoxygenation (administration of oxygen) reduced suction-induced hypoxia by 32%, and that number increased to 49% when combined with postoxygenation. Insufflation (delivery of oxygen through a double-lumen suction catheter or sidearm of an endotracheal tube adapter) increased suction-induced hypoxia by 63% and when combined with preoxygenation, by nearly 50%. Hyperoxygenation (administration of oxygen greater than what the patient is normally receiving) reduced hypoxia 30%. In addition, the reduction in hypoxia was 55% when hyperoxygenation and hyperinflation (inflating the lungs with a resuscitator bag or ventilator) were applied together. The most common FIO_2 applied in hyperoxygenation was 100%.

Study Strengths and Weaknesses

The authors noted the small samples used in the studies (ie, 322 subjects from 15 studies) and the inconsistencies between the techniques and terminology of the interventions.

Clinical Implications

The analysis revealed that preoxygenation alone and preoxygenation combined with hyperinflation decrease suction-induced hypoxia. Hyperinflation in this study was most commonly defined as a 150% tidal volume of 3–6 breaths via the ventilator rather than hyperinflation with a manual resuscitation bag. It also noted the importance of postoxygenation. The analysis did not demonstrate any improvement in hypoxemia with insufflation.

7. Metheny NA, Chang Y, Ye JS, Edwards SJ, Defer J, Dahms TE, Stewart BJ, Stone KS, Clouse RE. Pepsin as a marker for pulmonary aspiration. *Am J Crit Care*. 2002;11:150–154.

Study Sample

The authors examined 30 acutely ill, tube-fed patients receiving mechanical ventilaton.

Comparison Studied

The purpose of this research was to determine the frequency with which pepsin (found in gastric juice) is suctioned in tracheal secretions of tube-fed, mechanically ventilated patients and detected by immunoassay.

Study Procedures

A convenience sample of 136 specimens of suctioned tracheal secretions was collected in this exploratory study. Multiple samples were obtained from 26 of the 30 patients included in the study. An immunoassay with rooster polyclonal antibodies to human pepsin was used. The assay is highly specific, and all were performed by a biochemist. Additional data was also collected at the time of suctioning including whether the tube feeding was on, the type of feeding, and the position of the head of the bed.

Key Results

The results of the 136 specimens included; mean volume of 2.4 ± 0.2 mL normal saline was used with 52 specimens, and 23 were visibly bloody. Additionally the head of the bed was flat for 43 of the 136 specimens with tube feeding in progress with 85 of the 136. The remaining 51 specimens

were collected before tube feedings were started or when the feedings were on hold. Of the 136 specimens collected, 14 tested positive for pepsin with 5 subjects accounting for the results. The head of bed was flat for 13 out of the 14 positive pepsin specimens. These 13 positive results were from 4 patients with spinal cord injury.

Study Strengths and Weaknesses

The major weakness of this study is the small sample size.

Clinical Implications

The 14 positive pepsin samples suggest that gastric aspiration occurred in 5 of the 30 tube-fed, mechanically ventilated ICU patients. The findings also indicate that the immunoassay may be a better method for detecting aspiration than the questionable use of blue dye and the lack of specificity of glucose testing of aspirates. Additional work needs to be done to compare clinical outcomes with the presence or absence of pepsin in pulmonary secretions along with bedside availability of the test.

8. Grap MJ, Munro CL, Elswick RK, Sessler CN, Ward KR. Duration of action of a single, early oral application of chlorhexidine on oral microbial flora in mechanically ventilated patients: a pilot study. *Heart Lung*. 2004;33:83–91.

Study Sample

Thirty-four intubated patients admitted to the emergency department, surgical trauma ICU, and the neuroscience ICU were enrolled in this study.

Comparison Studied

The purpose of this pilot study was to describe the effect of an early postintubation oral application of 2 mL of 0.12% chlorhexidine gluconate (CHG) on oral microbial flora and ventilator-associated pneumonia.

Study Procedures

All trauma and surgical patients admitted to the emergency department, surgical trauma intensive care unit, and neuroscience intensive care unit were assessed for inclusion and randomized to the treatment group (single oral application of CHG by swab or spray) or to the control group (usual care). Subjects remained in the study for 72 hours after intubation or until extubation before 72 hours. Oral cultures for specific respiratory pathogens were obtained before intervention, 12 hours after study enrollment, and every 24 hours up to and including 72 hours. Sputum cultures and other data for measurement of ventilator-associated pneumonia were collected and tested using the Clincial Pulmonary Infection Score (CPIS) before the intervention, at 48 hours, and at 72 hours.

Key Results

Of the 34 patients enrolled, 23 patients were in the treatment group (11 CHG spray, 12 CHG swab), and 11 patients were in the control group. Ten patients had positive cultures at some-time during the study period (3 CHG spray, 3 CHG swab, and 4 control) with 5 of the 10 positive on admission. Reduction in oral culture scores were found in 2 patients (1 CHG swab and 1 CHG spray). The mean CPIS for the treatment group, although not statistically significant, increased only slightly (5.17 to 5.57 at 48 hours), whereas the mean CPIS for the control group increased from 4.7 to 6.6.

Study Strengths and Weaknesses

The major weakness of this study is the small sample size.

Clinical Implications

VAP pathogens may be present in the oral cavity earlier than previously documented. Although a statistically significant reduction was not seen with CHG treatment, a larger study may help to clarify the role of CHG in pulmonary infections. Although this pilot study examined post intubation application of CHG, additional research in the use of CHG before intubation may be important.

OTHER REFERENCES

1. AARC Clinical Practice Guideline. Endotracheal suctioning of mechanically ventilated adults and children with artificial airways. *Respir Care.* 1993;38:500–504.

2. AARC Clinical Practice Guideline. Management of airway emergencies. *Respir Care.* 1995;40:749–760.

3. AARC Clinical Practice Guideline. Removal of the endotracheal tube. *Respir Care.* 1999;44:85–90.

4. AARC Clinical Practice Guideline. Resuscitation and defibrillation in the healthcare setting. *Respir Care.* 2004;49:1085–1099.

5. Ackerman MH. The effect of saline lavage prior to suctioning. *Am J Crit Care.* 1993;2:326-330.

6. Ackerman M, Mick D. Installation of normal saline before suctioning in patients with pulmonary in prospective randomized trial. *Am J Crit Care.* 1998;7:261–266.

7. A Collective Task Force: American College of Chest Physicians; the American Association of Respiratory Care; & the American College of Critical Care. Evidence-based guidelines for weaning and discontinuing ventilatory support. *Chest.* 2001;120:375S–395S.

8. Ahrens T, Sona C. Capnography application in acute and critical care. *AACN Clin Issues.* 2003;14:123–132.

9. Akgul S, Akyolcu N. Effects of normal saline on endotracheal suctioning. *J Clin Nurs.* 2002;11:826–830.

10. American Association of Critical-Care Nurses. Ventilator-associated pneumonia [AACN practice alert]. Available at: http://www.aacn.org/AACN/practiceAlert.nsf/Files/VAP/$file/VAP.pdf. Accessed January 23, 2006.

11. American Heart Association. *Advanced Cardiac Life Support Procedure Manual.* Dallas, Tex:. American Heart Association. 2001.

12. American Society of Anesthesiology. *1995 Standards for Basic Anesthetic Monitoring.* 60th ed. Dallas, Tex: American Society of Anesthesiologists. 1995:384–385.

13. American Society of Anesthesiologists Task Force. Practice guidelines for management of the difficult airway. *Anesthesiology.* 2003;98:1269–1277.

14. American Thoracic Society and the Infectious Diseases Society of America. Guidelines for the management of adults with hospital-acquired, ventilator-associated, and healthcare-associated pneumonia. *Am J Respir Crit Care Med.* 2005;171:388–416.

15. Bach A, Boehrer H, Schmidt H, Geiss HK. Nosocomial sinusitis in ventilated patients. Nasotracheal versus orotracheal intubation. *Anaesthesia.* 1992;47:335–339.

16. Bach JR. Mechanical insufflation-exsufflation. Comparison of peak expiratory flows with manually assisted and unassisted coughing techniques. *Chest.* 1993;104:1553–1562.

17. Bach JR, Saporito LR. Criteria for extubation and tracheostomy tube removal for patients with ventilatory failure: a different approach to weaning. *Chest.* 1996;110:1566–1571.

18. Bailey C, Kattwinkel J, Teja K, Buckely T. Shallow versus deep endotracheal suctioning in young rabbits: pathologic effects on the tracheobronchial wall. *Heart Lung.* 1988;17:10–14.

19. Banner MJ, Blanch PB, Gabrielli A. Tracheal pressure control provides automatic and variable inspiratory pressure assist to decrease the impose resistive work of breathing. *Crit Care Med.* 2002;30:1106–1111.

20. Banner MJ, Kirby RR, Blanch PB. Differentiating total work of breathing into its component parts: essential for appropriate interpretation. *Chest.* 1996;109:1141–1143.

21. Barnason S, Graham J, Wild CM, Jensen LB, Rasmussen D, Schulz P, Woods S, Carder B. Comparison of two endotracheal tube securement techniques on unplanned extubation, oral mucosa, and facial skin integrity. *Heart Lung.* 1998;27:409–417.

22. Barnes TA, MacDonald D, Nolan J, et al. Airway devices. *Ann Emerg Med.* 2001;37:S145–S151.

23. Baun MM. Physiologic determinants of a clinically successful method of endotracheal suction. *West J Nurs Res.* 1984;6:213–228.

24. Beard B, Monaco FJ. Tracheostomy discontinuation: impact of tube selection on resistance during tube occlusion. *Respir Care.* 1993;38:267–270.

25. Bernhard WN, Cottrell, JE, Sivakumaran C, Patel K, Yost L, Turndorf H. Adjustment of intracuff pressure to prevent aspiration. *Anesthesiology.* 1979;50:363–366.

26. Berra L, De Marchi L, Panigada M, Yu Z, Baccarelli A, Kolobow T. Evaluation of continuous aspiration of subglottic secretion in vivo study. *Crit Care Med.* 2004;32:2071–2078.

27. Blackwood B. Normal saline instillation with endotracheal suctioning: primum non nocere (first do not harm). *J Adv Nurs.* 1999;29:928–934.

28. Bodai MM, Flones MJ. Cumulative effects of three sequential endotracheal suctioning episodes in the dog model. *Heart Lung.* 1984;15:148–154.

29. Boots RJ, Howe S, George N, Harris FM, Faoagali J. Clinical utility of hygroscopic heat and moisture exchangers in intensive care patients. *Crit Care Med.* 1997;25:1707–1712.

30. Bostick J, Wendelgass ST. Normal saline instillation as part of the suctioning procedure: effects on PaO$_2$ and the amount of secretions. *Heart Lung.* 1987;16: 532–540.

31. Bourjeily G, Fadlallah H, Supinski G. Review of tracheostomy usage: complications and decannulation procedures. *Clin Pulm Med.* 2002;9;273–278.

32. Boynton JH, Hawkins K, Eastridge BJ, O'Keefe GE. Tracheostomy timing and the duration of weaning in patients with acute respiratory failure. *Crit Care.* 2004;8:R261–R267.

33. Burns SM, Carpenter R, Smith, C, et al. Identifying inadvertent airway intubation during gastric tube insertion using a disposable colormetric CO$_2$ detector and variables that affect placement. Poster presented at: Annual Meeting of the Society for Critical Care Medicine; January 16, 2005; Phoenix, Ariz.

34. Burns SM, Carpenter R, Turwit JD. Report on the development of a procedure to prevent placement of feeding tubes into the lungs using end-tidal CO$_2$ measurements. *Crit Care Med.* 2001;29:936–939.

35. Burns SM, Spilman M, Wilmoth D, et al. Are frequent inner cannula changes necessary? a pilot study. *Heart Lung.* 1998;27:58–62.

36. Campbell DL, Ecklund M. Development of a research-based oral care procedure for patients with artificial airways. *NTI News.* May 7, 2002: B1–B16.

37. Celik S, Oztekin D, Akyolcu N, Isserver H. Sleep disturbance: the patient care activities applied at the night shift in the intensive care unit. *J Clin Nurs.* 2005;14: 102–106.

38. Center for Disease Control. Guidelines for preventing health-care-associated pneumonia, 2003. *MMWR.* 2004;53:1–36.

39. Cereda M, Villa F, Colombo E, Greco G, Nacoti M, Pesenti A. Closed system endotracheal suctioning maintains lung volume during volume-controlled mechanical ventilation. *Intensive Care.* 2001;27: 648–654.

40. Chang DW. In-hospital transport of the mechanically ventilated patient—2002 revision and update. AARC Clinical Practice Guideline. Available at: http://www.rcjournal.com/online_resources/cpgs/tmvpcpg-update.html. Accessed December 5, 2003.

41. Chase DZ, Campbell G, Byram D, Tribett D, Ananian L, Chulay M. Hemodynamic changes associated with endotracheal suctioning. *Heart Lung.* 1989;18:292–293.

42. Chastre J, Fagon J. State of the art: ventilator-associated pneumonia. *Am J Resp Crit Care Med.* 2002;165:867–903.

43. Chulay M. Arterial blood gas changes with a hyperinflation and hyperoxygenation suctioning intervention in critically ill patients. *Heart Lung.* 1988;17:654–661.

44. Chulay M, Graeber GM. Efficacy of a hyperinflation and hyperoxygenation suctioning intervention. *Heart Lung.* 1988;17:15–22.

45. Chulay M, Guzzetta C, Dossey B. AACN Handbook of Critical Care Nursing. Stamford, Conn: Appleton & Lange; 1997:119–153.

46. Collard H, Saint S, Matthay M. Prevention of ventilator-associated pneumonia: an evidence-based systematic review. *Ann Intern Med.* 2003;138: 494–501.

47. Connolly MA. Communicating with ventilator dependent patients. *Dimens Crit Care Nurs.* 1991;10: 115–122.

48. Conrardy PA, Goodman LR, Lainge F, Singer MM. Alteration of endotracheal tube position: flexion and extension of the neck. *Crit Care Med.* 1976;4:7–12.

49. Cook DJ, Meade MO, Perry AG. Qualitative studies on the patient's experience of weaning from mechanical ventilation. *Chest.* 2001;120:469S–473S.

50. Cooper JD, Grillo HC. Analysis of problems related to cuffs on endotracheal tubes. *Chest.* 1972;62:21–27.

51. Coppolo DP, May JJ. Self-extubations: a 12-month experience. *Chest.* 1990;98:165–169.

52. Cox CE, Carson SS, Holmes GM, Howard A, Carey T. Increase in tracheostomy for prolonged mechanical ventilation in North Carolina, 1993–2002. *Crit Care Med.* 2004;32:2219–2226.

53. Crimlisk JT, Horn MH, Wilson DJ, Marino B. Artificial airways: a survey of cuff management practices. *Heart Lung.* 1996;25:225–235.

54. Dane TEB, King EG. A prospective study of complications after tracheostomy for assisted ventilation. *Chest.* 1975;67:398–404.

55. Davis K, Branson RD, Porembka D. A comparison of the imposed work of breathing with endotracheal and tracheostomy tubes in a lung model. *Respir Care.* 1994;39:611–616.

56. DeBoer S, Seaver M, Amdt K. Verification of endotracheal tube placement: a comparison of confirmation techniques and devices. *J Emer Nurs.* 2003;29: 444–450.

57. Demers RS, Saklad M. Minimizing the harmful effects of mechanical aspiration. *Heart Lung.* 1973;2: 542–554.

58. Deutschman CS, Wilton P, Sinow J, Dibbell D Jr, Konstantinides FN, Cerra FB. Paranasal sinusitis associated with nasotracheal intubation: a frequently unrecognized source of sepsis. *Crit Care Med.* 1986; 14:111.

59. Dezfulian C, Shohania K, Collard HR, Kim HM, Matthay MA, Saint S. Subglottic secretion drainage for preventing ventilator-associated pneumonia: a meta-analysis. *Am J Med.* 2005;118:11–18.

60. Diehl J, El Atrous S, Touchard D, Lemaire F, Brochard L. Changes in the work of breathing induced by tracheostomy in ventilator-dependent patients. *Am J Respir Crit Care Med.* 1999;159:383–388.

61. Dobrum P, Canfield T. Cuffed endotracheal tubes, mucosal pressure and tracheal wall blood flow. *Am J Surg.* 1977;133:563–568.

62. Donald KJ, Robertson VJ, Tsebelis K. Setting an effective safe suction pressure: the effect of using a manometer in the suction circuit. *Intensive Care.* 2000;26:15–19.

63. Elpern EH, Okonek, MB, Bacon M, Gerstung C, Skrzynski M. Effect of the Passy-Muir tracheostomy speaking valve on pulmonary aspiration in adults. *Heart Lung.* 2000;29:287–293.

64. Elpern EH, Stutz L, Peterson S, Gurka DP, Skipper A. Outcomes associated with enteral tube feedings in a medical intensive care unit. *Am J Crit Care.* 2004;13: 221–227.

65. El-Solh AA, Pertrantoni C, Bhat A, et al. A reservoir of respiratory pathogens for hospital-acquired pneumonia in institutionalized elders. *Chest.* 2004;126: 1575–1582.

66. Ely EW, Inouye SK, Bernard GR, et al. Delirium in mechanically ventilated patient: validity and reliability for the intensive care unit (CAM-ICU). *JAMA.* 2001;286:2703–2710.

67. Ely EW, Gautam S, Margolin R, et al. The impact of delirium in the intensive care unit on hospital length of stay. *Intensive Care.* 2001;27:1892–1900.

68. Ely EW, Margolin R, Francis J, et al. Evaluation of delirium in critically ill patients: validation of the confusion assessment method for the intensive care unit (CAM-ICU). *Crit Care Med.* 2001;29:1370–1379.

69. Ely EW, Shintani A, Truman B, et al. Delirium as a predictor of mortality in mechanically ventilated patients in the intensive care unit. *JAMA.* 2004;291: 1753–1762.

70. Engoren M, Arslanian-Engoren C, Fenn-Buderer N. Hospital and long-term outcome after tracheostomy for respiratory failure. *Chest.* 2004;125:220–227.

71. Ernst A, Silvestri GA, Johnstone D. Interventional pulmonary procedures. *Chest.* 2003;123:1693–1717.

72. Fiastro JF, Habib MP, Quan SF. Pressure support compensation for inspiratory work due to endotracheal tubes and demand continuous positive airway pressure. *Chest.* 1988;93:499–505.

73. Fenstermacher D, Hong D. Mechanical ventilation—What have we learned? *Crit Care Nurs Q.* 2004;27: 258–294.

74. Fernadez M, Piacentini E, Blanch L, Fernandez R. Changes in lung volume with three systems of endotracheal suctioning with and without pre-oxygenation in patients with mild-to-moderate lung failure. *Intensive Care.* 2004;30:2210–2215.

75. Ferdinande P, Kim DO. Prevention of postintubation laryngotracheal stenosis. *Acta Otorhinolaryngol Belg.* 1995;49:341–346.

76. Finucane BT, Santora AH. *Principles of Airway Management.* 3rd ed. New York, NY: Springer-Verlag; 2003.

77. Fontaine DK. Sleep and the critically ill patient. In: Kinney MR, Packa DR, Dunbar SB, eds. *AACN Clinical Reference for Critical Care Nursing.* 3rd ed. St Louis, Mo: CV Mosby; 1993:351–364.

78. Fornataro-Clerici L, Zajac DJ. Aerodynamic characteristics of tracheostomy speaking valves. *J Speech Hear Res.* 1993;36:529–532.

79. Freytag CC, Theis FL, Konig W, Welte T. Prolonged application of closed-in-line suction catheters increases microbial colonization of the lower respiratory tract and bacterial growth on the catheter surface. *Infection.* 2004;31:31–37.

80. Frutos-Vivar F, Esteban A, Apezteguia C, et al. Outcome of mechanically ventilated patients who require a tracheostomy. *Crit Care Med.* 2005;33:290–314.

81. Gateley S, Cason C. Effectiveness of four methods of supplementing oxygen in minimizing suction-induced hypoxia. *Heart Lung.* 1985;14:11–17.

82. Goodnough SKC. Effects of oxygen and hyperinflation on arterial oxygen tension after endotracheal suctioning. *Heart Lung.* 1985;14:11–17.

83. Grap MJ, Munro C, Ashtiani B, Bryant S. Oral care interventions in critical care: frequency and documentation. *Am J Crit Care.* 2003;12:113–119.

84. Grap MJ, Munro CL, Elswick RK, Sessler CN, Ward KR. Duration of action of a single, early oral application of chlorhexidine on oral microbial flora in mechanically ventilated patients: a pilot study. *Heart Lung.* 2004;33:83–91.

85. Gray JE, MacIntyre NR, Kronenberger WG. The effects of bolus normal saline instillation in conjunction with endotracheal suctioning. *Respir Care.* 1990;35:785–790.

86. Griou E, Buu-Hoi A, Stephan F, et al. Airway colonization in long-term mechanically ventilated patients. Effects of semi-recumbent position and continuous subglottic suctioning. *Intensive Care.* 2004; 30:225–233.

87. Grmec S. Comparison of three different methods to confirm tracheal tube placement in emergency intubation. *Intensive Care.* 2002;28:701–704.

88. Grillo HC. The management of tracheal stenosis following assisted respiration. *J Thorac Cardiovasc Surg.* 1969;57:52–70.

89. Grillo HC, Cooper JD, Geffin B, Pontoppidan H. A low-pressure cuff for tracheostomy tubes to minimize tracheal injury. A comparative clinical trial. *J Thorac Cardiovasc Surg.* 1971;62:898.

90. Guyton DC, Barlow MR, Besselievre TR. Influence of airway pressure on minimum occlusive endotracheal tube cuff pressure. *Crit Care Med.* 1997;25:91–94.

91. Hagler DA, Traver GA. Endotracheal saline and suction catheters: sources of lower airway contamination. *Am J Crit Care.* 1994;3:444–447.

92. Halm MA, Sabo JA. Restraints: ritual or necessity? *AACN News.* July 2001:12–15.

93. Happ MB. Communicating with mechanically ventilated patients: state of the science. *AACN Clin Issues.* 2001;12:247–258.

94. Harris J, Miller T. Preventing nosocomial pneumonia: evidence-based practice. *Crit Care Nurse.* 2000;20:51–66.

95. Heffner JE. The role of tracheotomy in weaning. *Chest.* 2001;120:477S–484S.

96. Henneman E. Ask the expert: how often should ET tubes be repositioned and retaped? *Crit Care Nurse.* 1992;12:75–76.

97. Henneman EA. Patients with acute respiratory failure. In: Clochesy JM, Breu C, Cardin S, Whittaker AA, Rudy EB, eds. *Critical Care Nursing.* 2nd ed. Philadelphia, Pa: WB Saunders Co; 1996:630–655.

98. Heyland DK, Dhaliwal R, Drover JW, Gramlich L, Dodek R, the Canadian Critical Care Clinical Practice Guidelines Committee. Canadian clinical practice guidelines for nutritional support in mechanically ventilated, critically ill adult patients. *J Parenter Enteral Nutr.* 2003;27:355–373.

99. Heyland DK, Drover JW, Dhaliwal R, Greenwood J. Optimizing the benefits and minimizing the risks of enteral nutrition in the critically ill: role of small bowel feeding. *J Parenter Enteral Nutr.* 2002;26:S51–S55.

100. Houston S, Hougland P, Anderson JJ, LaRocco M, Kennedy V, Gentry LO. Effectiveness of 0.12% chlorhexidine gluconate oral rinse in reducing prevalence of nosocomial pneumonia in patients undergoing heart surgery. *Am J Crit Care.* 2002;11:567–570.

101. Hsu C, Chen K, Chang C, Jerng J, Yu C, Yang P. Timing of tracheostomy as a determinant of weaning success in critically ill patients: a retrospective study. *Crit Care.* 2005;9:R46–R52.

102. Hussey JD, Bishop MJ. Pressures required to move gas through the native airway in the presence of a fenestrated vs. a non-fenestrated tracheostomy tube. *Chest.* 1996;110:494–497.

103. Ibrahim EH, Mehringr L, Prentice D, et al. Early versus late enteral feedings of mechanically ventilated patients: results of a clinical trial. *J Parenter Enteral Nutr.* 2002;26:174–181.

104. Iregui M, Vaughan W, Kollef M. Nonpharmacological prevention of hospital-acquired pneumonia. *Seminars in Respiratory and Crit Care Med.* 2002;23:489–495.

105. Jaber S, Chanques G, Matecki S, et al. Post-extubation stridor in intensive care unit patients. *Intensive Care.* 2003;29:69–74.

106. Jacobi J, Fraser GL, Coursin DB, et al. Clinical practice guidelines for the sustained use of sedatives and analgesics in the critically ill adult. *Crit Care Med.* 2002;30:119–141.

107. Joint Commission on Accreditation of Healthcare Organizations. *Specific Manual for National Hospital Quality Measures—ICU (2005).* Available at: http://www.jcaho.org/pms/core+measures /icu+manual.htm. Accessed February 14, 2005.

108. Joint Commission on Accreditation of Healthcare Organizations. Preventing ventilator-related deaths and or injuries. *Sentinel Alert.* 2002. Available at: http://www.jcaho.org/about+us/news+letters/ sentinel+event+alert/print/sea_25.htm. Accessed April 11, 2005.

109. Kacmarek RM, Mack CW, Dimas S. *The Essentials of Respiratory Care.* 3rd ed. St. Louis, Mo: Mosby-Year Book, Inc; 1990.

110. Kaplow R, Bookbinder M. A comparison of four endotracheal tube holders. *Heart Lung.* 1994;23:59–66.

111. Kearl RA, Hooper RG. Massive air leaks: an analysis of the role of endotracheal tubes. *Crit Care Med.* 1993;21:518–521.

112. Kim PW, Roghmann MC, Perencevich EN, Harris AD. Rates of hand disinfection associated with glove use, patient isolation, and changes between exposure to various body site. *Am J Infection Control.* 2003;31:97–102.

113. King BR, Baker MD, Braitman LE, et al. Endotracheal tube selection in children: a comparison of four methods. *Ann Emerg Med.* 1993;22:530–534.

114. King K, Mandava B, Kamen JM. Tracheal tube cuffs and tracheal dilation. *Chest.* 1975;67:458–462.

115. Kinoch D. Instillation of normal saline during endotracheal suctioning: effects on mixed venous oxygen. *Am J Crit Care.* 1999;8:170–172.

116. Kleiber C, Krutzfield N, Rose EF. Acute histological changes in the tracheobronchial tree associated with different suction catheter insertion techniques. *Heart Lung.* 1988;17:10–14.

117. Koeman M, Chlorhexidine 2% preparation reduces the incidence of ventilator-associated pneumonia. Medscape Medical News Web site. Available at: http://www.medscape.com/viewarticle/492864_print. Accessed November 14, 2004.

118. Kollef MH. Prevention of hospital-associated pneumonia and ventilator-associated pneumonia. *Crit Care Med.* 2004;32:1396–1405.

119. Kollef MH. The prevention of ventilator-associated pneumonia. *N Engl J Med.* 1999;340:627–634.

120. Kollef MH, Shapiro SD, Boyd V, et al. A randomized clinical trial comparing an extended-use hygroscopic condenser humidifier with heated-water humidification in mechanically ventilated patients. *Chest.* 1998; 113:759–767.

121. Kollef MH, Skubas NJ, Sundt TM. A randomized clinical trial of continuous aspiration of subglottic secretions in cardiac surgery patients. *Chest.* 1999;116: 1339–1346.

122. Kunis KA, Puntillo KA. Ventilator-associated pneumonia in the ICU. *Am J Nurs.* 2003;103:64AA–64GG.

123. Kuzenski BM. Effect of negative pressure on tracheobronchial trauma. *Nurs Res.* 1978;27:260–263.

124. Lambolt N. Design and function of tracheal suction catheters. *Acta Anaesthesiol Scand.* 1982;26:1–3.

125. Leur JP, Zwaveling JH, Loef BG, Schans CP. Endotracheal suctioning versus minimally invasive airway suctioning in intubated patients: a prospective randomized controlled trial. *Intensive Care.* 2003;29: 426–432.

126. Levy H, Griego L. A comparative study of oral endotracheal tube securing methods. *Chest.* 1993;104: 1537–1540.

127. Lewis FR, Schlobohm RM, Thomas AN. Prevention of complications from prolonged tracheal intubation. *Am J Surg.* 1979;135:452–457.

128. Lin SM, Liu CY, Wang SH, et al. The impact of delirium on the survival of mechanically ventilated patients. *Crit Care Med.* 2004;32:2254–2259.

129. Loeser EA, Hodges M, Gliedman J, Stanley TH, Johansen RK, Yonetani D. Tracheal pathology following short-term intubation with low- and high-pressure endotracheal tube cuffs. *Anesth Analg.* 1978;57:577–579.

130. Lorente L, Lecuona M, Martin MM, Garcia C, Mora ML, Sierra A. Ventilator-associated pneumonia using a closed versus an open tracheal suction system. *Crit Care Med.* 2005;33:115–119.

131. Lovett PB, Flaxman A, Sturmann K. The insecure airway: a comparison of knots and commercial devices for securing endotracheal tubes [Abstract]. *Acad Emerg Med.* 2003;10:485–486.

132. Lucarelli MR, Shirk MB, Julian MW, Crouser ED. Toxicity of food drug and cosmetic Blue No. 1 dye in critically ill patients. *Chest.* 2004;125:793–795.

133. Ludy JE, Sole ML, Ludy M. Ventilatory assistance. In Sole ML, Klein DG, Moseley MJ, eds. *Introduction to Critical Care Nursing.* 4th ed. St. Louis, Mo: Elsevier, Inc; 2005:159–214.

134. Maccioli GA, Dorman T, Brown BR, et al. Clinical practice guidelines for the maintenance of patient physical safety in the intensive care unit: use of restraining therapies—American College of Crit Care Med Task Force 2001–2002. *Crit Care Med.* 2003;31: 2665–2676.

135. Maithel S, Blackburn GL. Editorial: Feeding the critically ill patient. *J Parenter Enteral Nutr.* 2003;27: 383–384.

136. Mancinelli-Van Atta J, Beck SL. Preventing hypoxemia and hemodynamic compromise related to endotracheal suctioning. *Am J Crit Care.* 1992;3:62–79.

137. Manzano JL, Lubillo S, Henriquez D, Martin JC, Perez MC, Wilson DJ. Verbal communication of ventilator dependent patients. *Crit Care Med.* 1993;21: 512–517.

138. Maury E, Guglielminotti J, Alzieu M, et al. How to identify patients with no risk for postextubation stridor? *J Crit Care.* 2004;19:23–28.

139. McClave SA, DeMeo MT, DeLegge MH, et al. North American summit on aspiration in the critically ill patient: a consensus statement. *J Parenter Enteral Nutr.* 2002;26:S80–S85.

140. McGinnis GE, Shively JG, Patterson RL, Magovern GJ. An engineering analysis of intratracheal tube cuffs. *Anesth Analg.* 1971;50:558.

141. Lynn-McHale Wiegand DJ, Carlson KK. *AACN Procedure Manual for Critical Care.* 5th ed. Philadelphia, Pa: Elsevier; 2005.

142. Medina M, Beydoun HK, Hsu WW, Brandstetter RD. Reducing unplanned extubations: the benefit of combined chest and arm restraints with sedation. *Chest.* 1993;273(s).

143. Metheny NA. Bedside methods for detecting aspiration in tube-fed patients. *Chest.* 1997;111:724–731.

144. Metheny NA, Chang Y, Ye JS, et al. Pepsin as a marker for pulmonary aspiration. *Am J Crit Care.* 2002;11:150–154.

145. Metheny NA, Scallom ME, Edwards SJ. Effect of gastrointestinal motility and feeding tube site on aspiration risk in critically ill patients: a review. *Heart Lung.* 2004;33:131–145.

146. Mevio E, Benazzo M, Quaglieri S, Mencherial S. Sinus infection in intensive care patients. *Rhinol.* 1996;34:1035–1040.

147. Miller RL, Cole RP. Association between reduced cuff leak volume and postextubation stridor. *Chest.* 1996;110:1035–1040.

148. Motta GJ, Trigillia D. The effect of an antimicrobial drain sponge dressing on specific bacterial isolates at tracheostomy sites. *Ostomy Wound.* 2005;51:60–66.

149. Nash M, Har-Ef G, Einhorn R. Advances in tracheotomy tube technology. *Surg Rounds.* 1996; November: 470–483.

150. Oh H, Seo W. A meta-analysis of the effects of various interventions in preventing endotracheal suction-induced hypoxemia. *J Clin Nurs.* 2003;12:912–924.

151. O'Keefe SJ, Foody W, Gill S. Transnasal endoscopic placement of feeding tubes in the intensive care unit. *J Parenter Enteral Nutr.* 2003;27:349–354.

152. Pacheco-Fowler V, Gaonkar T, Wyer PC, Modak S. Antiseptic-impregnated endotracheal tubes for the prevention of bacterial colonization. *J Hosp Infect.* 2004;57:170–174.

153. Parthasarathy S, Tobin MJ. Effect of ventilator mode on sleep quality in critically ill patients. *Am J Respir Crit Care Med.* 2002;166:1423–1429.

154. Parthasarathy S, Tobin MJ. Sleep in the intensive care unit. *Intensive Care.* 2004;30:197–206.

155. Pesiri AJ. Two-year study of the prevention of unintentional extubation. *Crit Care Q.* 1994;17:35–39.

156. Pesiri AJ, Stewart K, Kobe E, Stewart W. Protocol for prevention of unintentional extubation. *Crit Care Nurs Q.* 1990;12:87–90.

157. Pfeifer L, Orser L, Gefen C, McGuinees R, Hannon C. Preventing ventilator-associated pneumonia: what all nurses should know. *Am J Nurs.* 2001;101:24AA–24GG.

158. Pisani MA, McNicoll L, Inouye SK. Cognitive impairment in the intensive care unit. *Clin Chest Med.* 2003;24:727–737.

159. Puntillo KA, White C, Morris A, et al. Patients' perceptions and responses to procedural pain: results from the Thunder II Project. *Am J Crit Care.* 2001;10:238–251.

160. Rabitsch W, Kostler WJ, Fiebiger W, et al. Closed suctioning system reduces cross-contamination between bronchial system and gastric juices. *Anesth Analg.* 2004;99:886–892.

161. Raymond SJ. Normal saline instillation before suctioning: helpful or harmful? a review of the literature. *Am J Crit Care.* 1995;4:267–271.

162. Rello J, Ollendorf D, Oster G, et al. Epidemiology and outcomes of ventilator-associated pneumonia in a large US database. *Chest.* 2002;122:2115–2121.

163. Richard I, Girard M, Perrouin-Verbe B, Hiance D, Mauduyt de la Greve I, Mathe JF. Laryngotracheal stenosis after intubation or tracheostomy in patients with neurological disease. *Arch Phys Med Rehabil.* 1966;77:493–496.

164. Richmond AL, Jarog DL, Hanson VM. Unplanned extubation in adult critical care: quality improvement and education payoff. *Crit Care Nurse.* 2004;94:31–37.

165. Ridling DA, Martin LD. Endotracheal suctioning with or without instillation of isotonic chloride solution in critically ill children. *Am J Crit Care.* 2003;12:212–219.

166. Rubenfeld GD. Implementing effective ventilator practice at the bedside. *Curr Opin Crit Care.* 2004;10:33–39.

167. Rumbak MJ, Newton M, Truncale T, Schwartz SW, Adams J, Hazard PB. A prospective, randomized study comparing early percutaneous dilational tracheotomy to prolonged translaryngeal intubation (delayed tracheotomy)in critically ill medical patients. *Crit Care Med.* 2004;32:1689–1694.

168. Salahudin N, Zafar A, Sukhyani L, et al. Reducing ventilator-associated pneumonia rates through a staff education programme. *J Hosp Infect.* 2004;57:223–227.

169. Sandhu RS, Pasquale MD, Miller K, et al. Measurement of endotracheal tube cuff leak to predict postextubation stridor and need for reintubation. *J Am Coll Surg.* 2000;190:682–687.

170. Schleder B. Taking charge of ventilator-associated pneumonia. *Nurs Manage.* 2003;34:27–33.

171. Schleder B, Stott K, Lloyd RC. The effects of a comprehensive oral care protocol on patients at risk for ventilator-associated pneumonia. *J Advocate Health Care.* 2002;4:27–29.

172. Schweickert WD, Gehlbach BK, Pohlman AS, Hall JB, Kress JP. Daily interruption of sedative infusions and complications of critical illness in mechanically ventilated patients. *Crit Care Med.* 2004;32:1272–1276.

173. Sengstack P, Begley E. Acute care: the in's and out's of tracheostomy tubes. *Advances for Nurses.* 1999;1:11–14.

174. Shah C, Kollef MH. Endotracheal tube intraluminal volume loss among mechanically ventilated patients. *Crit Care Med.* 2004;32:120–125.

175. Skinner MW, Waldron RJ, Anderson MB. Normal laryngoscopy and intubation. In: Hanowell LH, Waldron RJ, eds. *Airway Management.* Philadelphia, Pa: Lippincott-Raven; 1996:81–96.

176. Smulders K, van der Hoeven H, Weers-Pothoff I, Vandenbroucke-Grauls C. A randomized clinical trial of intermittent subglottic secretion drainage in patients receiving mechanical ventilation. *Chest.* 2002;121:858–862.

177. Society of Otorhinolaryngology and Head-Neck Nurses. Practice guidelines: tracheostomy. *ORL Head Neck Nurs.* 1994;12:26–29.

178. Solazzi RW, Ward RJ. Analysis of anesthetic mishaps. The spectrum of medical liability cases. *Int Anesthesiol Clin.* 1984;22:43–59.

179. Sole ML, Byers JF, Ludy JE, Zhang Y, Banta CM, Brummel K. A multisite survey of suctioning techniques and airway management practices. *Am J Crit Care.* 2003;12:220–232

180. Sole ML, Poalillo FE, Byers JF, Ludy JE. Bacterial growth in secretions and on suctioning equipment of orally intubated patients: a pilot study. *Am J Crit Care.* 2002;11:141–149.

181. St. John RE. Airway management. *Crit Care Nurse.* 2004;24:93–96.

182. St. John RE, Malen JF. Contemporary issues in adult tracheostomy management. *Crit Care Nurs Clin N Am.* 2004;16:413–430.

183. St John RE. The pulmonary system. In: Alspach JG, ed, *Core Curriculum for Critical Care Nursing.* 5th ed. Philadelphia, Pa: WB Saunders Co; 1998;1–136.

184. Stauffer JL, Olson DE, Petty TL. Complications and consequences of endotracheal intubation and tracheostomy. *Am J Med.* 1981;70:65–76.

185. Stauffer J, Silvestri R. Complications of endotracheal intubation and tracheostomy. *Am J Med.* 1982;27:417–434.

186. Stewart CE. *Advanced Airway Management.* Upper Saddle River, NJ: Pearson Education, Inc; 2003:34–150.

187. Stone KS, Vorst EC, Lanham B, Zahn S. Effects of lung hyper-inflation on mean arterial pressure and post-suctioning hypoxemia. *Heart Lung.* 1989;14: 377–385.

188. Stone SJ, Pickett JD, Jesurum JT. Bedside placement of postpyloric feeding tubes. *AACN Clin Issues.* 2000;11:517–530.

189. Tasota FJ. Myth vs. reality: instillation of normal saline with suctioning. *AACN News.* 2002;19.

190. Tayal VS. Tracheostomies. *Emerg Med Clin North Am.* 1994;12:707–727.

191. Thompson L. Suctioning adults with an artificial airway. *The Joanna Briggs Institute for Evidence Based Nursing and Midwifery.* 2000;4:1–6.

192. Trout S, Aaron J, Zapta-Sirvent RL, Hansbrough JF. Influence of head and neck position on endotracheal tube position on chest X-ray examination: a potential problem in the infant undergoing intubation. *J Burn Care Rehabil.* 1994;15:405–407.

193. Ufberg JW, Bushra JS, Patel D, Wong E, Karras DJ, Kueppers F. A new pepsin assay to detect pulmonary aspiration of gastric contents among newly intubated patients. *Am J Emerg Med.* 2004;22:612–613.

194. Van Hooser DT. *Airway clearance with closed-system suctioning.* American Association of Critical-Care Nurses Web site. Available at: http://aacn.org /pdfLibra.NSF/Files/Airwayweb/$file/Airwayweb .pdf. Accessed Novemeber 17, 2005.

195. Van Saene HK, Ashworth M, Petros AJ, Sanchez M, de la Cal MA. Do not suction above the cuff. *Crit Care Med.* 2004;32:2160–2162.

196. Vassal R, Anh NGD, Gabillet JM, Guidet B, Staikowsky F, Offenstadt B. Prospective evaluation of self-extubations in a medical intensive care unit. *Intensive Care.* 1993;19:340–342.

197. Vincent JL. Ventilator-associated pneumonia. *J Hosp Infect.* 2004;57:272–280.

198. Ward CG, Gorham K, Hammond J, Varas R. Securing endotracheal tubes in patients with facial burns or trauma. *Am J Surg.* 1990;159:339–340.

199. Weilitz PB, Dettenmeier PA. Test your knowledge of tracheostomy tubes. *Am J Nurs.* 1994;94:46–50.

200. Whited RE. A prospective study of laryngotracheal sequela in long-term intubation. *Laryngoscope.* 1984; 94:367–377.

201. Williams ML. An algorithm for selecting a communication technique with intubated patients. *Dimens Crit Care Nurs.* 1992;11:222–229.

202. William R, Rankin N, Smith T, Galler D, Seakins P. Relationship between the humidity and temperature of inspired gas and the function of the airway mucosa. *Crit Care Med.* 1996;24:1920–1929.

203. Wilson D. Care of the chronic mechanically ventilated patient. In: Clochesy JM, Breu C, Cardin S, Whittaker AA, Rudy EB, eds. *Critical Care Nursing.* 2nd ed. Philadelphia, Pa: WB Saunders Co; 1996:689–713.

204. Wood DE, Mathisen DJ. Late complications of tracheotomy. *Clin Chest Med.* 1991;12:597–609.

205. Yaremchuk K. Regular tracheostomy tube changes to prevent formation of granulation tissue. *Laryngoscope.* 2003;113:1–10.

206. Yokoyama M, Kaga K, Suzuki M, Ishimoto S. Innominate artery erosion complicating use of tracheal tube with adjustable flange. *ORL J Otorhinolaryngol Relat Spec.* 1995;57:293–295.

207. Zack J, Garrison T, Trovillion E, et al. Effect of an education program aimed at reducing the occurrence of ventilator-associated pneumonia. *Crit Care Med.* 2002;30:2407–2411.

208. Zarotsky KE, D'Amelio LF. Bedside percutaneous tracheostomy: implications for critical care nurses. *Crit Care Nurse.* 1995;15:37–38,40–43.

209. Zeitouon SS, De Barros AL, Diccini S. A prospective, randomized study of ventilator-associated pneumonia in patients using a closed vs. open suction system. *J Clin Nurs.* 2003;12:484–489.

Equipment Guidelines for Intubation and Suctioning

Equipment	Infant (Premature to 1 Year)	Small Child (2–5 Years)	School-Age Child (6–12 Years)	Adolescent to Adult
Airway size				
Oral	00–2	2–3	3–4	4–5
Nasal (French)	12	16–20	20–24	24–36
Handheld resuscitator size	Child	Child	Child/Adult	Adult
Mask size	Preemie–Infant/Child	Child	Small Adult	Adult
Laryngoscope blade size	0–1 (Straight)	2 (Straight)	2–3 (Straight or curved)	4–5 (Straight or curved)
Endotracheal tube size (mm ID)	2.5–4.0	4.0–5.0	5.0–6.5	7.0–9.0
Tracheostomy tube size				
Jackson size	00–1	1–2	3–4	4–10
Inner diameter (mm ID)	2.5–3.5	3.0–5.5	4.0–6.5	5.0–9.0
Suction catheter size (French) Note: Catheter outer diameter should not exceed one-half the internal diameter of the tube.	5–6	6–8	8–10	10–16
Combitube esophageal/tracheal double-lumen airway size (French)		For patients 4′ to 5′6″ tall 37 Fr	For patients 5′ tall and above 41 Fr	

These guidelines should be used as an estimate only; actual sizes depend on the size and individual needs of the patient.
Always follow manufacturer recommendations.

Comparison of Artificial Airways

Type	Indications	Advantages	Disadvantages	Complications	Comments
Nasopharyngeal airway (nasal trumpet) (Figure 1B-1)	When frequent nasotracheal suctioning is indicated on a nonintubated patient • Most useful on lethargic, or semiresponsive patients who are breathing spontaneously but who are unable to effectively cough and clear their secretions from the hypopharynx. • May be used instead of an oral airway when that type of airway is not feasible (eg, oral trauma, intact gag reflex).	Allows for frequent suctioning without damage to nasal mucosa from the suction catheter: • Easy to insert • Minimal training required • Can be used and removed as needed	Uncomfortable for the patient, especially if left in for more than 1 or 2 days: • Easily dislodged • If the tube is too long, it may enter the esophagus. • May injure the nasal mucosa with bleeding and possible clots aspirated into trachea.	Bleeding, nasal-mucosal damage, laryngospasm, vomiting, gastric distention (if tube extends into the esophagus): • Longer use may be associated with increased risk of sinusitis, otitis, bleeding (common during initial insertion but usually minimal).	Adult sizes (ID mm) Large: 8.0 to 9.0 Medium: 7.0 to 8.0 Small: 6.0 to 7.0 The most common French sizes are 28, 30, and 32 Fr. • Use water soluble lubricant or anesthetic jelly for insertion. • Gently insert close to the midline along the floor of the nostril into the posterior pharynx behind the tongue. • Secure airway to nose with adhesive or twill tape. • Tube should be changed to the other nostril every 24 hours to avoid pressure necrosis of the nasal mucosa. • Use caution not to insert the airway too deep as it may enter the larynx or esophagus.

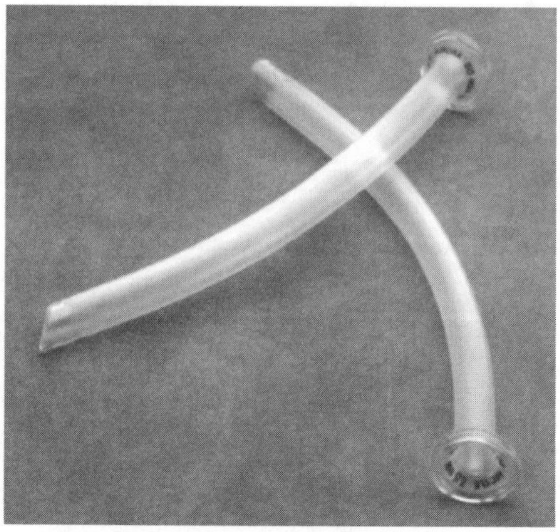

FIGURE 1B-1: Nasopharyngeal airway (nasal trumpet).

Type	Indications	Advantages	Disadvantages	Complications	Comments
Oropharyngeal (oral) airway (Figure 1B-2)	• Oral airways are rigid or slightly flexible devices that displace the base of the tongue from the posterior pharyngeal wall. • Used as an intermediate, short-term method to maintain an open airway in unconscious patients until a more stable airway can be inserted • Permits bag-valve-mask ventilation • Also used to prevent patient from biting on an orotracheal tube and facilitates suctioning inside the mouth	• Easy to insert by trained personnel	• Will cause gagging in the awake patient; therefore, should not be used unless the gag reflex is absent or blunted by anesthesia. • Makes oral care difficult • Should not be used routinely with orotracheal intubation	• If the airway is too long, it may press the epiglottis against the entrance to the larynx, producing complete airway obstruction. • Oral mucosal breakdown • Gagging with possible vomiting, aspiration, and laryngospasm • Patient discomfort • Dental injuries, soft tissue ulceration, and pressure necrosis of the lip, tongue, palate, and posterior pharyngeal wall (lower lip ulcers are especially common).	Comes in pediatric and adult sizes. Adult sizes Large: 100 mm (size 5) Medium: 90 mm (size 4) Small: 80 mm (size 3) • Styles include: Guedel (tubular) and Berman (channels along its sides) • It is important to suction the mouth and pharynx prior to placing an oral airway. • Important not to push the tongue posteriorly during insertion, obstructing the airway • During use, it is critical to inspect the lips and oral mucosa for potential pressure areas and maintain oral hygiene. • Remove, clean, and reposition daily as feasible.

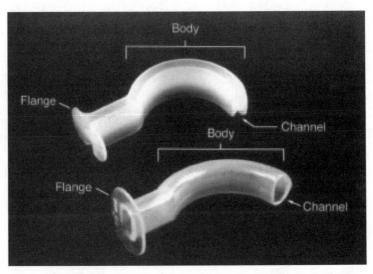

FIGURE 1B-2: Oropharyngeal (oral) airway.

Type	Indications	Advantages	Disadvantages	Complications	Comments
Combitube	• Utilized to provide an emergency airway while resuscitating a profoundly unconscious patient who requires artificial airway support, and when endotracheal intubation is not readily available or has failed to successfully establish an airway • Used for prehospital, surgical, and emergency care • Tube is available in two sizes, based on patient height (see Appendix 1A for sizing)	• Double-lumen design allows for rapid airway establishment through either esophageal or tracheal placement. • Can be inserted blindly (by trained personnel), which eliminates the need for laryngoscope • Pharyngeal balloon holds device firmly in place and helps prevent escape of gas through nose or mouth. • Full-length lumen allows for suctioning of gastric contents with no interruption of ventilation in the event the Combitube airway is placed in the esophagus. • Esophageal cuff inflates to seal esophagus so gas does not enter the stomach and gastric contents are not aspirated. • Requires no stabilization or securing device following placement.	• Will cause gagging in awake patient with intact gag reflex • Should not be used in patients with known esophageal disease • Contraindicated in patients who have ingested caustic agents. • See manufacturer recommendations	• Combitube contains latex and may cause allergic reaction in those patients and caregivers with known sensitivity to latex. • Medications delivered by endotracheal tube cannot be used with a Combitube in the esophageal position. • Improper placement and resultant hypoventilation • Sore throat • Dysphagia • Bleeding • Pharyngeal perforation • Esophageal laceration or rupture	• Must be replaced with an endotracheal tube if continued airway management (in-hospital) is required. • Multiple steps required for proper insertion, placement, assessment, and cuff inflation. As with any airway device, always follow manufacturer instructions for use. • Proper assessment of tube location with verification by both auscultation and other additional methods (ie, end-tidal carbon dioxide or colorimetric CO_2 detection) is important. • Ongoing assessment of ventilation effectiveness is critical while Combitube is in place. • When removing Combitube, ensure that personnel qualified in endotracheal intubation are present.

Type	Indications	Advantages	Disadvantages	Complications	Comments
Oral endotracheal tube (Figure 1B-3)	• Modern tracheal tubes are disposable and individually packaged for single use in sterile, transparent plastic that maintains the required radius of curvature. • Airway management required for short term or when mechanical ventilation is necessary • Used in patients with sinus problems, nasal fractures, or at risk for sinusitis.	• Allows for direct visualization of the vocal cords • Ease and speed of tube placement in most individuals • Low mortality rate associated with placement	• Patient discomfort secondary to placement in mouth and inability to speak • Greater potential for poor nutrition than tracheotomy • Aesthetically more objectionable than tracheotomy • Placement in a semiconscious patient may result in vomiting and aspiration of gastric contents • Difficult to insert in patients with limited neck mobility	• Oral bleeding • Broken teeth • Aspiration • Esophageal intubation • Vocal cord injury • Right mainstem intubation (most frequent complication) • Cuff leak or failure • Tube obstruction (secretions)	• Most commonly used in ICU setting • Awake patient often requires IV sedation prior to insertion. • Larger size endotracheal tubes ($\geq$ 8 mm ID) allow for easy passage of bronchoscope. • Some patients require addition of oral airway to protect from tube biting.

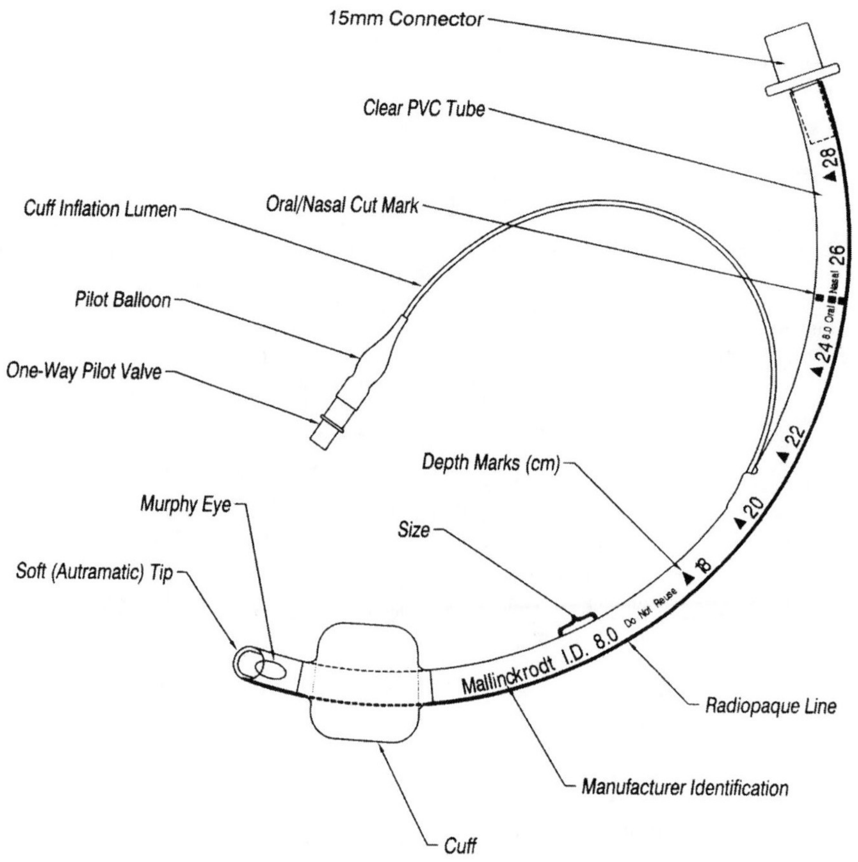

FIGURE 1B-3: Oral endotracheal tube.

Type	Indications	Advantages	Disadvantages	Complications	Comments
Nasal endotracheal tube	• Airway management required for short term or when mechanical ventilation is necessary • Breathing patient who requires an artificial airway • Can be used in patient with cervical spine injuries if in-line stabilization is used (eg, C-spine collar)	• Does not require neck extension • Can be used in an awake patient • Facilitates oral care • May be easier for patients to communicate (can mouth words) • Patients may be able to take small sips of liquids • Reduced risk of right mainstem intubation	• Technically more difficult to insert, requires highly skilled clinician • Spontaneous breathing is required for blind nasal intubation	• Nasal bleeding • Sinusitis • Otitis • Esophageal intubation • Vocal cord injury • Cuff leak or failure • Tube obstruction (secretions)	• Contraindicated in patients with a coagulopathy, when cerebrospinal fluid is present (leaking), and with intranasal disorders. • The smaller ID tube used with nasal intubation may make suctioning more difficult, along with increasing airflow resistance and work of breathing, and difficulty in passing fiber-optic bronchoscope.
Laryngeal mask airway (large bore tube with a distal inflatable molded mask)	• May be used as an alternative to the face mask for maintaining control of the airway during anesthetic procedures • Also indicated as an emergency airway when standard endotracheal intubation is not available or has failed • Patient should be unconscious during insertion	• Blind insertion through the mouth into the hypopharynx without need for direct visualization of the vocal cords • Decreased trauma because insertion does not require laryngoscope or pass through the vocal cords	• Temporary • Does not protect against aspiration • The LMA provides a low-pressure seal and cannot be used for patients where high peak pressures are anticipated	• Most common complications are air leaks and aspiration.	• The LMA is considered an appropriate short-term airway by the American Heart Association ACLS 2000 program. • Comes in reusable and disposable models along with a variety of sizes from neonate to adult depending on manufacturer. Several manufacturers offer similar types of laryngeal-sealing airway devices with different designs and features.
Tracheostomy tube	When a definitive airway cannot be established with an oral or nasal endotracheal tube (eg, upper airway trauma) When long-term airway management is indicated	• Provides a stable airway • Avoids laryngeal and upper airway complications of translaryngeal intubation • Provides greater patient comfort than endotracheal intubation • Facilitation of feeding, mouth care, suctioning, and speech • Elimination of right mainstem intubation • Decreases airway resistance and mechanical dead space (shorter tube) • Improved mobility for less intensive patient care environment (transfer out of ICU to ward, subacute, or long-term facility)	• Requires use of operating room in most cases. However, there is increasing interest in percutaneous technique that allows placement in the ICU at the bedside. • Permanent scar • Potential for more severe complications (eg, tracheal stenosis) • Increased frequency of aspiration • Persistent open stoma for several days after decannulation, reducing cough efficiency	• Hemorrhage • Subcutaneous emphysema • Pneumothorax, pneumomediastinum • Stoma infection • Aspiration • Granuloma formation • Tube obstruction • Tracheoesophageal fistula • Tracheoinnominate artery fistula • Airway bacterial colonization • Tracheal stenosis • Tracheal malacia	• Many sizes/types available with special features to meet individual patient needs (see Appendix 1C). • Percutaneous tracheotomy involves inserting either a single or multiple dilator through the skin and into the trachea between the 2nd and 3rd tracheal ring to expand the tissue and create a stoma tract. Complication rates are the same or slightly less than traditional surgical technique. This technique should not be performed with uncorrected coagulopathy, midline neck mass, nonintubated patients, and in children.

Types of Tracheostomy Tubes

Tube Type	Description	Advantages	Disadvantages	Comments
Plastic/Silicone (Figures 1C-1, 1C-2, 1C-3, 1C-4, 1C-5, 1C-6, 1C-9)	• Plastic tracheostomy tubes are the most commonly used type of tube in critical care. They are available with or without a cuff. Tubes may be fenestrated or nonfenestrated. • These tubes are considered "disposable"—they are left in for finite periods, whereas metal tubes must be cleaned but last for extended time periods. • Available in variety of sizes. The Jackson tube size scheme does not correspond exactly either to the outer or inner diameter of the tube, rather, it is a general approximation for tube identification. • Specifications for tube sizes (eg, inner diameter [ID], outer diameter [OD], and tube length [mm]) can be obtained from the manufacturer and are located on the tracheostomy tube box and package insert. • Alternate materials sometimes used with certain tracheostomy tubes include wire reinforced silicone. • Types of tube cuffs available include air-filled, foam, and low profile, or tight-to-shaft (TTS). • Tracheostomy tube distal tips are sometimes modified or tapered to facilitate insertion during percutaneous tracheostomy.	• Tubes with disposable inner cannulas are easy to manage as they require no cleaning, just replacement. • Reusable inner cannula tubes are available with some manufacturers. • The inner cannula allows the outer cannula to be left in and an adequate airway maintained while the inner cannula is cleaned. • Standard air-filled cuffs are typically high-volume/low-pressure profile. • Tight-to-shaft cuffs when deflated have a low profile to the tube's outer cannula, which aids in insertion and may allow more airway space around tube during speech. • Foam cuffs passively inflate at atmospheric pressure and have the advantage of limiting intracuff pressure.	• Cost of any disposable item must be justified. Disposable inner cannulas are not manufactured to hold up to repeated cleaning and extended use. • Cleaning inner cannulas entails cost of labor and time, including health care worker and patient compliance in routine cleaning. • Single cannula tubes are available. If the tube becomes obstructed however, the entire tube (versus the inner cannula only in a dual cannula tube) must be removed. • Wire-reinforced silicone tubes can not be used in MRI imaging because of the metal material. • Tight-to-shaft cuffs have high-pressure/low-volume characteristics, and silicone material requires more frequent assessment due to leaks that occur over time. • When using a foam cuff, use of a one-way speaking valve is contraindicated due to natural orientation of the cuff passively inflated. • Certain brands of percutaneous tubes require a dedicated style of inner cannula for compatibility.	• Tubes are available with or without inner cannulas, which may be either disposable or nondisposable (ie, must be cleaned). • When inner cannulas are being replaced, the clinician must ensure that the correct size inner cannula is being used. (Smaller size inner cannulas will fit into a larger size outer cannula but will cause a dramatic change in the diameter of the airway). • Pediatric tubes are very narrow and do not have inner cannulas. • Inner cannulas are typically cleaned (or changed if disposable cannulas are being used) every 8–12 hours or prn in the hospital setting. The frequency of cleaning/changing catheters will vary based on the needs of the patient. • May be custom ordered for specific needs

Tube Type	Description	Advantages	Disadvantages	Comments
Metal (Figure 1C-10)	• Used primarily in long-term tracheostomy and laryngectomy patients. (Laryngectomy tubes are also available in plastic.) • Available in sizes 000–14 (Jackson).	• Can be used for long periods of time	• Requires a special adapter (15 mm) if not built into the inner cannula for connection to a handheld resuscitator bag, ventilator circuit, or one-way speaking valve.	• Not commonly used with ventilator patients because it does not have a cuff and requires 15-mm adapters to connect to ventilator • May be custom ordered for specific needs
Fenestrated (Figures 1C-7, 1C-8)	• Tracheostomy tubes with fenestrations (holes) in tube; air moves up from lungs through fenestrations, allowing vibration of the vocal cords and speech	• Used in patients to improve ease of speaking • Used as additional source of upper airway airflow during weaning from tracheostomy tube	• Tissue can grow into fenestrations causing plugging (granulation formation). • This extra tissue can occur on the outside of the skin by the stoma tract or may develop inside the trachea where the tube enters the airway. • Fenestrations can also plug with mucous, rendering the tube useless in terms of its ability to allow airflow through the vocal cords for speech.	• Location of the tube fenestration relative to the patient's tracheal anatomy may explain why some patients develop granulation tissue formation while others do not. • Consider use of nonfenestrated inner cannula on routine basis, (ie, during sleep) if feasible. May prevent tissue entering the fenestration.
Tracheostomy stoma buttons (Figure 1C-11)	• Short plastic or silastic tubes used to keep the stoma open • These tubes are used to provide airway opening in patients who otherwise do not require airway protection (eg, vocal cord paralysis, sleep apnea).	• Easy to maintain • May be used with certain speaking valves • There is a reduced chance of tracheal erosion (no foreign body in the trachea).	• Cannot be used in patients on mechanical ventilator • Difficult to size properly • They provide no additional protection against aspiration than a traditional, cuffed tube.	
Extra-long flexible tubes	• Provide airway management for patients with special needs (eg, abnormal tracheal anatomy) • Tubes are generally longer than standard tubes and are frequently used to bypass areas of tracheal injury or damage such as tracheal stenosis or malacia.	• Nonarcuate shape conforms better to tracheal anatomy than standard arcuate shaped tubes. • Some extra-long tubes have adjustable neck plate or flange for initial sizing.	• Cost • Most commonly available in extra-long tubes; do not have an inner cannula • Patients should not be sent home with adjustable neck flange tubes; tube must be converted to fixed position flange style requiring conversion to custom tube.	• May be custom ordered for special needs

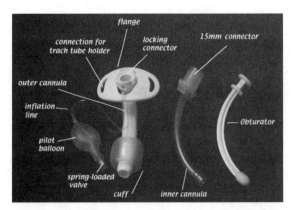

FIGURE 1C-1: Parts of a tracheostomy tube. (Reprinted from Critical Care Nursing Clinics of North America, St. John RE, Malen JF: Contemporary issues in adult tracheostomy management. Vol. 16: 403–413, © (2004) with permission from Elsevier)

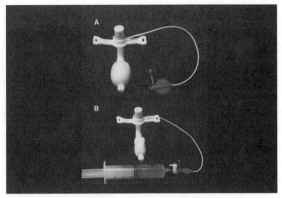

FIGURE 1C-2: Foam cuff single-cannula tracheostomy tube (A) Cuff inflated (B) cuff manually deflated. (Reprinted from Critical Care Nursing Clinics of North America, St. John RE, Malen JF: Contemporary issues in adult tracheostomy management. Vol. 16: 403-413, © (2004) with permission from Elsevier)

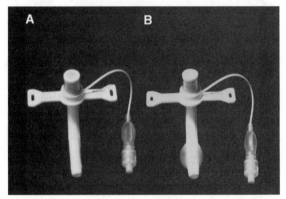

FIGURE 1C-3: Bivona tight-to-shaft single-cannula tracheostomy tube (A) Cuff deflated (B) high-pressure low-volume cuff inflated. (Reprinted from Critical Care Nursing Clinics of North America, St. John RE, Malen JF: Contemporary issues in adult tracheostomy management. Vol. 16: 403–413, © (2004) with permission from Elsevier)

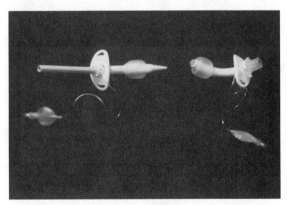

FIGURE 1C-4: Percutaneous tracheostomy tube (Left) with tapered distal tip (shown with percutaneous tube loading dilator) and modified high volume low-pressure cuff (right) standard cuffed tracheostomy tube. (Reprinted from Critical Care Nursing Clinics of North America, St. John RE, Malen JF: Contemporary issues in adult tracheostomy management. Vol. 16: 403–413, © (2004) with permission from Elsevier.)

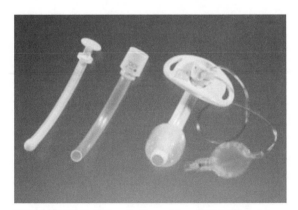

FIGURE 1C-5: Shiley dual-cannula cuffed tracheostomy tube with nondisposable (reuseable) inner cannula. (Photo courtesy of Nellcor, a unit of Tyco Healthcare, Pleasanton, Calif)

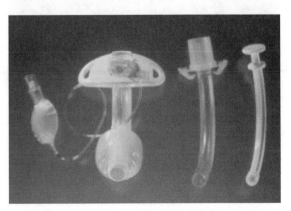

FIGURE 1C-6: Shiley dual-cannula cuffed tracheostomy tube with disposable inner cannula. (Photo courtesy of Nellcor, a unit of Tyco Healthcare, Pleasanton, Calif)

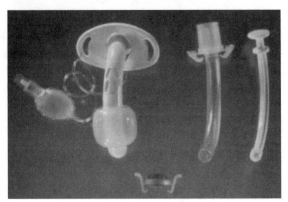

FIGURE 1C-7: Shiley dual-cannula cuffed fenestrated tracheostomy tube with multiple fenestrations. (Photo courtesy of Nellcor, a unit of Tyco Healthcare, Pleasanton, Calif)

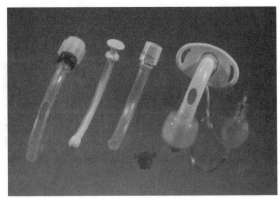

FIGURE 1C-8: Shiley dual-cannula cuffed fenestrated tracheostomy tube with single fenestrations. (Photo courtesy of Nellcor, a unit of Tyco Healthcare, Pleasanton, Calif)

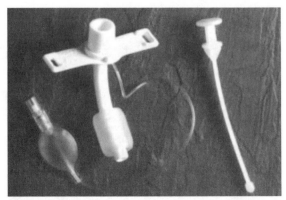

FIGURE 1C-9: Shiley single-cannula cuffed tracheostomy tube. (Photo courtesy of Nellcor, a unit of Tyco Healthcare, Pleasanton, Calif)

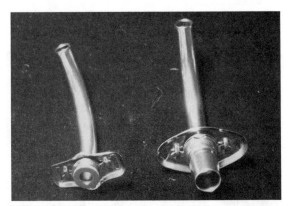

FIGURE 1C-10: Metal dual-cannula tracheostomy tube with and without 15-mm connector. (Reprinted from Critical Care Nursing Clinics of North America, St. John RE, Malen JF: Contemporary issues in adult tracheostomy management. Vol. 16: 403–413, © (2004) with permission from Elsevier)

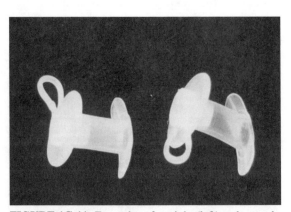

FIGURE 1C-11: Examples of straight (left) and curved (right) stoma stents. Stents are used to keep the stoma tract open (after removal of the tracheostomy tube) and allow access to the trachea for suctioning. Because the stent rests against the anterior tracheal wall, there is less physical restriction to breathe spontaneously around the sides of a capped tracheostomy tube. (Reprinted from Critical Care Nursing Clinics of North America, St. John RE, Malen JF: Contemporary issues in adult tracheostomy management. Vol. 16: 403–413, © (2004) with permission from Elsevier)

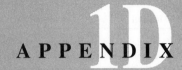

Communication Options for Patients With Artificial Airways

Method	Description	Advantages	Disadvantages	Comments
Touching, pointing, gesturing	Patient points to a desired item (eg, suction catheter) or makes symbol with their hand (eg, pulls at tube when they want it out)	• Simple, easy to understand basic needs	• Cannot be used for complex needs	• Requires patient dexterity and range of motion with hands or arms which may be limited due to physical condition or other reasons (ie, IVs, arterial line)
Writing	Patient communicates needs in writing. Similar technique—"magic slate" (words disappear when top sheet is lifted).	• Inexpensive and readily available	• Requires patient be able to write (and read) • Difficult for many patients secondary to position in bed, vision, lines, restraints, etc. (may lead to frustration) • Requires fine motor skill • Paper and pencil do not always enhance patient communication effectiveness. • Magic slates afford more privacy but may be difficult to read.	• Perhaps most widely used method
Eye blinking	Coded eye-blink system, for example: 1 = no 2 = yes 3 = pain, etc	• May be the only source of muscular control for patients with neurological diseases or injuries	• Time consuming for caregivers and patients • May be tiring • Requires coordinated cognitive awareness and functional eye control	
Alphabet boards and commonly used pictures, words, or phrase boards	Patients point to or nod agreement (eg, blink or nod) to desired words, letters, or pictures on a premade communication tablet or board.	• Boards with standard phrases and needs are available commercially. • Personalized boards are easy to make to record unique patient needs.	• Process may be extremely cumbersome for patients, especially when words must be spelled out, one letter at a time. • Process of communication is time-consuming for all involved.	• Alphabet boards assume patient can spell. • Often used with neurologically impaired patients (eg, Guillain Barre), when writing is impossible • Word boards may not be available in the patient's language.

Method	Description	Advantages	Disadvantages	Comments
Computers, electronic devices	Patients type out needs and questions on keyboard or touch screen. Also can include electronic voice output communication aids that combine prerecorded speech with labeled icons or pictures Typically used in long-term situations when patient is at a high level of functioning.	• Can be used effectively over a wide range of age groups • High degree of success can be achieved with practice in patients with normal mentation.	• Expensive • Patient generally must provide own computer • Need mechanisms to prevent theft • May require high degree of cognitive function and visual acuity	
Tone devices	Electric tone generators consisting of a handheld vibrator that is applied midway between the mandibular angle and the notch of the thyroid cartilage, thereby substituting for the larynx as an amplifier for speech ("electrolarynx")	• Can be successful when other devices are not possible	• Healthcare workers need frequent in-servicing on correct technique. • Expensive	• Enthusiasm for the device is often lost when improper positioning or application of pressure prevents successful results quickly.
Talking tracheostomy tubes	Several types available Cuffless tracheotomy tubes are available (depending on manufacturer/model) with a silver one-way speaking valves attached to interchangeable inner cannulas (used in stable patients who can leave the valve on for extended periods). Another type of tracheostomy tube utilizes an additional port to direct pressurized air or oxygen over the vocal cords and through the pharynx independent of the respiratory cycle.	• The valve is readily available (does not get lost!) • Proper patient selection allows intelligible whispered or spoken speech.	• Cuffless version not for use with patients requiring significant mechanical ventilatory support or a cuffed tracheostomy tube (silver one-way valve) • Misdirection of the pressurized gas flow through the tracheostomy stoma and occlusion of the tube's exit port with secretions and tissue • Patients must be able to articulate speech and form words with their mouth.	• Usually not used until at least 5 to 7 days after tracheostomy placement Continuous flow as gas over vocal cords may lead to drying of the glottis and inflammation with possible hoarseness.
Tracheostomy stoma buttons	A tracheostomy stoma button fits from the skin to just inside the anterior wall of the trachea. An optional one-way valve on the external end of the button allows for inspiration with less dead space, and expiration with speech. Adapters can be used to allow suctioning through the button. Can only be used in situations where the patient can tolerate being off the ventilator and breath spontaneously May be part of the decannulation process when the patient is stable and no longer needs the tracheostomy tube or to maintain stoma patency for future use	• Patient can breathe and clear secretions through their native airway without the added resistance of an intratracheal tube when the buttons are plugged. • A tracheostomy tube can be reinserted through the stoma tract that was preserved by the button.	• Requires practitioners be competent in the use of the buttons. • Difficult to accurately size a patient to a button which will not extend into the tracheal lumen • Certain buttons require straps or skin sutures to secure them in position. • If button fit is too loose in the stoma or the external fixation device is poorly applied, aspiration of the device during forced inspiration can occur.	• The patient's trachea and oral cavity must be suctioned well prior to removal of the tube and insertion of a button (the trachea should be resuctioned after insertion of the button). • Best tolerated by patients with small to moderate amounts of secretions and a strong cough (ie, can clear secretions through their mouth)

Method	Description	Advantages	Disadvantages	Comments
Speaking valves (Figures 1D-1, 1D-2)	A one-way valve is placed on the end of the tracheostomy tube allowing air movement into the trachea via the tube with exhaled air directed up past the vocal cords and out the nose and mouth. Air movement on expiration is directed around the sides of the tracheostomy tube. A fenestrated tracheostomy tube is sometimes used to add an additional passageway for exhaled airflow to be directed through the native airway.	• Can be used in patients on or off the ventilator, depending on valve • Useful in patients who are unable to tolerate complete occlusion of the trachea with a button • Contraindicated in certain patients such as those with laryngeal dysfunction • Patients with thick, copious secretions may have difficulty using	• Requires skilled clinicians to use with ventilator (may involve adjustment of ventilator settings) • May require special adapter to fit on ventilator tubing • Must be replaced periodically according to manufacturer guidelines	• Early involvement of speech pathologist may be helpful in identifying if speaking valve is indicated. • Caution: The cuff on the tracheostomy tube must be completely deflated when any type of speaking valve is used. • Speaking valves should not be used on foam-cuffed tubes as they naturally inflate based on atmospheric pressure. • The patient's trachea and oral cavity must be suctioned well before deflating the cuff. (The trachea should be resuctioned after deflating the cuff to clear any secretions that may have drained into the bronchus.) • Best tolerated by patients with small to moderate amounts of secretions and a strong cough (ie, can clear secretions through their mouth) • Use in ventilated patients requires collaborative planning by speech therapist, respiratory therapist, and nursing staff to maximize effectiveness • Valve should not be worn at bedtime or during other sleep periods. • Should be cleaned frequently according to manufacturers' recommendation to avoid buildup of secretions or damage to valve.

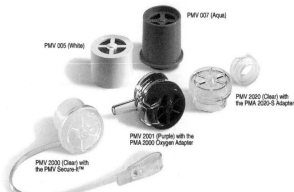

FIGURE 1D-1: Tracheostomy and ventilator swallowing and speaking valves. (Photo courtesy of Passy-Muir, Inc., Irvine, Calif)

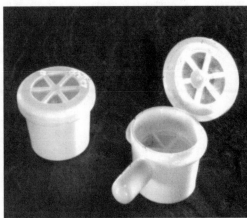

FIGURE 1D-2: One-way tracheostomy speaking valve without (left) and with (right) supplemental oxygen side port adapter for spontaneously breathing patients. (Photo courtesy of Nellcor, a unit of Tyco Healthcare, Pleasanton, Calif)

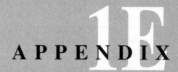
Terminology Associated With Various Types of Suctioning Procedures

Suction Method	Description	Advantages	Disadvantages	Comments
Open catheter suctioning	• Involves disconnecting the patient from the ventilator before suctioning • Following a brief suction period (< 10–15 sec) the patient is reconnected to the ventilator.	• Cost effective when patient requires suctioning infrequently • Provides less traction on the airway during activity for ventilator patients in a chronic, home, or rehabilitation center	• Patients do not receive oxygen during the procedure. • Puts staff at higher risk for exposure to patient secretions. • Cost is higher with single use catheter.	• Patients receiving supplemental PEEP (≥ 5 cm H_2O) must have a special valve attached to manual resuscitator bag during suctioning procedure. • A variety of types of suction catheters are available (eg, plastic and rubber). Certain catheters are available with directional or coudé (angled) tips to allow catheter positioning to the left lung if desired. • The red "rubber" catheters are softer and more flexible and may be more appropriate for patients with bleeding disorders or friable mucosa.
Closed catheter suctioning	• Uses an in-line suction catheter • Suctioning is performed without interruption of ventilation. • The suction catheter is housed in a sterile sleeve. The catheter is advanced through a diaphragm in the sleeve into the patient's ET or tracheostomy tube while maintaining airway stabilization.	• Closed circuit preventing caregiver exposure • Allows the patient to maintain high F_{IO_2} and PEEP during the procedure • Avoids suction-related lung volume loss • Numbered catheter allows depth control.	• Extra weight from in-line suction catheter may increase tension on the tracheal or tracheostomy tube. • The extra length of the suction tubing may provide additional access for the patient to reach and contribute to accidental extubation. Drape tubing out of reach. • Manufacturers make both endotracheal and tracheostomy (shorter catheter) versions. Ensure that correct catheter is chosen to prevent trauma. • Ensure that the trigger sensitivity is properly set. • Ensure that the catheter is withdrawn completely to	• The Centers for Disease Control and Prevention does not make recommendations for changing the closed in-line suction system or preference for open vs. closed suctioning. However, recent data suggests that these systems can be used in-line for greater than manufacturer's recommendations without increasing the incidence of ventilator-associated pneumonia. • Follow your individual facility's policy on changing ventilator circuits and closed in-line suction systems. • Theoretical concerns exist related to applying suction in a closed system, leading to atelectasis.

Suction Method	Description	Advantages	Disadvantages	Comments
			prevent increased airway pressure, and follow institution policy regarding locking suction control between use.	
Hyperoxygenation	• The process of delivering oxygen at a level higher than the patient's baseline FIO_2 level. • Hyperoxygenation should be performed prior to, during, or after suctioning.			• Has a solid research basis supporting its usefulness in preventing hypoxemia during suctioning • May use 100% button feature on certain ventilators.
Hyperventilation	• The process of delivering extra breaths to the patient before, during, or after suctioning; the extra breaths may be given with a handheld manual resuscitator bag or via the ventilator • The breath size may be identical or different than the volume the patient is currently receiving.		• Difficult to maintain consistent volumes when handheld resuscitators are used • If used alone, hypoxemia may occur during suctioning	• May be used alone or in combination with hyperoxygenation
Hyperinflation	• Can be provided with the ventilator or a handheld resuscitator bag • The process of delivering breaths to a patient before, during, or after the suctioning process; these breaths being delivered are at a higher tidal volume than the patient is receiving via the ventilator			• More complex in that it requires ventilator adjustments • Use of a handheld resuscitator bag limits possible tidal volume delivery even when a 2-handed technique is used.
Manual inflation	• The process of delivering a breath to the patient using a handheld resuscitation bag			• Used for suctioning when the patient is removed from the ventilator. Does not imply the use of hyperoxygenation or hyperventilation.
Preoxygenation	• The process of delivery of supplemental oxygen to the patient before, during, or after suctioning			• Used in both mechanically ventilated and nonventilated patients • May use 100% button feature on certain ventilators
Insufflation	• The concomitant delivery of oxygen during suctioning. • Oxygen is administered through the double lumen of a special suction catheter or the sidearm of an endotracheal tube adapter.	• Allows oxygen to be administered during suctioning	• Requires special equipment	• Recent meta-analysis showed an increased rate of hypoxia with insufflation applied.

Suction Method	Description	Advantages	Disadvantages	Comments
Normal saline instillation	• The instillation of sterile normal saline into the endotracheal tube during endotracheal suctioning		• Has been shown to result in hypoxemia and patient distress • May contaminate the lower airway with bacteria that has adhered to the tracheal tube wall during instillation	• Normal saline instillation may be effective in stimulating a cough. However, alternative strategies should be employed including adequate hydration, airway heat and humidity, and mucolytic agents and respiratory treatments. • Not likely to loosen secretions as humidification requires small particle fluid, not lavage • Normal saline has no mucolytic properties. • Consider use of vibrating chest vest, insufflator/exsufflator, repositioning, and/or chest physiotherapy as an adjunct to loosen and mobilize secretions.

High Risk Intubation/Reintubation

- History of difficult intubation
- Epiglottis
- Status after maxillary/facial surgery with jaws wired shut
- Status after cervical spine stabilization/surgery
- Status asthmaticus—first 2 days following intubation
- Neck infection with airway compromise
- Requiring PEEP = 10 cm H_2O and/or FIO_2 = 0.60
- Bronchopleural fistula
- Inhalation injuries
- Morbidly obese postoperative patient with respiratory compromise
- Any patient who has history of multiple intubations in past
- Patients who develop postextubation glottic edema and stridor
- Major neck procedure
- Congenital airway abnormalities
- Airway tumors
- Airway abnormalities including granulomas, stenosis, or malacia
- Facial or neck trauma

Invasive and Noninvasive Modes and Methods of Mechanical Ventilation

Lynelle N. B. Pierce, RN, MS, CCRN

Invasive and Noninvasive Modes and Methods of Mechanical Ventilation

CASE STUDY

JT was an 18-year-old man brought into the trauma center with multiple gunshot wounds. One bullet traversed his right upper thoracic cavity, injuring the right upper lobe of the lung and the pulmonary artery; the second bullet created a through-and-through wound of the left lower extremity. JT underwent emergency thoracic surgery: a right upper lobectomy and repair of the pulmonary artery. The lower extremity developed compartment syndrome, necessitating a fasciotomy that oozed large amounts of serosanguinous drainage. JT required massive volume resuscitation with crystalloids and blood component therapy to maintain hemodynamic stability and ensure adequate tissue oxygenation.

Postoperatively, JT was admitted directly to the surgical ICU. His ventilator settings were volume assist-control (A/C) rate, 16; fraction of inspired oxygen (FIO_2), 0.8; positive end-expiratory pressure (PEEP), 10 cm H_2O; and tidal volume (VT), 800—slightly over 12 mL/kg for this 64-kg man. An assessment of patient data revealed a chest radiograph with patchy, diffuse infiltrates suggestive of early acute respiratory distress syndrome (ARDS); peak inspiratory pressure (PIP), 50 cm H_2O; pH, 7.30; $PaCO_2$, 43; PaO_2, 53; SaO_2, 88%; bicarbonate (HCO_3^-), 20; and a base excess (BE), –5, demonstrating a metabolic acidosis and hypoxemia. The PIP was rising because, as ARDS developed, the pulmonary tissue was becoming less compliant from multiple episodes of hypotension secondary to acute reduction in circulating blood volume requiring massive volume resuscitation. His PIP was of concern because of the potential for ventilator-induced lung injury. The higher the airway pressures, the greater the risk of barotrauma—the disruption of the alveolus allowing air to dissect along facial planes and accumulate in the pleural space or other compartments or lead to subcutaneous emphysema. Volutrauma is lung parenchymal damage induced by local overdistention. When lung disease is heterogeneous, as in ARDS, volume is preferentially distributed to the healthier alveoli because they are easier to open. The result, local overdistention, causes injury.

The goals of therapy were then defined: to optimize oxygenation by ensuring an $SaO_2 \geq 90\%$, to optimize hemodynamics to ensure adequate tissue oxygenation and thus resolve the metabolic acidosis by achieving a hemoglobin (Hb) of 10 mg/dL and a cardiac index of 3.5 L/min, and to reduce the potentially lung-damaging PIP by maintaining the plateau pressure at ≤ 30 cm H_2O. To accomplish the goal of limiting the plateau pressure JT would be ventilated with small VT (as low as 4–5 mL/kg if necessary) and the $PaCO_2$ would be allowed to rise gradually (permissive hypercapnia). This therapeutic approach to reducing the PIP was possible because there were no contraindications (eg, increased intracranial pressure) to an elevated $PaCO_2$. Continuous IV sedation was used to help JT tolerate invasive devices, mechanical ventilation, and the hypercapnia.

JT was switched to pressure-control (PC) ventilation (chosen for its ability to ventilate the patient with a lower PIP) at a level of 28 cm H_2O, which resulted in VT, 7 mL/kg (450 mL); FIO_2 0.8; PEEP, 10 cm H_2O and a rate of 18. Pressure control delivers the set inspiratory pressure level immediately at the onset of inspiration and sustains this pressure throughout the inspiratory phase. The alveoli reach their critical opening pressure earlier in inspiration and are splinted open by the constant inspiratory pressure. With PC ventilation, the decelerating flow wave pattern creates a less turbulent flow of gases as they enter the lung, thereby improving their distribution in the lung. JT was also given 2 more units of packed red blood cells, resulting in a Hb of

10.5, and was put on dobutamine at 5 μg/kg per minute, resulting in a cardiac index of 3.4 L/min. Repeat arterial blood gas (ABG) analysis revealed pH 7.28; Pao_2, 66; $Paco_2$, 52; HCO_3^-, 22; BE, –3; and Sao_2 89%. The PIP was 38 cm H_2O pressure (plateau of 24 cm H_2O), as could be predicted when using an inspiratory pressure-control level of 28 cm H_2O over 10 cm H_2O baseline pressure, or PEEP. The concern of iatrogenic lung damage induced by mechanical ventilation with high PIP was reduced, and the hemodynamic goals achieved.

Concern persisted regarding the toxic levels of oxygen, Fio_2 0.8, on which JT remained. The oxygenation goal was $Sao_2 \geq 90\%$ on $Fio_2 \leq 0.5$ to avoid pulmonary oxygen toxicity. Therefore, it was decided to use inverse inspiratory-to-expiratory (I:E) ratio ventilation. Traditional I:E ratio is 1:2. Inverse-ratio ventilation prolongs the inspiratory phase of ventilation, allowing less compliant alveoli more time to fill during inspiration. The expiratory phase is reduced with the subsequent breath beginning before complete exhalation occurred, preventing the alveoli from reaching their critical closing volume and shutting at end expiration. Thus, more alveoli are recruited and remain open, intrapulmonary shunt is decreased, and oxygenation improves. Because complete exhalation does not occur before the next breath begins, some gases are trapped in the lung. This volume of gas creates pressure in the alveoli and is known as *auto-PEEP*. Because auto-PEEP forms during inverse-ratio ventilation at rapid respiratory rates the amount of set-PEEP must be reduced. To improve oxygenation the I:E ratio was inversed first to 1:1; when the patient remained hemodynamically stable it was further inversed to 1.5:1, then 2:1. Set-PEEP was reduced to 5 cm H_2O pressure and auto-PEEP was measured. Total PEEP (the amount of set-PEEP plus the auto-PEEP) was determined to be 15 cm H_2O (Figure 2-1).

Oxygenation was continuously monitored by pulse oximetry, and a pulmonary artery catheter was inserted for close monitoring of JT's cardiac performance and tissue perfusion. The level of PEEP was titrated to achieve an improvement in oxygenation without deterioration in the patient's hemodynamic status, which would result in inadequate tissue oxygenation. The goal was to use enough baseline pressure, PEEP, to recruit the unstable alveoli (increase the functional residual capacity [FRC]) and keep the lung open throughout the respiratory cycle, without overdistending the compliant

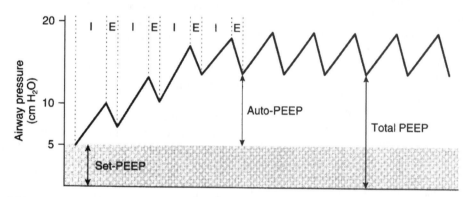

Figure 2-1: The phenomenon of auto-PEEP, caused by inversion of the I:E ratio. Insufficient expiratory time permits the trapping of gases in the lung. This trapped gas creates pressure, which is known as auto-PEEP. (From Pierce LNB. *Guide to Mechanical Ventilation and Intensive Respiratory Care.* Philadelphia, Pa: WB Saunders, Co; 1995. Used with permission.)

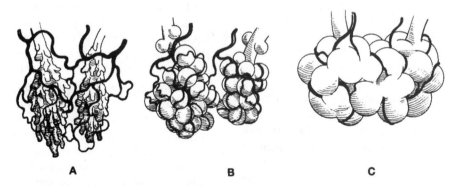

Figure 2-2: Effect of application of PEEP on the alveoli. (A) Atelectatic alveoli before PEEP application. (B) Optimal PEEP application has reinflated alveoli to normal volume. (C) Excessive PEEP application overdistends the alveoli and compresses adjacent pulmonary capillaries, creating dead space with its attendant hypercapnia. (From Pierce, LNB. *Guide to Mechanical Ventilation and Intensive Respiratory Care.* Philadelphia, Pa: WB Saunders, Co; 1995. Used with permission.)

alveoli (Figure 2-2). This approach was consistent with the strategy to prevent ventilator-induced lung injury (see Clinical Recommendations for Ventilatory Techniques: Lung Protection Strategies). As the SpO_2 gradually rose, the FIO_2 was titrated down, finally achieving an FIO_2 of 0.5.

Additional strategies to improve oxygenation that could have been employed include the use of a recruitment maneuver, which is the periodic application of sustained airway pressure. The sustained airway pressure opens, or recruits, alveoli that are collapsed. Such a maneuver is often followed by an increase in PEEP level that holds open the newly recruited alveoli. The use of the prone position could also have been used to improve ventilation/perfusion matching and distribution of gas in the lung and therefore oxygenation.

Over the course of the next week and a half JT's improved status allowed for a reversion of the inverse I:E ratio, thus eliminating the auto-PEEP. Set-PEEP was decreased to 5 cm H_2O pressure, and the FIO_2 was further reduced to 0.35. The PIP was now 27 cm H_2O, PC of 22 cm H_2O over 5 cm H_2O PEEP, rate of 12. Because the FRC of the lung had been increased by recruiting more alveoli using inverse I:E ratio ventilation, the patient's tidal volumes had gradually increased over the last week and a half to 8 mL/kg, and the permissive hypercapnia had gradually reversed. An ABG analysis showed pH, 7.34; PaO_2, 98; $PaCO_2$, 47; HCO_3^-, 24; BE, +1; and SaO_2, 99%.

When the I:E ratio was normalized JT was weaned to minimal analgesia and sedation levels and was alert and oriented most of the time. He began triggering assisted breaths and participated more in ventilating himself. Two options for ventilatory support were to decrease the PC level to 20, which resulted in a V_T of 7 mL/kg, or to decrease the rate to 10. These maneuvers would increase $PaCO_2$ and thus the patient's drive to breathe.

The patient's spontaneous breaths could be assisted with either pressure assist-control (A/C) or pressure control/pressure support (PC/PS). In pressure A/C, the breaths initiated by the patient would be assisted with the same level of inspiratory pressure delivered with the mandatory PC breaths. This method results in minimal additional work of breathing for the patient—only that which is required to trigger the ventilator—and the ventilator then fully assists the breath with the preset pressure level. In PC/PS the patient's spontaneous breaths would be augmented with a different level of inspiratory pressure assistance. This level could be set at a lower level of assistance than that afforded the mandatory PC breaths. The patient could then be titrated a greater degree of work to perform on the PS breaths. The third method of ventilatory support discussed was to switch the patient to a volume-targeted mode of ventilation such as synchronized intermittent mandatory ventilation (SIMV). The physician felt more comfortable with volume modes of ventilation, and so JT was placed on SIMV, 12; V_T, 650; FIO_2, 0.35; and PEEP, 5 cm H_2O.

Assessment of patient data revealed PIP 34 cm H_2O, plateau pressure, 27 cm H_2O; total RR, 25; spontaneous V_T,

3.1 to 3.6 mL/kg(190 to 210 mL/breath); and SpO_2, 94%. The team recognized that the patient would fatigue if this level of ventilatory work continued to be required. Therefore, the spontaneous breaths were augmented with enough PS (8 cm H_2O) to result in a V_T of 5 mL/kg; the patient's spontaneous V_T increased to 420 mL/kg, and his respiratory rate decreased to 16 from 18.

Over the course of the next few days JT was able to achieve the goal of 5 mL/kg on the spontaneous breaths on 5 cm H_2O PS as his ARDS further resolved and his respiratory muscles strengthened. An aggressive weaning plan was then instituted using spontaneous breathing trials, and the patient was weaned from ventilatory support on hospital day 16. (See Chapter 3, Weaning from Mechanical Ventilation.)

This case clearly exemplifies the complexity and multitude of options available for skillful management of mechanical ventilation in the ICU. The clinician must understand the rationale of each mode, what parameters should be monitored to evaluate patient response and effectiveness of therapy, and how the latest research guides management to prevent iatrogenic complications of this fascinating therapy.

GENERAL DESCRIPTION

A ventilator is a device that moves gas into the lungs, with expiration remaining a passive process just as it is when a patient is spontaneously breathing. Ventilatory support is indicated in acute hypercapnic or hypoxemic respiratory failure, from whatever cause, to provide adequate alveolar ventilation and thus carbon dioxide removal, or to improve arterial oxygenation. It is also indicated to permit sedation or neuromuscular blockade as in operative anesthesia and rarely for therapeutic hyperventilation in the presence of intracranial hypertension. Mechanical ventilation does not correct the underlying pathology. It supports oxygenation and ventilation until the underlying disease can be treated and is resolved sufficiently that the patient can independently manage the work of breathing.

Negative pressure ventilators, which date back to the early 1900s, mimic spontaneous respiration by developing negative pressure around the thoracic cavity. This negative pressure is transmitted to the interior of the thorax, and air, at atmospheric pressure, flows into the chest. In acute care, positive pressure ventilators support ventilation by supplying gas and positive pressure to the airway, forcing air into the lungs. Positive pressure ventilators, therefore, alter the normal physiologic pressure in the chest during spontaneous respiration. It is this creation of positive pressure in the thorax that leads to most of the complications related to mechanical ventilation such as barotrauma or decreased cardiac output. In general, positive pressure ventilation is delivered via an artificial airway (eg, an endotracheal tube or tracheostomy). As an outgrowth of developments to support nocturnal ventilation in patients with sleep apnea, techniques have been developed to deliver positive pressure ventilation via nasal or face mask systems. This type of ventilation is called *noninvasive posi-*

tive pressure ventilation (NPPV). Indications for the use of NPPV have expanded over the past 5 years. When the patient meets the criteria, it is being used in place of endotracheal intubation and mechanical ventilation (invasive ventilation). Clinicians who are very experienced in the use of NPPV are using this technique to wean patients from invasive ventilation, liberating them from ventilatory support (see Clinical Recommendations for Ventilatory Techniques: Noninvasuive Positive Pressure Ventilation).

Spontaneous breathing requires no conscious effort to pass through the 4 phases of a respiratory cycle: (1) inspiration, (2) end inspiration, (3) expiration, (4) initiation of a new inspiration. The ventilator is simply a machine that must "be told" how to carry out each phase by the operator adjusting ventilator settings. The 4 phases a ventilator must complete to provide a ventilatory cycle to the patient are inspiration, inspiratory-expiratory changeover, expiration, expiratory-inspiratory changeover (Figure 2-3). Phase variables are ventilator settings used to begin, sustain, and terminate each phase. An example of a phase variable, or setting, during expiration is the setting of PEEP.

The variable techniques by which the patient and ventilator interact to perform the ventilatory cycle are called *modes of mechanical ventilation.* Generally modes are either controlled or assisted. In controlled ventilation the ventilator initiates the breath and performs all the work of breathing (WOB). In assisted ventilation the patient initiates and terminates some or all of the breaths, with the ventilator giving variable amounts of support throughout the respiratory cycle. Hence, the modes of ventilation vary in degree of patient versus ventilator effort.

The mode chosen for a particular patient is determined by how much WOB the patient ought to perform. In full-ventilatory support the ventilator performs all the WOB. In partial ventilatory support, both the patient and ventilator contribute. With some modes, adjustments can be made in the ventilator settings to provide gradations from partial to full-ventilatory support over the course of ventilation.

Modes of positive pressure ventilation may be divided into volume-targeted and pressure-targeted ventilation. This classification stems from the limit variable or the target value set for inspiration. The limit variable is the preset value during inspiration that the ventilator maintains, but does not cause inspiration to end. In volume-targeted ventilation the limit variable during inspiration is the preset V_T. Volume-targeted modes such as A/C and SIMV have been the favored ventilatory support modes in adults for the past 30 years. In pressure-targeted ventilation (PS, PC, pressure A/C, airway pressure-release ventilation), pressure is the target variable and is held constant at a preset level throughout inspiration. Over the last 15 to 20 years, use of pressure-targeted modes has become more widespread. Volume-targeted and pressure-targeted modes can be integrated, as in SIMV+PS where during inspiration the mandatory (SIMV) breaths are delivered with a target volume, and the patient's spontaneous breaths are supported with a target pressure. Further, hybrid modes integrate volume- and pressure-targeted concepts in the same mode (eg, pressure-regulated volume control [PRVC], volume support [VS]).

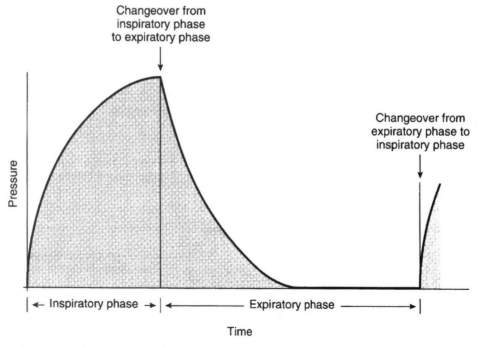

Figure 2-3: The 4 phases of the respiratory cycle on a ventilator. (From Pierce, LNB. *Guide to Mechanical Ventilation and Intensive Respiratory Care.* Philadelphia, Pa: WB Saunders, Co; 1995. Used with permission.)

The key difference between volume- and pressure-targeted modes is the assurance of either a set VT or a set PIP. In volume-targeted modes the patient is delivered the set VT: the amount of pressure required to deliver the breath is variable and depends on the compliance and resistance factors of the patient-ventilator system. In pressure-targeted modes the PIP throughout inspiration is established, and the VT delivered to the patient varies as it depends on the compliance and resistance factors of the patient's pulmonary system and the ventilator circuitry.

Large tidal volumes (10–15 mL/kg) were accepted during the use of conventional modes of mechanical ventilation for many years. These large VTs were a result of studies, primarily done on patients undergoing anesthesia, where it was found that ventilation with monotonous, low VTs resulted in microatelectasis. Periodic inflation of the lung with sigh volumes or the use of larger VTs resulted in less microatelectasis and improved compliance.

It is now known that the use of a large VT can damage the lung. Large VT ventilation is among the ways that inappropriate management of mechanical ventilation can produce lung damage, similar to ARDS, and is known as ventilator-induced lung injury (VILI). VILI may take the form of barotrauma, volutrauma, oxygen toxicity, atelectrauma (the recruitment and derecruitment of unstable alveoli) and biotrauma (the activation of inflammatory mediators).

As a result of new knowledge regarding iatrogenic lung damage induced by mechanical ventilation, lung-protective strategies of ventilation have arisen. Strategies to protect the lung during mechanical ventilation include the use of adequate PEEP to "open" recruitable alveoli (open-lung technique) and limiting alveolar pressures to 30 cm H$_2$O, which may require the use of VTs as small as 4 to 8 mL/kg to achieve this target maximum airway pressure (low VT ventilation).

The use of a small VT requires permitting the PaCO$_2$ to rise (permissive hypercapnia). New consideration is also being given to techniques such as high-frequency oscillatory ventilation (HFOV) for lung protection. HFOV may decrease lung injury because it limits the magnitude of pressure/volume excursions.

The number of modes continues to increase in efforts to improve the efficiency of mechanical ventilation. There is no one best mode for managing patients in respiratory failure, although each mode has its advantages and disadvantages. However, there is also a great need for research that supports the varying views.

ACCURACY

Rigorous system checks designed to prevent technical inaccuracies and system failures assure accuracy. Scheduled routine maintenance must also be performed at intervals specified by the manufacturer, usually between patient uses and after a specified number of hours of use. Calibrations of pressure, time, flow, volume, and oxygen concentration are performed between patients and after a defined number of hours of use. If a ventilator is in continual operation, facility standards should dictate when it should be rotated out of use for cleaning and calibration—usually every 7 days. If any malfunctions are detected during any of the system checks, the ventilator must not be connected to a patient before the malfunction is remedied.

Some microprocessor ventilators when first turned on will perform a power-on self-test (POST) procedure to detect and correct the cause of internal problems. During use, these microprocessor ventilators continue to evaluate their functioning, perform internal corrections, and notify the operator if unable to operate as programmed.

Preuse checks, simplified system checks done before connecting the patient to the ventilator, are performed with a test lung attached to the ventilator circuitry to assess whether the ventilator appropriately delivers breaths according to the prescribed settings. During this check the operator mimics a patient's spontaneous respiratory effort to determine if the ventilator responds appropriately.

While the ventilator is in use, patient-ventilator system checks should be performed on a scheduled, institution-specific basis. A check should also be performed before obtaining an ABG value or bedside pulmonary function data, after any changes in ventilator settings, as soon as possible after any patient deterioration, and at any time when the function of the ventilator is questionable.

Ventilators vary in size, capabilities, configuration, and ease of use. For rapid problem solving, clinicians must be familiar with the messages and the keyboard on the ventilator with which they are working. In general, ventilator panels are divided into fields that contain dials or touch pads, grouped according to function. A field may be either an area of display or control. The control fields are where the ventilator settings and alarm parameters are established. The display fields provide patient information such as exhaled VT, minute ventilation, and airway pressures. In addition, most modern ventilators display graphic waveforms called scalars or loops. These graphics provide visual information about pressure, time, flow, and volume as well as pulmonary mechanics.

Ventilators have a number of audible and visual alarms for patient safety that alert staff of changes in patient condition or possible malfunction. But alarms serve a purpose only if properly set and are intended only as backup to close patient observation. Patient events that trigger alarms include high airway pressure, low minute ventilation, and apnea. Technical alarms include low air or oxygen pressure and machine failure, which indicate the ventilator is unable to control the flow of gas to the patient. When the operator cannot correct a technical problem with a ventilator at the bedside, then the ventilator should be immediately removed from service and evaluated. Finally, ventilator accuracy is ensured by having only properly trained personnel performing routine ventilator checks and making adjustments in the ventilator settings. The changing of one ventilator setting may require an interdependent setting also be adjusted to ensure appropriate delivery of gas to the patient.

COMPETENCY

Validation of competency to care for the patient on a mechanical ventilator should be done during an employee's initial orientation. A nurse must demonstrate competency in knowledge and technical skills before independently managing a patient on a mechanical ventilator. As new therapies and technology are introduced in a clinical setting appropriate education is necessary. The frequency of education and competency validation is determined by how frequently the nurse cares for mechanically ventilated patients, by episodes of improper operation, and when new ventilatory management techniques and strategies are introduced in the clinical setting.

KNOWLEDGE

- Anatomy of the upper and lower pulmonary system
- Pulmonary physiologic concepts that allow the clinician to apply mechanical ventilation in a more rational manner including compliance and resistance
- Principles of gas exchange
- Principles of ABG interpretation
- Principles of positive-pressure ventilation: modes, settings, adjusting settings to optimize oxygenation and ventilation, effect on thoracic pressures and cardiovascular function and management of such effects, effect on airway pressures and assessment and management of high pressures
- Mechanics of positive-pressure ventilation; troubleshooting alarms; components of brief ventilator check (accuracy of settings and assessment of patient data of exhaled V_T, PIP, respiratory frequency, etc)
- Principles of artificial airway management
- Principles of pulse oximetry

SKILLS

1. Physical assessment of the cardiac and pulmonary systems
2. Artificial airway management, including suctioning
3. Application and management of a nasal or full face mask for NPPV
4. Performance of patient-ventilator system check

ETHICAL CONSIDERATIONS

Withdrawal of ventilatory support as a part of end-of-life care and the use of noninvasive (mask) ventilation in terminal respiratory failure are the two primary ethical considerations related to mechanical ventilation. The increased emphasis on positive and supportive palliative care provided by the healthcare team as well as appropriate use of healthcare resources has raised interest in and awareness of the importance of these topics.

Discontinuation of ventilatory support may be indicated when it is the patient's informed request or the request of an appropriate patient surrogate, when further ventilatory assistance has been deemed medically futile, and when further intervention serves no benefit. Under any of these circumstances efforts are then focused on reducing the patient's pain and suffering.

A patient who is competent has the right to decide what should be done. After the conditions of informed consent are fulfilled, the patient may choose whether to continue ventilator therapy. In fact, invasive or noninvasive ventilation is contraindicated when a competent patient or designated surrogate expresses that the therapy not be used. For the incapacitated or incompetent patient the decision to withdraw therapy rests with the surrogate decision maker. After being fully informed of the implications of the decision, the surrogate uses one of two principles to make a decision: substituted judgment or best interest. In substituted judgment, the decision is based on the patient having clearly communicated his or her wishes on earlier occasions. If the surrogate does not know what the patient would choose, the principle of best interest applies to the decision making. When the patient's wishes are not clear, healthcare providers must weigh the benefits and burdens of the therapy and then act in the best interest of the patient.

Once the decision has been made to withdraw ventilatory support the logistics of ventilator withdrawal become the focus. The desires of the family should be solicited and met. Whether ventilatory support is gradually weaned or rapidly removed, the comfort of the patient is paramount, which may require analgesics or sedatives or both. The use of sedatives and analgesics during removal of ventilatory support to treat discomfort, anxiety, and dyspnea associated with the disease process and with respiratory distress raise additional ethical considerations as their use may contribute to earlier death. This is known as the concept of double effect: an action is justified if certain criteria are satisfied; for example, one does not will the evil outcome, the act itself is not evil, the evil does not follow directly from the good (the narcotic is given to relieve the discomfort, not to directly cause death), and there is proportional good involved.

Another ethical consideration is the use of NPPV in terminal respiratory failure. The first issue is the application by the health care provider of NPPV as an aggressive measure to patients who have indicated they do not want intubation and mechanical ventilation when their disease becomes terminal, but still desire aggressive treatment. The second issue is the application of mask ventilation to patients with terminal disease in an effort to reduce symptoms and prolong life a few extra hours to allow completion of life-closure tasks. The use of artificial means such as NPPV to support life in conditions where the disease is terminal is considered unethical by some. These individuals argue that NPPV under these conditions prolongs dying, uses valuable resources, could delay the care of other patients, and may be against the patient's wishes. The ethical principles that apply are nonmaleficence—to do no further harm—and justice—the fair allocation of medical resources. There are no simple answers to these ethical dilemmas.

OCCUPATIONAL HAZARDS

The potential exists for transmission of infectious agents into the patient's room. Bacteria from the patient do appear in the moist environment of the expiratory side, but transmission is reduced by attaching a disposable bacteria filter to the ventilator's expiratory inlet. Spray when suctioning or when emptying condensate in the collection chambers can be reduced through the use of closed suction systems and closed water trap systems that reduce environmental contamination. Personal protective apparel should be worn when the potential for contamination with body fluids exists.

In addition, the potential for electrical hazards exists. All electrical equipment should be checked routinely for damage. In the interest of patient safety, the ventilator should be plugged into an outlet that immediately operates on a backup generator in the event of electrical failure.

FUTURE RESEARCH

The field is wide open for the researcher interested in studying various aspects of modes of mechanical ventilation. The recognition that the lung is damaged by inappropriate application of mechanical ventilation highlights the need for further research on ways to minimize the risk of VILI. Low V_T ventilation results in lower plateau pressures but can also result in atelectasis. Research is needed on the various recruitment maneuvers recommended for opening these alveoli. Experimental literature suggests that spontaneous breathing and ventilatory pattern (rate, inspiratory:expiratory ratio, and flow curves) may influence the incidence and severity of ventilator-induced lung injury, but further evidence is required to define an optimal pattern. Related to the use of permissive hypercapnia, research is needed to further explore the effect of high $PaCO_2$ on weaning and whether there is any effect on weaning time because of excessive $PaCO_2$. High-frequency ventilation warrants further investigation in controlled clinical trials, using endpoints recommended in today's lung-protective strategies.

Prospective, randomized studies are necessary to evaluate the differences between set-PEEP and auto-PEEP in promoting oxygenation without furthering lung injury or compromising delivered tidal volumes. Human studies are also warranted to evaluate the effect of flow triggering on the work of breathing and ability to wean.

Research is also needed to describe the understanding of and application of lung protective strategies and modes of ventilation by the people caring for the mechanically ventilated patient. New strategies and modes continue to emerge, and the management of the mechanically ventilated patient is becoming increasingly complex. There is a tremendous need for educators and members of the biotechnical industry to discern the understanding of those providing care.

SUGGESTED READINGS

Burns SM. Ventilatory management—volume and pressure modes. In: Lynn-McHale DJ, Carlson, KK, eds. *AACN Procedure Manual for Critical Care.* 4th ed. Philadelphia, Pa: WB Saunders Co; 2001:178–195.

Campbell RS, Davis BR. Pressure-controlled versus volume-controlled ventilation: does it matter? *Resp Care.* 2002; 47;416–424.

Chatburn RL, Primiano FP. A new system for understanding modes of mechanical ventilation. *Resp Care.* 2001; 46:604–621.

Gattinoni L, Chiumello D, Russo R. Reduced tidal volumes and lung protective ventilatory strategies: where do we go from here? *Current Opin Crit Care.* 2002;8:45–50.

Hess DR, Kacmarek RM. *Essentials of Mechanical Ventilation.* New York, NY: McGraw-Hill, 2002.

Hill N. *Noninvasive Positive Pressure Ventilation: Principles and Applications.* Armonk, NY: Futura Publishing Company, 2001.

Kacmarek RM. Ventilator-induced lung injury. *Int Anesthesiol Clin.* 1999;37:47–64.

Pierce LNB. *Guide to Mechanical Ventilation and Intensive Respiratory Care.* Philadelphia, Pa: WB Saunders Co; 1995.

Slutsky AS. Consensus conference on mechanical ventilation-January 28-30, 1993 at Northbrook, Ill. Parts 1 and 2. *Intensive Care Med.* 1994;20:64–79,150–162. (See the published erratum in *Intensive Care Med.* 1994;20:378.)

CLINICAL RECOMMENDATIONS

Volume-Targeted Ventilatory Modes

The rating scales for the Level of Recommendation range from I to IV, with levels indicated as follows: I, manufactuer's recommendations only; II, theory based, no research data to support recommendations; recommendations from expert consensus group may exist; III, laboratory data only, no clinical data to support recommendations; IV, limited clinical studies to support recommendations; V, clinical studies in more than 1 or 2 different populations and situations to support recommendations; VI, clinical studies in a variety of patient populations and situations to support recommendations.

Period of Use	Recommendation	Rationale for Recommendation	Level of Recommendation	Supporting References	Comments
Selection of Patients	Apply continuous mandatory ventilation (CMV) only to patients with no respiratory effort (under anesthesia), are chemically paralyzed, or when deeply sedated.	CMV delivers a fixed ventilatory pattern regardless of the patient's breathing pattern. While the patient can try to breath spontaneously the machine will not respond. Therefore, CMV requires sedation, sedation with paralysis, or hyperventilation beyond the apneic threshold. These conditions must be maintained or the patient who attempts to breathe will experience sensations of air hunger, work of breathing (WOB) will be significantly increased, and gas exchange and hemodynamics may be adversely affected.	II: Theory based, no research data to support recommendation from expert consensus groups may exist	See Other References: 131	Some ventilator manufacturers use the term *CMV* to indicate the assist/control (A/C) mode. Their rationale involves redefining CMV to mean *controlled mandatory ventilation*, in which every breath is of a mandatory tidal volume (V_T).
	Use A/C when it is desirable to deliver constant V_T thus consistent alveolar ventilation, and to allow the patient to assist yet perform minimal work. The goal is to allow the ventilator to perform the bulk of the work of breathing (WOB).	During A/C, when the patient initiates a breath the ventilator delivers a breath of the preset V_T. Research demonstrates that the WOB required by the patient is minimal (when the flow rate and sensitivity are set properly) but can be considerable if the patient's flow demands are not met. This type of ventilation is desirable when the patient is too weak to perform the WOB (eg, when emerging from anesthesia, pulmonary compliance is decreased, or a low oxygen cost of breathing is desired).	V: Clinical studies in more than 1 or 2 different patient populations/situations to support recommendations	See Other References: 105, 109, 160	A/C combines the security of controlled ventilation ensuring ventilatory support with each breath, while allowing the patient to assist. Assisting reduces discomfort and patient ventilator dysynchrony.
	Use SIMV for a wide range of ventilatory support needs when the patient has normal respiratory drive and it is desirable to allow the patient to assist, thus contributing more to the WOB. Also use as a method for discontinuing mechanical ventilation.	During SIMV the patient receives a preset number of breaths of a preset V_T while being able to breathe spontaneously between the mandatory breaths. Level of ventilatory support varies from full to partial and depends on the number of SIMV breaths prescribed. Weaning with	VI: Clinical studies in a variety of patient populations and situations to support recommendations	See Other References: 35, 40, 41	

Period of Use	Recommendation	Rationale for Recommendation	Level of Recommendation	Supporting References	Comments
Selection of Patients *(cont.)*		SIMV is achieved by gradually reducing the number of SIMV breaths, thus requiring the patient to take on more of the WOB.			
Application of Device and Initial Use	Minimize work of breathing by ensuring sensitivity is set to allow patient to trigger the ventilator with ease, setting flow rate high enough to meet patient ventilatory demand, and using a decelerating ramp flow pattern.	A/C and IMV can be set to provide full-ventilatory support, ie, ventilatory muscles may be completely rested if settings are appropriate and the patient is slightly hyperventilated (ventilated above spontaneous V_T and flow rate). With assisted modes, data show that the patient generates muscular effort of varying degrees during *both* assisted and spontaneous breaths. The work of chest inflation is shared between the ventilator and the respiratory muscles. Improperly set sensitivity and flow rate settings can substantially increase the work for the patient.	VI: Clinical studies in a variety of patient populations and situations to support recommendations	See Other References: 8, 54, 105, 109, 110, 160	Continuous flow systems further decrease the patient's WOB as compared to pressure-triggered systems and the work required to open the demand valve. Flow-triggering (flow-by) therefore decreases the WOB associated with initiating a breath (see "Prevention of Complications" below).
Ongoing Monitoring	Monitor peak inspiratory pressure (PIP) in volume modes because it is variable.	Ventilator delivers a preset V_T. Amount of pressure required to deliver the set volume depends on patient's lung compliance and patient ventilator resistance factors.	IV: Limited clinical studies to support recommendations	See Other References: 25, 26, 66, 72, 84, 88, 133	
	Monitor exhaled V_T to ensure it closely matches the set V_T.	Although V_T is preset on the ventilator control panel, delivery is not guaranteed. Sites of potential air loss include around the cuff or via an intrapleural air leak.			
	Monitor arterial blood gas (ABG) during A/C to ensure patient does not develop respiratory alkalosis. Use of SIMV *may* result in lower pH and higher $PaCO_2$. Improved effect of SIMV over A/C is unlikely in patients with preexisting respiratory alkalosis.	Patient may increase respiratory rate (RR) because of anxiety, pain, or neurologic factors. Increased RR may lead to hyperventilation because each patient initiated breath results in delivery of a preset V_T. Use of SIMV at a lower rate allows patient greater control over ventilation. Patients with brain injury whose respiratory alkalosis is presumed to be central in origin will likely develop alkalosis in either mode.	VI: Clinical studies in a variety of patient populations and situations to support recommendations	See Annotated Bibliography: 6 See Other References: 36, 41, 78, 98	If hyperventilation occurs, reevaluate ventilator settings and consider sedation. Do not add mechanical dead space to promote CO_2 rebreathing as patient response is to increase minute ventilation (V_E) and WOB to compensate. If respiratory alkalosis persists, consider changing SIMV to PS, where the patient has greater control, providing the patient can tolerate an increase in the WOB.

Period of Use	Recommendation	Rationale for Recommendation	Level of Recommendation	Supporting References	Comments
Ongoing Monitoring *(cont.)*					When pH returns to normal using SIMV vs CMV, evidence shows it is generally at the expense of an increase in WOB.
Prevention of Complications	Reduce amount of work required of patient to trigger a breath by using a continuous flow or a flow-triggered system rather than a pressure-triggered system. If no flow-triggered system is available, add a small amount of pressure support (PS) to improve the delivery of fresh gas to the patient.	In a pressure-triggered system the patient must draw back a preset amount of negative pressure (the pressure sensitivity) before the ventilator delivers fresh gas. A time delay occurs before fresh gas is delivered (lag time), resulting in insufficient gas flow to meet the patient's ventilatory demand during early inspiration. Lag time varies between ventilator models.	IV: Limited clinical studies to support recommendations	See Other References: 30, 34, 61, 67, 71, 110, 139, 140, 157	Some pressure-triggered or older ventilator systems require as much as 6 to 8 cm H_2O pressure drop from end expiratory pressure to initiate the gas flow. The time delay to delivery of fresh gas can be as long as 0.3 to 0.7 sec in these systems.
		In a flow-triggered (flow-by) system a base flow of gas travels continuously through the ventilator circuitry; trigger sensitivity is based on a sensed reduction in flow. To maintain a constant supply of fresh gas, the ventilator increases flow of gases in the circuit as it senses the patient's inspiratory flow demand. Flow is immediately available to the patient (no lag time) and it is easily obtained.			Not all ICU ventilators are capable of flow triggering. However, this will likely change with ventilator upgrades due to the identified advantages of flow triggering.
	Use full ventilatory support for as short a time as possible, gradually allowing patient to participate in WOB as tolerated.	Reduce atrophy of respiratory muscles. Putting respiratory muscles to rest for as little as 48 hours can result in reduced diaphragm mass, strength, and endurance.	III: Laboratory data only, no clinical data to support recommendations	See Other References: 5, 94, 166	The extent to which respiratory muscle atrophy develops during prolonged full-ventilatory support in humans is unknown.
	Minimize adverse hemodynamic effects of positive pressure ventilation by maintaining adequate preload, minimizing increases in mean airway pressure, and, when possible, allowing spontaneous respirations.	The degree to which cardiac output is affected during positive pressure ventilation depends on mean airway pressure (Paw), the extent to which the pressure is transmitted to the pleural space, and the patient's volume status. The primary cause of cardiac output reduction is positive pressure in the thorax, which reduces venous return (preload) to	VI: Clinical studies in a variety of patient populations and situations to support recommendations	See Annotated Bibliography: 6 See Other References: 16, 29, 33, 39, 82, 113, 121, 125, 142, 156	Paw may be reduced by using SIMV, as spontaneous breaths are interspersed between mandatory breaths, resulting in a Paw over time that is lower than on a mode where all breaths are mandatory volume breaths. Reduction in cardiac output is most pronounced with hypovolemia. In patients with

Period of Use	Recommendation	Rationale for Recommendation	Level of Recommendation	Supporting References	Comments
Prevention of Complications (*cont.*)		the heart. During sponta-neous respirations intrapleural pressure becomes negative, promoting venous return.			normal cardiac function, data indicate that a reduction in Paw may result in improvement in cardiac output, because preload return is enhanced. With reduced chest wall compliance (eg, in ascites, muscle splinting, chest burns) the percentage of airway pressure transmitted to the pleural space increases. Conversely, when lung compliance is reduced, the percentage is reduced, although if the chest wall remains compliant the effect is modest. With a dilated failing left ventricle, cardiac function may improve when the patient is placed on controlled versus assisted mode possibly because of decreased atrial filling secondary to an increase in mean thoracic pressure. The decrease in preload improves left ventricular performance in heart failure. (For strategies to reduce Paw see also Ventilatory Techniques: Lung Protection Strategies below.)
	Maintain PIP at $\leq$ 40 cm H_2O pressure to reduce incidence of pulmonary barotrauma. If PIP reaches 40 cm H_2O, implement measures to decrease PIP to include use of SIMV, decelerating flow wave curve, or a pressure-targeted mode of ventilation.	Conditions that increase plateau pressure above 40 cm H_2O may result in alveolar lung units becoming overdistended beyond the limits of their elastic capacity leading to injury.	VI: Clinical studies in a variety of patient populations and situations to support recommendations	See Annotated Bibliography: 3, 10 See Other References: 2, 114, 127, 145, 153	See also "Ventilatory Techniques: Lung Protection Strategies" below.
Quality Control Issues	The nurse or the respiratory therapist should perform a patient-ventilator system check at least every 2 hours.	The patient-ventilator system check will evaluate accuracy of settings, allow for analysis of patient data such as PIP and exhaled V_T, and ensure assessment of patient tolerance and synchrony with chosen mode of support.	II: Theory based, no research data to support recommendations; recommendations from expert consensus groups may exist	See Other References: 3, 25	

CLINICAL RECOMMENDATIONS

Pressure-Targeted Ventilatory Modes

The rating scales for the Level of Recommendation range from I to IV, with levels indicated as follows: I, manufactuer's recommendations only; II, theory based, no research data to support recommendations; recommendations from expert consensus group may exist; III, laboratory data only, no clinical data to support recommendations; IV, limited clinical studies to support recommendations; V, clinical studies in more than 1 or 2 different populations and situations to support recommendations; VI, clinical studies in a variety of patient populations and situations to support recommendations.

Period of Use	Recommendation	Rationale for Recommendation	Level of Recommendation	Supporting References	Comments
Selection of Patients	Use pressure targeted ventilation at low levels (5 to 10 cm H_2O) to overcome patient work associated with an endotracheal tube and the ventilator circuit.	An endotracheal tube creates airflow resistance that produces an undesirable workload, which may cause discomfort and compromise ventilatory function. Low level PS compensates for extra WOB through endotracheal tube and a demand valve.	V: Clinical studies in more than 1 or 2 different patient populations and situations to support recommendations	See Other References: 23, 52, 70	The smaller the inner diameter of the endotracheal tube, the higher the resistance to gas flow through the tube and, therefore, the greater the WOB.
	Titrate level of inspiratory pressure to reduce patient's WOB (as evidenced by reduction in tachypnea and abnormal breathing patterns) and to achieve desired V_T and V_E.	As pressure ventilation is titrated upward, ventilatory muscles are unloaded and the WOB is decreased. Signs of fatigue and excessive WOB (eg, tachypnea, abnormal breathing patterns) diminish. PS ventilation changes the quality of work to reduce the ventilatory requirement to produce a change in volume.	VI: Clinical studies in a variety of patient populations and situations to support recommendations	See Annotated Bibliography: 9 See Other References: 7, 11, 20, 22, 49, 79, 85, 101, 102, 152, 155, 158	As WOB is decreased with pressure-targeted ventilation, it is accompanied by changes in the breathing pattern and accessory muscle recruitment that can be observed at the bedside.
	Use pressure modes to improve patient ventilator synchrony.	Pressure-targeted modes set pressure as the independent variable, allowing volume and flow to synchronize with the patient's ventilatory effort. Pressure modes always use a decelerating flow wave pattern, which provides rapid flow at the initiation of the breath and variable flow throughout the breath, meeting the patient's inspiratory flow demand throughout inspiration. Patient effort is therefore reduced and comfort increased. Further, during PS ventilation the patient can vary frequency and inspiratory time to maintain acid base status.	IV: Limited clinical studies to support recommendations	See Other References: 99, 102, 103, 104, 134, 155	
	Use PS for weaning from mechanical ventilation.	Refer to Chapter 3, Weaning from Mechanical Ventilation.			

Period of Use	Recommendation	Rationale for Recommendation	Level of Recommendation	Supporting References	Comments
Selection of Patients *(cont.)*	Use in patients in whom it is desirable to control peak inspiratory pressure (PIP). Use pressure targeted ventilation in patients with noncompliant lungs who demonstrate high airway pressure on conventional volume targeted ventilation.	Early initiation of pressure targeted ventilation results in lower PIP and improved pulmonary compliance, thereby potentially limiting injury to the lung from high distending pressures.	V: Clinical studies in more than 1 or 2 different patient populations and situations to support recommendations	See Annotated Bibliography: 4, 10 See Other References: 72, 150	With PS ventilation the patient must have a reliable respiratory drive because every breath is patient triggered. Spontaneous inspiratory efforts are augmented with a clinician selected amount of inspiratory pressure. PC ventilation assists the breath during inspiration just as PS does; however, a rate is set at which the ventilator will deliver the pressure targeted breaths. Sensitivity can be set so that the patient cannot assist (pure control ventilation) or so the patient can initiate additional breaths above the set rate (pressure A/C). In pressure A/C, patient initiated breaths are augmented with the set inspiratory pressure level or with a second set pressure level (called PC/PS). Volume targeted ventilation, administered with a decelerating flow wave pattern, may result in similar lung mechanics and gas exchange as pressure targeted ventilation, which is always delivered with a decelerating flow wave pattern.
	Use pressure control inverse inspiratory:expiratory (I:E) ratio ventilation or airway pressure release ventilation (APRV) in patients with noncompliant lung disease and persistent oxygenation problems despite a high FIO_2 and levels of PEEP.	Oxygenation can be improved without the undesirable effect of increasing peak alveolar or end expiratory pressure (provided no unknown auto-PEEP develops). Prolonged inspiratory time ventilation results in an increase in Paw. Maintaining a higher Paw improves the stability of the alveoli over the course of the respiratory cycle. An increase in the number of stable alveolar units results in an increase in the functional residual capacity and, thus, an improvement in oxygenation.	VI: Clinical studies in a variety of patient populations and situations to support recommendations	See Annotated Bibliography: 2 See Other References: 1, 28, 37, 68, 92, 136, 144, 148, 150	Inspiratory:expiratory ratios of 1:1, 1.5:1, 2:1, are called inverse I:E ratios. In noncompliant lungs, the short inspiratory time during conventional ventilation allows unstable alveoli to collapse during the relatively longer expiratory phase. The inspiratory effect of prolonged inspiratory phase ventilation is to allow unstable lung units more time to fill and an equilibration of volume between the alveoli. Dead space ventilation and the percentage of shunt both decrease because gas is more evenly distributed in the lung. The relatively com-

Period of Use	Recommendation	Rationale for Recommendation	Level of Recommendation	Supporting References	Comments
Selection of Patients (*cont.*)					pliant alveoli are not overdistended by gases that preferentially flow to them, as may occur during an inflation period of standard duration. It is believed that alveoli that close and then "snap" open during the course of one respiratory cycle experience injury related to this stress.
	Patients should be sedated to prevent spontaneous breathing efforts during PC inverse ratio ventilation.	If the patient is allowed to breathe during the inversed ventilatory cycle, disrupted airway pressure dynamics may lead to deterioration in oxygenation and contribute to lung injury.			The simultaneous shortening of the expiratory phase prevents unstable alveoli from collapsing at end expiration, because the next inspiration typically begins before they reach their closing volume. Rapid rates create air trapping in the lung, which creates pressure known as auto-PEEP.
	Low sedation is required with APRV as spontaneous breathing is allowed.	In APRV the patient is ventilated at a high-level CPAP for a prolonged time (typically 5–6 seconds). This is followed by a rapid release to a lower pressure level (0–5 cm H_2O). The patient may breathe small breaths at any time throughout the respiratory cycle.			
Application of Device and Initial Use	Ensure no leaks are present in the circuitry or around cuff of artificial airway.	If an air leak occurs, the ventilator may fail to cycle to expiration because the flow rate that terminates inspiratory flow will not be reached. This will result in application of positive pressure throughout the respiratory cycle, much as in continuous positive airway pressure (CPAP).	II: Theory based, no research data to support recommendations; recommendations from expert consensus groups may exist	See Other References: 99, 132	
Ongoing Monitoring	Closely monitor exhaled tidal volumes.	With pressure-targeted ventilation the V_T is variable. It is determined by patient effort, the amount of applied inspiratory pressure, and the compliance and resistance of the system (patient and ventilator). Therefore, there is a potential for suboptimal alveolar ventilation in a patient with unstable ventilatory drives (PS), or rapidly changing lung impedances or circuitry resistance factors.	V: Clinical studies in more than 1 or 2 different patient populations/ situations to support recommendations	See Other References: 19, 72, 132, 133, 135, 164	

Period of Use	Recommendation	Rationale for Recommendation	Level of Recommendation	Supporting References	Comments
Ongoing Monitoring *(cont.)*	During inverse-ratio ventilation, as expiratory time is decreased, monitor for the development of dynamic hyperinflation, or auto PEEP.	Auto-PEEP has the same physiological effects of PEEP and adds a cumulative effect to the operator chosen or set PEEP. Regional alveolar overdistention and barotrauma may occur with excessive total PEEP. Further, during pressure-targeted ventilation an increase in total PEEP will result in a decrease in V_T because the change in pressure over the inspiratory phase is reduced.	IV: Limited clinical studies to support recommendations	See Annotated Bibliography: 2 See Other References: 14, 28, 32, 47, 130	Auto-PEEP *cannot* readily be detected by reading the pressure manometer on the ventilator without performing a special maneuver. To measure auto-PEEP, the exhalation valve must be occluded for several seconds just before the next breath would begin. This allows the ventilator pressure manometer to read both circuit pressure (set-PEEP) and airway pressure (auto-PEEP).
Prevention of Complications	Reduce amount of work required of patient to trigger a breath by using a continuous flow or flow-triggered system rather than a pressure-triggered system. If no flow-triggered system is available, add a small amount of PS to improve the delivery of fresh gas to the patient.	Reduce amount of work required to trigger a breath by using a flow-triggered system In a flow-triggered (flow-by) system a base flow of gas travels continuously through the ventilator circuitry; trigger sensitivity is based on a sensed reduction in flow. To maintain a constant supply of fresh gas, the ventilator increases flow of gases in the circuit as it senses the patient's inspiratory flow demand. Flow is immediately available to the patient (no lag time) and it is easily obtained.	V: Clinical studies in more than 1 or 2 different patient populations and situations to support recommendations	See Other References: 30, 34, 61, 67, 71, 104, 110, 139, 140, 157	Some pressure-triggered or older ventilator systems require as much as 6–8 cm H_2O pressure drop from end-expiratory pressure to initiate the gas flow. The time delay to delivery of fresh gas can be as long as 0.3–0.7 sec in these systems
	Closely monitor patient's hemodynamic status. Use a pulmonary artery catheter if the patient is on PC inverse I:E ratio ventilation.	With pressure-targeted ventilation the mean airway and intrathoracic pressures rise, potentially resulting in a decrease in cardiac output and oxygen delivery.	IV: Limited clinical studies to support recommendations	See Other References: 1, 28, 33, 108, 111	The patient will not benefit from an improved PaO_2 if cardiac output, and therefore oxygen delivery, decreases. The clinician should be prepared to support cardiac output with volume and, potentially, inotropic agents.
Quality Control Issues	When using PS, administer medications with metered dose inhalers as opposed to in-line nebulizers.	Patients on PS ventilation must generate a negative pressure to trigger the ventilator. Use of an in-line, continuous flow nebulizer makes it more difficult, or impossible, for the patient to generate this negative pressure. The ventilator will erroneously sense the increased flow created by the nebulizer as the patient's V_E and will not sound an alarm, resulting in failure to detect apnea.	II: Theory based, no research data to support recommendations; recommendations from expert consensus groups may exist	See Other References: 12	

CLINICAL RECOMMENDATIONS

Ventilatory Techniques: Lung Protection Strategies

The rating scales for the Level of Recommendation range from I to IV, with levels indicated as follows: I, manufactuer's recommendations only; II, theory based, no research data to support recommendations; recommendations from expert consensus group may exist; III, laboratory data only, no clinical data to support recommendations; IV, limited clinical studies to support recommendations; V, clinical studies in more than 1 or 2 different populations and situations to support recommendations; VI, clinical studies in a variety of patient populations and situations to support recommendations.

Period of Use	Recommendation	Rationale for Recommendation	Level of Recommendation	Supporting References	Comments
Selection of Patients	Patients with acute lung injury (ALI) and acute respiratory distress syndrome (ARDS)	ARDS affects lung function in a nonhomogeneous distribution. Less involved areas of the lung receive a disproportionate share of the V_T. Conventional ventilatory strategies that use high V_T, FIO_2, and levels of PEEP may result in high peak inspiratory and alveolar pressures that increase the risk of barotrauma. Volutrauma (stretching and alveolar damage to the lung) may also result from regional alveolar overdistention. Both barotrauma and volutrauma worsen lung injury.	VI: Clinical studies in a variety of patient populations and situations to support recommendations	See Annotated Bibliography: 1 See Other References: 3, 44, 58, 59, 69, 106, 107, 115, 127	
	Patients with acute respiratory failure (ARF) with asthma and chronic obstructive airway disease	Acute respiratory failure in asthma and chronic airway disease is associated with significant expiratory obstruction and hyperinflation of the lung. The increased expiratory lung volume causes an increased pressure in the lung that can cause volutrauma and barotrauma.	IV: Limited clinical studies to support recommendations	See Other References: 145, 163	
Application of Device and Initial Use	Maintain stable alveolar units by applying an adequate level of PEEP to recruit alveoli, increase the functional residual capacity, and keep recruited alveoli open throughout the respiratory cycle.	Excessive PEEP stretches alveoli and leads to injury. Too little PEEP allows recruited alveoli to collapse during exhalation requiring the next positive pressure breath to "snap open" the alveolus before it can fill. Repetitive alveolar collapsing and opening contributes to parenchymal injury (shear stress) during positive pressure breathing. Providing enough PEEP to prevent repeated small airway and alveolar opening and closing reduces alveolar injury. This is known as the "open lung" strategy.		See Annotated Bibliography: 1, 3 See Other References: 45, 91, 100, 122, 135, 138, 144, 145, 161	Determining the amount of PEEP to recruit and maintain alveoli above the opening pressure of the lung is a challenge. Some authors suggest developing a pressure volume (PV) curve of the lung and adjusting PEEP to levels above the lower inflection point on the curve, which correlates to the opening pressure of the lung. However, others say that alveolar recruitment occurs along the entire inspiratory limb of the PV curve. Titrate PEEP by monitoring oxygena-

Period of Use	Recommendation	Rationale for Recommendation	Level of Recommendation	Supporting References	Comments
Application of Device and Initial Use *(cont.)*					tion and hemodynamics. A PEEP of 10–20 cm H_2O may be required. As possible, titrate FIO_2 down to 0.5, while ensuring $SpO_2 > 90\%$. Then incrementally decrease PEEP to lowest level while maintaining SpO_2 of 90%–95%
	Further minimize pulmonary edema formation and avoid ventilator induced lung injury by limiting the plateau (alveolar) pressure to 30 cm H_2O.	Ventilation with high peak inspiratory and plateau airway pressures increases vascular filtration pressure and microvascular permeability. High pressures also produce stress fractures of capillary endothelium, epithelium, and basement membranes and cause lung rupture. Mechanical damage leads to leakage of fluid, protein, and blood into the tissue and air spaces or air leakage into tissue spaces.	VI: Clinical studies in a variety of patient populations and situations to support recommendations	See Annotated Bibliography: 3 See Other References: 18, 40, 42, 43, 44, 45, 57, 88, 91, 106, 126, 127, 152, 162	The mode of ventilation may vary; however, many believe that pressure control is an attractive option for a lung protective strategy because the peak pressure cannot rise above the preset value.
	To accomplish the goal of limiting plateau pressure the patient should be ventilated with V_T 6 mL/kg of ideal body weight. If plateau pressure remains > 30 cm H_2O, the V_T should be further reduced and the $PaCO_2$ should be permitted to rise (permissive hypercapnia) unless the presence, or risk, of raised intracranial pressure (ICP) or other contraindication exists that would demand a more normal CO_2. Rapid rises in $PaCO_2$ should be avoided. Slow reduction of V_T may allow renal compensation of the respiratory acidosis.	To limit plateau pressure in the lung to protect the lung from further injury, maintenance of a normal CO_2 may be sacrificed. Control elevation in the $PaCO_2$ to prevent complications related to rapid induction of respiratory acidosis.	VI: Clinical studies in a variety of patient populations and situations to support recommendations	See Annotated Bibliography: 3, 7 See Other References: 3, 48, 60, 86, 93	Potential harmful effects of low V_T ventilation include progressive atelectasis and derecruitment. Although high V_T (12 mL/kg) should be avoided, intermediate ventilation (8–10 mL/kg) could be considered if plateau pressure remains in the safe range.
	Minimize FIO_2 to ≤ 0.6 while maintaining arterial oxygen saturation of $\geq 90\%$.	Exposure to a high FIO_2 increases alveolar PO_2 (PaO_2). High PaO_2 increases microvascular permeability to protein, can lead to absorption atelectasis and surfactant inactivation, and may impede tracheal mucus flow due to ciliary abnormalities and goblet cell hyperplasia. Hyperoxia can also lead to excess oxi-	VI: Clinical studies in a variety of patient populations and situations to support recommendations	See Other References: 38, 53, 77, 81	

Period of Use	Recommendation	Rationale for Recommendation	Level of Recommendation	Supporting References	Comments
Application of Device and Initial Use *(cont.)*		dant production, lipid per-oxidation, protein oxidant damage, and cell death.			
	Determine the recruit-ment potential of the patient through periodic applications of high sus-tained airway pressure, ie, recruiting maneuvers.	Opening of collapsed alve-oli may be achieved through a recruitment maneuver. A variety of approaches have been tried such as the application of continuous positive airway pressure of 35–40 cm H_2O for 40 seconds, intermittent higher tidal volumes, inter-mittent higher PEEP, extended sigh, or PC of 30 above 15–20 cm H_2O PEEP for 1–2 minutes as tolerated. The actual open-ing pressure of the alveoli is determined by the transpulmonary pressure, which varies depending on patient characteristics and stage of ARDS.	IV: Limited clinical studies to support recommendations	See Annotated Bibliography: 1 See Other References: 55, 72, 107, 129, 137	Potential problems with recruitment maneuvers include barotrauma sec-ondary to high pressure across the lung and hypotension secondary to increased intrathoracic pressure transmitted to the capillary bed. PEEP may need to be increased after the maneuver to maintain the effects. The optimal way to perform recruitment maneuvers remain unknown, and no data are available that demonstrate that they improve outcome.
Prevention of Complications	Monitor for adverse effects of respiratory acidemia.	Acute hypercapnia has potential deleterious effects—intracranial hyper-tension in patients with increased ICP, pulmonary hypertension, intracellular acidosis, increased sympa-thetic activity, and may possibly lead to GI hemorrhage by decreasing gastric pH.	IV: Limited clinical studies to support recommendations	See Other References: 27, 50, 77, 143, 151, 154	

CLINICAL RECOMMENDATIONS

Ventilatory Techniques: Noninvasive Positive Pressure Ventilation

The rating scales for the Level of Recommendation range from I to IV, with levels indicated as follows: I, manufactuer's recommendations only; II, theory based, no research data to support recommendations; recommendations from expert consensus group may exist; III, laboratory data only, no clinical data to support recommendations; IV, limited clinical studies to support recommendations; V, clinical studies in more than 1 or 2 different populations and situations to support recommendations; VI, clinical studies in a variety of patient populations and situations to support recommendations.

Period of Use	Recommendation	Rationale for Recommendation	Level of Recommendation	Supporting References	Comments
Selection of Patients	COPD patients with ARF as an early intervention to prevent deterioration to the point of requiring endotracheal intubation. Use when at least two are present: Moderate to severe dyspnea with use of accessory muscles and paradoxical abdominal motion, moderate to severe acidosis (pH 7.30–7.35) and hypercapnia ($PaCO_2$ 45–60 mm Hg), or respiratory frequency > 25 breaths/min. If patient is alert, NPPV should be therapy of first choice unless exclusion criteria present (see comments).	NPPV has been investigated extensively in COPD patients with hypercapnic ARF. It is highly effective in improving gas exchange abnormalities, decreasing the need for intubation, reducing length of hospital stay, and lowering mortality.	VI: Clinical studies in a variety of patient populations and situations to support recommendations	See Other References: 17, 21, 80, 89, 120, 128	With noninvasive ventilation there is adequate ventilatory support without the need to perform endotracheal intubation, eliminating its associated complications and reducing the incidence of nosocomial pneumonia. Patients can eat and speak and are free from the discomfort of an artificial airway. Exclusion criteria: apnea, cardiovascular instability, somnolence, high aspiration risk, viscous/copious secretions, recent facial or gastroesophageal surgery, craniofacial trauma, fixed nasopharyngeal abnormality, extreme obesity.
	Use mask CPAP for patients with acute cardiogenic pulmonary edema.	CPAP rapidly improves oxygenation by reexpanding fluid filled alveoli, increasing the functional residual capacity, and therefore improving lung compliance. These effects reduce the work of breathing and improve respiratory rate. Favorable effect has also been demonstrated in need for intubation, reduced ICU length of stay, and improved hospital mortality.	VI: Clinical studies in a variety of patient populations and situations to support recommendations	See Other References: 15, 96	Caution use of CPAP in patients with good ventricular performance and low filling pressures because venous return may be reduced resulting in a decreased cardiac output.
	Use NPPV to avoid intubation in immunocompromised patients with early acute hypoxemic respiratory failure.	Early use of NPPV results in improved oxygenation, lower intubation rates, and lower mortality. Patients experience less serious complications.	VI: Clinical studies in a variety of patient populations and situations to support recommendations	See Other References: 5, 74	

Period of Use	Recommendation	Rationale for Recommendation	Level of Recommendation	Supporting References	Comments
Selection of Patients *(cont.)*	Patients with hypoxemic respiratory failure who are hemodynamically stable, without severely impaired mental status, and not in need of an artificial airway for secretion management or aspiration protection. Conditions could include pneumonia, atelectasis, trauma, aspiration, post-operative respiratory failure.	NPPV can improve gas exchange, lower the need for intubation, and reduce ICU length of stay in patients with acute hypoxemic respiratory failure. Mask ventilation can be used to administer PEEP and recruit underventilated alveoli, increase the functional residual capacity (FRC), and thus improve oxygenation. NPPV is associated with fewer serious complications such as sinusitis and pneumonia. The wide variety of diagnoses in this category makes it difficult to apply results to individual diagnostic groups.	IV: Limited clinical studies to support recommendations	See Other References: 6, 46, 65, 89, 112, 164	The patient must have a patent natural airway, a spontaneous drive to breathe, and can assist in the management of secretions because the lack of artificial airway access reduces control of the airway for suctioning secretions or protecting from aspiration. Use mask CPAP with caution in patients with basilar skull fracture. A case of pneumocephalus was reported in a trauma patient with unrecognized basilar skull fracture.
	Patients with acute or chronic respiratory disorders who are unable to meet extubation criteria but are otherwise good candidates for NPPV	When the respiratory muscles are unable to independently manage the workload, NPPV provides effective ventilator assistance without the risks of prolonged intubation and with improved patient comfort. This new approach shortens duration of invasive mechanical ventilation. Results have been inconsistent for reducing ICU and hospital LOS, need for tracheostomy, and pneumonia.	V: Clinical studies in more than one or two different populations/situations to support recommendations	See Annotated Bibliography: 5 See Other References: 63, 76, 123	Exert caution when selecting patients for early extubation. Ensure patient is good candidate for NPPV.
	Patients who fail planned or unplanned extubation	To avoid reintubation and thereby the associated complications Noninvasive ventilation may provide an adequate level of support for respiratory distress with a lower level of complications. It provides ventilatory assistance without the resistance of the artificial airway. There is a trend toward lower success rates in unplanned extubation.	IV: Limited clinical studies to support recommendations	See Other References: 83, 87	Carefully select patients and closely monitor until stabilized.

Period of Use	Recommendation	Rationale for Recommendation	Level of Recommendation	Supporting References	Comments
Selection of Patients *(cont.)*	Patients for whom intubation and mechanical ventilation would not normally be considered (for example, do-not-intubate patients, patients with late stage disease or terminal conditions) in whom it is believed that their respiratory failure results from an acute condition that could be reversed by using brief mechanical ventilatory support	Patients who decline intubation could possibly benefit from noninvasive support administered concurrently with therapies to treat an acute respiratory process. In patients with poor prognoses, noninvasive ventilatory support may allow time to make resuscitate/do not resuscitate decisions and for life closure tasks.	IV: Limited clinical studies to support recommendations	See Other References: 10, 13, 56, 117	Concern arises regarding possible use of noninvasive ventilation when further intervention is futile. Refer to "Ethical Considerations."
Application of Device and Initial Use	Carefully size nasal or oronasal mask to ensure proper fit and patient comfort.	Select the proper mask interface to ensure success. Oronasal masks may lower CO_2 more effectively and may benefit mouth breathers. However they may generate feelings of claustrophobia making patients unable to tolerate NPPV and may be harder to fit and therefore generate leaks. Nasal masks add less dead space; allow for speech, expectoration, and oral intake without mask removal; and are sensed as more comfortable by the patient. When a nasal mask is applied, patients must breathe solely through the nares (see also Prevention of Complications).	VI: Clinical studies in a variety of patient populations and situations to support recommendations	See Other References: 90, 124	Masks come in a variety of sizes and materials. Most are clear and made of soft materials with either air or soft silicone cushion seals. Some are made with a swivel adapter. Masks are secured to the head with adjustable straps, or head caps, that attach to prongs on the mask.
	Deliver NPPV using a combination of low level PEEP (5 cm H_2O) to improve FRC (or offset auto PEEP in COPD), and PS adjusted to correct gas exchange abnormalities.	Low level PEEP improves the FRC and oxygenation and offsets auto PEEP in COPD, which significantly reduces inspiratory workload. PS can be adjusted to achieve desired exhaled V_T and to sufficiently unload the respiratory muscles. The use of a pressure-targeted mode enables the peak pressure in the mask to be limited, which may reduce leaks and gastric insufflation and improve synchrony especially in the presence of leaks.	IV: Limited clinical studies to support recommendations	See Other References: 9, 62, 64, 89, 118, 159	NPPV can be delivered with volume- or pressure-targeted modes or as CPAP. Various names for NPPV modes are found in the literature, including bi-level positive airway pressure called BiPAP (Respironics Inc, Murrysville, Pa). Possibly as an extension of this trade name, some authors erroneously refer to NPPV as BiPAP.

Period of Use	Recommendation	Rationale for Recommendation	Level of Recommendation	Supporting References	Comments
Application of Device and Initial Use *(cont.)*	Deliver NPPV with a bi-level ventilator, originally designed for home use for sleep apnea, but has been newly configured for acute care, or via a standard critical care ventilator.	Either type can be used for short-term applications. Bi-level devices have been designed to deliver NPPV and are more leak tolerant.	II: Theory based, no research data to support recommendations; recommendations from expert consensus groups may exist	See Other References: 95, 119, 141	
Ongoing Monitoring	Monitor for gastric distention and place a gastric tube for decompression as necessary.	When administering positive pressure ventilation with a face mask, air may be swallowed or forced down the esophagus.	II: Theory based, no research data to support recommendations; recommendations from expert consensus groups may exist	See Other References: 116, 133	To reduce the possibility of gastric insufflation, use peak mask pressures ≤ 30 cm H_2O.
Prevention of Complications	Use minimum strap tension to achieve a seal and alter mask position to prevent areas of pressure and skin breakdown. At the first sign of pressure and before skin breakdown occurs, apply a patch of wound care dressing to prevent further problems.	The nasal or oronasal masks used to administer noninvasive ventilation must have a tight seal to ensure the patient receives the full benefit of ventilatory support. Nasal bridge skin erythema or breakdown is the most common complication of NPPV. Compliance with therapy diminishes when patient discomfort increases.	VI: Clinical studies in a variety of patient populations and situations to support recommendations	See Other References: 75, 95, 119, 146, 164	A mask with a transparent dome is preferable because it allows visualization of the airway and secretions.
	Use artificial tears to moisten the eyes and a humidification system for the inspired gases.	Leakage of gases around the nasal portion of the mask may dry the eyes, leading to conjunctivitis. Mucous membranes of the nose may become dry from inspiration of high volume, dry gases.	IV: Limited clinical studies to support recommendations	See Other References: 13, 31, 119	It is not necessary to heat the inspired gases because the upper airways that normally heat inspired gases are not bypassed. Nasal dryness may respond to normal saline nasal spray or drops. If dryness fails to respond to these measures a pass-over type humidifier can be added to the ventilator circuit.
Quality Control Issues	Use a system that detects air leaks and compensates for them by increasing flow.	Increases assurance that patient will receive adequate V_T	IV: Limited clinical studies to support recommendations	See Other References: 95, 116, 141	When an air leak occurs check to see if exhaled V_T is compromised, reposition the mask, apply wound care dressing to seal leaks, reduce the amount of PEEP or PS as tolerated, or try another mask.

Period of Use	Recommendation	Rationale for Recommendation	Level of Recommendation	Supporting References	Comments
Quality Control Issues *(cont.)*	When delivering two levels of positive airway pressure (PS and PEEP) via circuitry that requires the patient to breathe through a single tube, use a nonrebreathing valve and low-level end expiratory positive airway pressure (EPAP) to prevent CO_2 rebreathing.	CO_2 rebreathing may occur in single tube systems when 2 levels of airway pressure are used, even at the lowest level of PEEP. This side effect of the technique has prevented $PaCO_2$ from dropping in hypercapnic patients.	IV: Limited clinical studies to support recommendations	See Other References: 51, 97, 141	*Caution:* Placing the nonrebreathing valve in the circuitry increases expiratory resistance and may decrease V_T.

ANNOTATED BIBLIOGRAPHY

1. **Amato MBP, Barbas CSV, Medeiros DM, et al. Effect of a protective-ventilation strategy on mortality in the acute respiratory distress syndrome.** *New Engl J Med.* **1998; 338:347–354.**

Study Sample

The study sample consisted of 53 patients with early acute respiratory distress syndrome (ARDS).

Comparison Studied

Comparison was made between conventional ventilation and protective ventilation. Conventional ventilation was based on a strategy of maintaining the lowest positive end-expiratory pressure (PEEP) for acceptable oxygenation, with a tidal volume (Vt) of 12 mL/kg and normal arterial carbon dioxide pressure ($PaCO_2$) level (35–38 mm Hg). Protective ventilation involved end-expiratory pressures set above the lower inflection point of the pressure-volume curve, a Vt of 6 mL/kg, driving pressure of 20 cm H_2O above PEEP, permissive hypercapnia, and preferential use of pressure limited ventilatory modes. The primary end point was survival at 28 days. Secondary end points included survival to hospital discharge, occurrence of clinically detectable barotraumas, and weaning rate adjusted for APACHE II score.

Study Procedures

After enrollment, all patients underwent a standardized regimen of ventilatory-hemodynamic procedures for at least 30 minutes, the control period. After the patient was stabilized, laboratory, hemodynamic, and respiratory measurements were obtained. Then a pressure-volume curve was developed to identify the lower inflection point. The patient was then randomly assigned to one of the two groups. The assigned ventilatory strategy was maintained until extubation or death.

Key Results

The study was stopped during the fifth interim analysis, after 53 patients had been enrolled because of a significant survival difference. After 28 days, 38% of the protective ventilation group had died, as compared to 71% in the conventional ventilation group ($P < .001$). Differences in weaning rates mirrored the results for survival ($P = .005$). The protective ventilation group also had a lower rate of clinical barotraumas (7% vs. 42%, $P = .02$) despite the use of higher PEEP and higher mean airway pressures. The difference in survival to discharge was not significant.

Study Strengths and Weaknesses

Stringent algorithms were used for infectious problems, hemodynamic management, nutrition, sedation, dialysis and general care to minimize bias. However, due to the complexity of the procedures used in the protocol it was impossible to blind the researchers to control and treatment groups. Because the protective ventilation strategy involved many concurrent maneuvers, it is difficult to determine the key ventilatory variable responsible for treatment effect.

Clinical Implications

The protective ventilation new approach to mechanical ventilation in ARDS may reduce ventilator induced pressure injury, increase the changes of earlier weaning, and improve long term survival.

2. **Armstrong BW, MacIntyre NR. Pressure-controlled, inverse ratio ventilation that avoids air trapping in the adult respiratory distress syndrome.** *Crit Care Med.* **1995;23:279–285.**

Study Sample

The study sample consisted of 14 patients with ARDS who were receiving mechanical ventilation with volume-control (VC) conventional ratio ventilation followed by pressure-control inverse ratio ventilation (PC-IRV).

Comparison Studied

Oxygenation in patients ventilated with conventional ventilation was compared to PC-IRV used to increase the mean airway pressure and therefore improve oxygenation.

Study Procedures

Data from a 12-hour crossover period from VC conventional ratio ventilation to PC-IRV was analyzed retrospectively. Variables analyzed were respiratory rate (RR), Vt, minute ventilation (Ve), peak inspiratory pressure (PIP), mean airway pressure (Paw), inspiratory:expiratory (I:E) ratio, FIO_2, arterial blood gas (ABG) values, and cardiovascular data. After initiation of PC-IRV, data were reassessed at subsequent times during the 12-hour period.

Key Results

On PC-IRV there was a significant reduction in PIP and significant increases in Paw and PaO_2. Cardiac output decreased but other hemodynamic variables remained stable.

Study Strengths and Weaknesses

Limitations include the retrospective nature of the study. Also data over the study period was not averaged. Of particular note was that data during the PC period included an assessment performed when the patient was at their "best oxygenation," which may skew the data. Patients on PC-IRV were paralyzed, but it was not clear whether patients on VC were. Strength of the study is that VT was constant on both modes.

Clinical Implications

Oxygenation is primarily a function of Paw. PC-IRV can be used to increase the Paw without producing auto-PEEP, which effects lung inflation pressures and delivered VT and is difficult to monitor. Cardiac performance and tissue oxygen delivery must be monitored with a pulmonary artery catheter when using techniques that increase Paw.

3. **Brower RG, Matthay MA, Morris A, et al. Ventilation with lower tidal volumes as compared with traditional tidal volumes for acute lung injury and the acute respiratory distress syndrome. The Acute Respiratory Distress Syndrome Network. *N Engl J Med.* 2000 May 4;342(18):1301–1308.**

Study Sample

A total of 861 patients with acute lung injury and ARDS were enrolled in the study which was stopped early because mortality was lower in the treatment group ($P = .007$).

Comparison Studied

Traditional ventilation was compared to ventilation with lower tidal volume. Traditional ventilation involved an initial VT of 12 mL/kg and a plateau pressure of 50 cm H_2O or less, whereas lower tidal volume ventilation involved an initial VT of 6 mL/kg or less and a plateau pressure of 30 cm H_2O or less. The first primary outcome was death prior to discharge and breathing without assistance; the second primary outcome was number of ventilator free days between days 1 and 28. Other outcomes were number of days without organ or system failure and the occurrence of barotrauma.

Study Procedures

Patients who met study criteria were randomly assigned to receive mechanical ventilation involving either traditional tidal volumes or lower tidal volumes using a centralized interactive voice system. The volume assist/control mode was used for all patients. Initial VT was based on predicted body weight calculations. In the group treated with traditional VT, the initial VT was 12 mL/kg. This was subsequently reduced or increased in stepwise increments to maintain the plateau pressure at 45 to 50 cm H_2O. In the group treated with lower

VT, the VT was reduced by 6 mL/kg. Tidal volume was adjusted in stepwise increments to maintain plateau pressure 25 to 30 cm H_2O. Data were collected at baseline, and on days 1, 2, 3, 4, 7, 14, 21, and 28.

Key Results

Mortality was lower in the group treated with lower tidal volumes than in the group treated with traditional tidal volumes (31.0% vs 39.8%, $P = .007$) and the number of ventilator days was also lower in the treatment group ($P = .007$). The mean tidal volumes on days 1 to 3 were 6.2 +/– 0.8 and 11.8 +/– 0.8 mL/kg of predicted body weight ($P < .001$), respectively, and the mean plateau pressure were 25 +/– 6 and 33 +/– 8 cm H_2O ($P < .001$), respectively. There was no significant difference in duration of mechanical ventilation between the two groups. The number of days without nonpulmonary organ or system failure was significantly higher in the low VT group ($P = .006$). The incidence of barotrauma was similar in the two groups.

Study Strengths and Weaknesses

A strength is the study power being a multicenter (10 university centers), randomized, controlled trial. Protocol did not control for amount of PEEP applied. Intervention group required higher levels of PEEP.

Clinical Implications

In patients with acute lung injury and ARDS, mechanical ventilation with lower tidal volume (6 mL/kg ideal body weight) than is traditionally used results in decreased mortality and decreases the number of ventilator days. In these patients high priority should be given to mechanical ventilation strategies that prevent excessive lung stretch.

4. **Davis K, Branson RD, Campbell RS, Porembka DT. Comparison of volume control and pressure control ventilation: is flow waveform the difference? *J Trauma.* 1996;41:808–814.**

Study Sample

The study population consisted of 25 postsurgical or posttrauma patients with ARDS requiring mechanical ventilation with the following indications: PEEP level, $\geq$ 10 cm H_2O; RR, $\geq$ 8 breaths per minute; oxygen concentration, $\geq$ .5; PIP, $\geq$ 40 cm H_2O; and requiring sedation and paralysis.

Comparison Studied

Ventilatory pressures, oxygenation and ventilation parameters, and hemodynamic variables measured during pressure-control (PC) and volume-control (VC) ventilation using square and decelerating flow waveforms to determine if flow waveform makes a difference.

Study Procedures

In random sequence ventilator mode was changed from VC with a square flow waveform, PC with a decelerating flow waveform, or VC with a decelerating flow waveform. Tidal volume, VE, and airway pressures were continuously measured at the proximal airway. After 2 hours in each mode, ventilatory, hemodynamic, gas exchange, and respiratory mechanics data were collected.

Key Results

Both PC and VC ventilation with a decelerating flow waveform provided better oxygenation at a lower PIP and higher Paw than VC ventilation with a square flow waveform. There were no differences between VC ventilation and PC ventilation used with the decelerating flow waveform.

Study Strengths and Weaknesses

A strength of this study is that during the study period FIO_2, respiratory frequency, I:E ratio, PEEP, and VT were held constant. Limitations include the short period of study at each flow waveform because it has been suggested that the effect of PC ventilation becomes more pronounced over time. Findings cannot be extrapolated to patients who are breathing spontaneously or who have other forms of disease.

Clinical Implications

Volume-control ventilation with a decelerating flow waveform may be used to improve oxygenation and reduce the PIP in ARDS while providing the security of consistent volume delivery. High-pressure alarm limits should be set tight to prevent excessive airway pressures and barotrauma.

5. **Ferrer M, Esquinas A, Arancibia F, et al. Noninvasive ventilation during persistent weaning failure: a randomized controlled trial. *Am J Resp Crit Care Med.* 2003;168:70–76.**

Study Sample

Forty-three mechanically ventilated patients who had failed a weaning trial for 3 consecutive days. Trial was stopped after a planned interim analysis.

Comparison Studied

Comparison was made between extubation and noninvasive ventilation (noninvasive ventilation) with once daily weaning attempts (conventional ventilation).

Study Procedures

Intubated patients who met criteria and in whom the spontaneous breathing trial failed during 3 consecutive days were randomly assigned, using a computer-generated table for each center either for: (1) extubation and noninvasive ventilation (NIV) treatment (NIV group) or (2) reconnection to the ventilator and once-daily weaning attempts (conventional weaning group). The NIV group were continuously ventilated after extubation for up to 24 hours using the spontaneous/timed mode. Then NIV was gradually withdrawn until patients could permanently sustain spontaneous breathing. Face mask was first choice but nasal masks were used. In the conventional weaning group, spontaneous breathing trials were performed until patients could be extubated. Successful weaning was defined as the ability to sustain spontaneous breathing for at least 3 consecutive days.

Key Results

Compared with the conventional weaning group, the NIV group had statistically significant shorter periods of invasive ventilation ($P = .003$), ICU days ($P = .002$), hospital stay ($P = .026$), less need for tracheostomy ($P < .001$) and increased ICU ($P = .045$) and 90-day survival ($P = .044$). The incidence of nosocomial pneumonia ($P = .042$) and of septic shock ($P = .045$) was higher in the conventional weaning group. Though not statistically significant the incidence of reintubation was approximately half the conventional-weaning group and NIV resulted in fewer tracheostomies.

Study Strengths and Weaknesses

This study was a prospective, randomized clinical trial in 2 centers; however, it was impossible to blind the researchers to which group the patient was randomized. Patients in the conventional ventilation group received more sedation. Patients assigned to NIV were weaned gradually over a period of time, whereas patients in the conventional ventilation group were weaned using only daily T-piece trials.

Clinical Implications

NIV is effective in shortening the duration of mechanical ventilation in patients with persistent weaning failure. Caution needs to be taken when removing the artificial airway of patients unable to ventilate independently. Criteria for choosing patients who are appropriate for NIV should be adhered to closely. Careful bedside monitoring is required throughout the transition from invasive to NIV.

6. **Groeger JS, Levinson MR, Carlon GC. Assist control versus synchronized intermittent mandatory ventilation during acute respiratory failure. *Crit Care Med.* 1989;17:607–612.**

Study Sample

A total of 40 critically ill patients without chronic obstructive lung disease in a special care unit at a cancer center formed the study sample.

Comparison Studied

Hemodynamic, metabolic, and ventilatory measurements during ventilation with both synchronized intermittent mandatory ventilation (SIMV) and A/C were used with a crossover protocol to determine if one mode proved to be advantageous over the other. Hemodynamic data collected included blood pressure (BP), heart rate and rhythm, mean BP and, in 34 patients, pulmonary capillary wedge pressure (PCWP), mean pulmonary artery pressure (PAP), and cardiac output. Metabolic data collected included basal energy expenditure and resting energy expenditure. Ventilatory data included V_E; PEEP; mean, peak, and plateau airway pressures; and oxygenation variables obtained from an arterial blood gas analysis.

Study Procedures

Patients were first placed on SIMV and then switched to A/C using the same ventilator settings. Data were obtained 30 minutes after the patient was placed on each mode.

Key Results

Respiratory rate was significantly higher on SIMV; however, V_E was the same for both modes. Alveolar ventilation, as reflected by the $PaCO_2$, was significantly lower during SIMV. Mean airway pressure was significantly higher on A/C. Blood pressure was always lower during A/C than SIMV, falling by more than 10 mm Hg in the total group. Cardiac output, PAP, central venous pressure, and left ventricular stroke work were all higher with SIMV than during A/C. Resting energy expenditure and volume of oxygen consumption were significantly higher during SIMV than A/C, but the magnitude was not clinically significant.

Study Strengths and Weaknesses

Researchers report that the patients were receiving continuous IV sedation; however, no analysis was performed on whether sedation had an effect. Strengths include that patients were given time to equilibrate on the mode before measures were taken, no interventions were performed during that period that may effect ventilation or oxygenation, and patients were eliminated from analysis if a change in temperature greater than 0.5°C occurred during the study period.

Clinical Implications

Alveolar ventilation is higher on A/C than SIMV resulting in a lower $PaCO_2$. Therefore, patients with shallow V_T and rapid breathing would benefit from A/C. Patients experience less adverse hemodynamic effects when ventilated with SIMV than with A/C. Acutely ill patients may be able to regulate their V_E with a reduced work of breathing on A/C rather than SIMV.

7. Hickling KG, Henderson SJ, Jackson R. Low mortality associated with low volume pressure limited ventilation with permissive hypercapnia in severe adult respiratory distress syndrome. *Intensive Care Med.* **1990;16:372–377.**

Study Sample

A total of 53 patients with ARDS formed the study sample.

Comparison Studied

The study compared the outcome of patients with severe ARDS managed with limitation of PIP, low V_T, spontaneous breathing using SIMV from the start of ventilation, and permissive hypercapnia without bicarbonate to buffer acidosis against Acute Physiology and Chronic Health and Evaluation (APACHE)-II predicted mortality for all adult patients managed in the same ICU during 1992.

Study Procedures

Patients with ARDS were routinely ventilated with SIMV using V_T 7 mL/kg initially and reducing it as necessary to keep the PIP less than 30 cm H_2O when possible, and always below 40 cm H_2O. Ventilator rate was generally begun at 14 to 20 breaths per minute and then gradually reduced, disregarding hypercapnia and tachypnea. PEEP was used to maintain $SaO_2 > 90\%$. Some patients were ventilated with pressure support (PS).

Key Results

Hospital mortality for subjects in the study was significantly lower than the mean APACHE-II predicted mortality rate.

Study Strengths and Weaknesses

This study was poorly controlled in terms of fluid replacement, sedation, levels of PEEP employed, and levels of oxygen administered. The comparison group was retrospective, whereas a concurrent control group would make this study much stronger.

Clinical Implications

"Resting" the lung during ARDS management by avoiding regional lung overdistention may improve both recovery of the lung and patient outcome in ARDS.

8. Mercat A, Graini L, Teboul JL, Lenique F, Richard C. Cardiorespiratory effects of pressure-controlled ventilation with and without inverse ratio in the adult respiratory distress syndrome. *Chest.* **1993;104:871–875.**

Study Sample

A total of 10 patients with ARDS formed the study sample.

Comparison Studied

Volume control with I:E ratio of 1:2, PC with I:E ratio of 1:2, and PC-IRV with I:E ratio of 2:1 were compared for gas exchange, hemodynamics, and airway pressures.

Study Procedures

The 3 ventilatory modes were tested in random order. Each ventilatory mode was applied for 1 hour before gas exchange, hemodynamic, and airway pressure measurements were taken.

Key Results

No significant differences in Pao_2 were observed among the 3 modes. The peak airway pressure was significantly lower in PC-IRV than in PCV and VCV, but plateau pressure did not differ in the 3 modes. The mean airway pressure was highest, and the cardiac index and oxygen delivery were lowest with PC-IRV. $Paco_2$ was significantly lower during PC-IRV.

Study Strengths and Weaknesses

In all modes the Fio_2, V_T, RR, and total PEEP were kept constant. All patients were sedated, paralyzed, and ventilated with the same type of ventilator. Modes were applied for a short duration, even though it can take several hours to see the full benefit of PC-IRV.

Clinical Implications

When applying PC-IRV, monitoring must be in place as the patient's hemodynamic status may be adversely affected, resulting in a reduction in oxygen delivery. The increase in Pao_2 with PC-IRV seen by some authors may be related to the formation of auto-PEEP. PCV and PC-IRV are useful modes to apply when a reduction in peak airway pressure is desired.

9. Pierce JD, Gerald K. Differences in end-tidal carbon dioxide and breathing patterns in ventilator-dependent patients using pressure support ventilation. *Am J Crit Care.* **1994;3:276–281.**

Study Sample

The study population was formed of adult patients (n = 12) who had been mechanically ventilated for at least 5 days and had failed at least 2 ventilator weaning attempts. Days on mechanical ventilation ranged from 7 to 63.

Comparison Studied

Researchers studied the differences in end-tidal carbon dioxide ($ETCO_2$) and breathing patterns at varying PS ventilation levels in ventilator-dependent patients.

Study Procedures

Breathing patterns were measured using a plethysmograph and a ventilator. Capnography was measured via the exhalation port. Variables measured included RR, V_T, V_E, $ETCO_2$, and chest and abdominal movement to evaluate for chest-abdominal asynchrony. Recordings were taken at 10-minute intervals at the PS levels of 0, 10, 15, and 20 cm H_2O, in an increasing, stepwise fashion.

Key Results

As the level of PS was increased the RR, $ETCO_2$, and asynchronous movement of chest and abdomen decreased. Tidal volume increased with the higher levels of PS.

Study Strengths and Weaknesses

Findings are applicable to patients who have been mechanically ventilated for durations that vary widely from very brief to quite prolonged.

Clinical Implications

Pressure support can be titrated upward to improve the patient's V_T and carbon dioxide excretion. Using higher PS levels can reduce the work of breathing as evidenced by chest-abdominal synchrony and a reduction in RR.

10. Rappaport SH, Shpiner R, Yoshihara G, et al. Randomized, prospective trial of pressure-limited versus volume-controlled ventilation in severe respiratory failure. *Crit Care Med.* **1994;22:22–32.**

Study Sample

A total of 27 patients receiving care in a medical ICU for acute, severe hypoxemic respiratory failure were the study sample.

Comparison Studied

The study compared volume-controlled and pressure-limited ventilation to identify differences in disease course and outcome associated with early institution of pressure-limited or volume-controlled ventilation. Variables measured were PIP, Paw, $ETCO_2$, CO_2 minute excretion, inspiratory and expiratory VT, pause pressure, static thoracic compliance, inspiratory resistance, and PaO_2/FIO_2 values. APACHE-II scores were recorded daily.

Study Procedures

Patients were randomly assigned to either pressure-limited or volume-controlled ventilation. Variables were collected at 1-minute intervals via a connection between the ventilator and a 286 computer for up to 72 hours or until extubation or death. Data were screened to remove data collected when the patient was not ventilated during a steady state, such as during suctioning. The remaining data was averaged over 6-hour periods, generating a maximum of 12 values for each variable in patients monitored for the full 72 hours.

Key Results

Patients randomized to pressure-limited ventilation demonstrated statistically significant lower PIP, a more rapid increase in static compliance, and fewer days of mechanical ventilation than patients on volume-controlled ventilation. Sedation requirements were equivalent between the two groups. No patients on either mode developed barotrauma.

Study Strengths and Weaknesses

Groups were well matched for severity of illness as measured by the APACHE-II scores and the PaO_2/FIO_2 scores.

Clinical Implications

Pressure-limited ventilation may have a beneficial role when used as the primary ventilatory modality in patients with ARDS.

OTHER REFERENCES

1. Abraham E, Yoshihara G. Cardiorespiratory effects of pressure controlled inverse ratio ventilation in severe respiratory failure. *Chest.* 1989;96:1356–1359.
2. Al-Saady N, Bennett ED. Decelerating inspiratory flow waveform improves lung mechanics and gas exchange in patients on intermittent positive pressure-ventilation. *Intensive Care Med.* 1985;11:68–75.
3. Amato MBP, Barbas CSV, Medeiros DM, et al. Beneficial effects of the "open lung approach" with low distending pressures in acute respiratory distress syndrome. *Am J Respir Crit Care Med.* 1995;152:1835–1846.
4. American Association of Respiratory Care Mechanical Ventilation Guidelines Committee. AARC clinical practice guideline: patient-ventilator system checks. *Respir Care.* 1992;37:882–886.
5. Antonelli M, Conti G, Bufi M, et al. Noninvasive ventilation for treatment of acute respiratory failure in patients undergoing solid organ transplantation: a randomized trial. *JAMA.* 2000;283:235–241.
6. Antonelli M, Conti G, Rocco M, et al. A comparison of noninvasive positive-pressure ventilation and conventional mechanical ventilation in patients with acute respiratory failure. *N Engl J Med.* 1998;339:429–435.
7. Annat GJ, Viale JP, Dereymez CP, Bouffard YM, Delafosee BX, Motin JP. Oxygen cost of breathing and diaphragmatic pressure-time index: measurement in patients with COPD during weaning with pressure support ventilation. *Chest.* 1990;98:411–444.
8. Anzueto A, Tobin MJ, Moore G, Peters JI, Seidenfeld JJ, Coalson JJ. Effect of prolonged mechanical ventilation on diaphragmatic function: a preliminary study of a baboon model. *Am Rev Respir Dis.* 1987;135:A201.
9. Appendini L, Patessio A, Zanaboni S, et al. Physiologic effects of positive end-expiratory pressure and mask pressure support during exacerbations of chronic obstructive pulmonary disease. *Am J Respir Crit Care Med.* 1994;149:1069–1076.
10. Averill FJ, Adkins G. Use of bi-level positive airway pressure (BIPAP) in patients with acute respiratory failure. *Chest.* 1993;104:143S.
11. Banner MJ, Kirby RR, MacIntyre NR. Patient and ventilator work of breathing and ventilatory muscle loads at different levels of pressure support ventilation. *Chest.* 1991;100:531–533.
12. Beaty CD, Ritz RM, Benson MS. Continuous in-line nebulizers complicate pressure support ventilation. *Chest.* 1989;96:1360–1363.
13. Benhamou D, Girault C, Faure C, et al. Nasal mask ventilation in acute respiratory failure. Experience in elderly patients. *Chest.* 1992;102:912–917.

14. Benson MS, Pierson DJ. Auto-PEEP during mechanical ventilation of adults. *Respir Care.* 1988;33: 557–568.

15. Bersten AD, Holt AW, Vedig AE, et al. Treatment of severe cardiogenic pulmonary edema with continuous positive airway pressure delivered by face mask. *N Engl J Med.* 1991;325:1825–1830.

16. Biondi JW, Schulman DS, Mathay RA. Effects of mechanical ventilation on right and left ventricular function. *Clin Chest Med.* 1988;9:55–71.

17. Bott J, Carroll MP, Conway JH, et al. Randomized controlled trial of nasal ventilation in acute ventilatory failure due to chronic obstructive airway disease. *Lancet.* 1993;341:1555–1558.

18. Brochard L. Pressure-limited ventilation. *Respir Care.* 1996;41:447–455.

19. Brochard L. Pressure support ventilation. In: Tobin MJ, ed. *Principles and Practice of Mechanical Ventilation.* New York, NY: McGraw-Hill; 1994:239–257.

20. Brochard L, Harf A, Lorino H, Lemaire F. Inspiratory pressure support prevents diaphragmatic fatigue during weaning from mechanical ventilation. *Am Rev Respir Dis.* 1989;139:513–21.

21. Brochard L, Mancebo J, Wysocki M, et al. Noninvasive ventilation for acute exacerbations of chronic obstructive pulmonary disease. *N Engl J Med.* 1995; 333:817–822.

22. Brochard L, Pluskwa F, Lemaire F. Improved efficacy of spontaneous breathing with inspiratory pressure support. *Am Rev Respir Dis.* 1987;136:411–415.

23. Brochard L, Rua F, Lorino H, Lemaire F, Harf A. Inspiratory pressure support compensates for the additional work of breathing caused by the endotracheal tube. *Anesthesiology.* 1991;75:739–745.

24. Burns SM. Weaning from Mechanical Ventilation. In: Burns SM ed. *Care of Mechanically Ventilated Patient,* 2nd ed. Boston, Mass: Jones and Bartlett; 2006:95–160.

25. Campbell RS. Managing the patient-ventilator system: system checks and circuit changes. *Respir Care.* 1994;39:227–236.

26. Campbell RS, Davis BR. Pressure-controlled versus volume-controlled ventilation: does it matter? *Respir Care.* 2002;47:416–424.

27. Carvalho CRR, Barbas CSV, Medeiros DM, et al. Temporal hemodynamic effects of permissive hypercapnia associated with ideal PEEP in ARDS. *Am J Respir Crit Care Med.* 1997;156:1458–1466.

28. Chan K, Abraham, E. Effects of inverse-ratio ventilation on cardiorespiratory parameters in severe respiratory failure. *Chest.* 1992;102:1556–1561.

29. Chapin JC, Downs JB, Douglas ME, et al. Lung expansion, airway pressure transmission and positive end-expiratory pressure. *Arch Surg.* 1979;114: 1193–1197.

30. Christopher KL, Neff TA, Bowman JL, et al. Demand and continuous flow intermittent mandatory ventilation systems. *Chest.* 1985;887:625–630.

31. Confalonieri M, Aiolfi S, Scartabellati A. Use of non-invasive positive pressure ventilation in severe community-acquired pneumonia [abstract]. *Am J Respir Crit Care Med.* 1995;151:A424.

32. Conoscenti C, Menashe P, Meduri GU, Gottleib J. Intrinsic PEEP during inverse ratio ventilation [abstract]. *Am Rev Respir Dis.* 1987;135:A55.

33. Cournand A, Motley HL, Werko, L, et al. Physiological studies of the effects of intermittent positive pressure breathing on cardiac output in man. *Am J Physiol.* 1948;152:162–174.

34. Cox D, Niblett DJ. Studies on continuous positive airway pressure breathing systems. *Br J Anaesth.* 1984;56:905–911.

35. Cullen P, Modell JH, Kirby R, et al. Treatment of flail chest: use of intermittent mandatory ventilation and positive end-expiratory pressure. *Arch Surg.* 1975; 110:1099–1103.

36. Culpepper JA, Rinaldo JE, Rogers RM. Effect of mechanical ventilator mode on tendency towards respiratory alkalosis. *Am Rev Resp Dis.* 1985;132: 1075–1077.

37. Davis K, Johnson DJ, Branson RS, et al. Airway pressure release ventilation. *Archives of Surg.* 1993;128: 1348–1352.

38. Davis WB, Rennard SI, Bitterman PB, et al. Pulmonary oxygen toxicity. Early reversible changes in human alveolar structures induce by hyperoxia. *N Engl J Med.* 1983;309:878–883.

39. Downs JB, Douglas ME, Santelippo PM, et al. Ventilatory pattern, intrapleural pressure, and cardiac output. *Anesth Analg.* 1977;56:88–96.

40. Downs JB, Klein EF, Desautels D, et al. Intermittent mandatory ventilation: a new approach to weaning patients from mechanical ventilation. *Chest.* 1973;64: 331–335.

41. Downs JB, Perkins HM, Modell JH. Intermittent mandatory ventilation: an evaluation. *Arch Surg.* 1974;109:519–523.

42. Dreyfuss D, Bassett G, Soler P, Sauman G. Intermittent positive-pressure hyperventilation with high inflation pressures produces pulmonary microvascular injury in rats. *Am Rev Respir Dis.* 1985;132:880–884.

43. Dreyfuss D, Saumon G. The role of tidal volume, FRC and end-inspiratory volume in the development of pulmonary edema following mechanical ventilation. *Am Rev Respir Dis.* 1993;148:1194–1203.

44. Dreyfus D, Saumon G. Ventilator-induced lung injury. *Am J Respir Crit Care Med.* 1998;157: 294–323.

45. Dreyfuss D, Soler P, Bassett G, Saumon G. High-inflation pressure pulmonary edema. *Am Rev Respir Dis.* 1988;137:1159–1164.

46. Duncan SR, Negrin RS, Mihn FG, et al. Nasal continuous positive airway pressure in atelectasis. *Chest.* 1987;92:621–624.

47. Duncan SR, Rizk NW, Raffin TA. Inverse ratio ventilation, PEEP in disguise [letter]. *Chest.* 1987;92: 380–392.

48. Eisner MD, Thompson T, Hudson LD, et al. Efficacy of low tidal volume ventilation in patients with different clinical risk factors for acute lung injury and the acute respiratory distress syndrome. *Am J Resp Crit Care Med.* 2001;164:231–236.

49. Ershowsky P, Krieger B. Changes in breathing pattern during pressure support ventilation. *Respir Care.* 1987;32:1011–1016.

50. Feihl F, Perret C. Permissive hypercapnia: how permissive should we be? *Am J Respir Crit Care Med.* 1994;150:1722–1737.

51. Ferguson GT, Gilmartin M. CO_2 rebreathing during BiPAP ventilatory assistance. *Am J Respir Crit Care Med.* 1995;151:1126–1135.

52. Fiastro JF, Habib MP, Quan SF. Pressure support compensation for inspiratory work due to endotracheal tubes and demand CPAP. *Chest.* 1988;93: 499–502.

53. Fisher AB. Oxygen therapy: side effects and toxicity. *Am Rev Respir Dis.* 1980;122:61–69.

54. Flick GR, Bellamy PE, Simmons DH. Diaphragm contraction during assisted mechanical ventilation. *Chest.* 1989;96:130–135.

55. Foti G, Cereda M, Sparacino ME, et al. Effects of periodic lung recruitment maneuvers on gas exchange and respiratory mechanics in mechanically ventilated acute respiratory distress syndrome (ARDS) patients. *Intensive Care Med.* 2000;26:501–507.

56. Freichels TA. Palliative ventilatory support: use of noninvasive positive pressure ventilation in terminal respiratory insufficiency. *Am J Crit Care.* 1994;3: 6–10.

57. Fu Z, Costello ML, Tsukimoto K, et al. High lung volume increases stress failure in pulmonary capillaries. *J Appl Physiol.* 1992;73:123–133.

58. Gattinoni L, Pesanti A, Avalli L, Rossi F, Bombino M. Pressure volume curve of total respiratory system in acute respiratory failure: computed tomographic scan study. *Am Rev Respir Dis.* 1987;136:730–736.

59. Gattinoni L, Pesanti A, Torresin A, et al. Adult respiratory distress syndrome profiles by computer tomography. *J Thorac Imaging.* 1986;3:25–30.

60. Gentilello LM, Anardi D, Mock C, et al. Permissive hypercapnia in trauma patients. *J Trauma.* 1995;39: 846–853.

61. Gibney RTN, Wilson RS, Pontoppidan H. Comparison of work of breathing on high gas flow and demand valve continuous positive airway pressure systems. *Chest.* 1982;82:692–695.

62. Girault D, Bonmarchand G, Richard JC, et al. Physiologic assessment of ventilatory mode during noninvasive ventilation in acute hypercapnic respiratory failure (AHRF): assist-control ventilation (ACV) [abstract]. *Am J Respir Crit Care Med.* 1995;151: A426.

63. Girault C, Daudenthun I, Chevron V, et al. Noninvasive ventilation as a systematic extubation and weaning technique in acute or chronic respiratory failure: a prospective, randomized controlled study. *Am J Respir Crit Care Med.* 1999;160:86–92.

64. Girault C, Richard JC, Chevron V, et al. Comparative physiologic effects of noninvasive assist-control and pressure support ventilation in acute hypercapnic respiratory failure. *Chest.* 1997; 111:1639–1648.

65. Gregoretti C, Burbi L, Berardino M, et al. Noninvasive mask ventilation (NIMV) in trauma and major burn patients. *Am Rev Respir Dis.* 1992;145:A75.

66. Grossbach I. Troubleshooting ventilator- and patient-related problems, Part I. *Crit Care Nurse.* 1986;6: 58–70.

67. Gurevitch MJ, Gelmont D. Importance of trigger sensitivity to ventilator response delay in advanced chronic obstructive pulmonary disease with respiratory failure. *Crit Care Med.* 1989;17:354–359.

68. Gurevitch MJ, Van Dyke J, Yound ES, et al. Improved oxygenation and lower peak airway pressures in severe adult respiratory distress syndrome. Treatment with inverse-ratio ventilation. *Chest.* 1986;89:211–213.

69. Haake R, Schlichtig R, Ustad DR, Henschen RR. Barotrauma, pathophysiology, risk factors, and prevention. *Chest.* 1987;91:608–613.

70. Haberthur C, Elsasser S, Eberhard L. et al. Total versus tube-related additional work of breathing in ventilator-dependent patients. *Acta Anaesthesiologica Scandinavica.* 2000;44:749–757.

71. Henry WC, West GA, Wilson, RS. A comparison of the oxygen cost of breathing between a continuous-flow CPAP system and a demand-flow CPAP system. *Resp Care.* 1983;28:1273–1281.

72. Hess DR, Bigatello LM. Lung recruitment: the role of recruitment maneuvers. *Resp Care.* 2002;47:308–317.

73. Hickling K. Low volume ventilation with permissive hypercapnia in the adult respiratory distress syndrome. *Clin Intensive Care.* 1992;3:67–78.

74. Hilbert G, Gruson D, Vargas F, et al. Noninvasive ventilation in immunosuppressed patients with pulmonary infiltrates, fever, and acute respiratory failure. *N Engl J Med.* 2001; 344:481–487.

75. Hill N. Complications of noninvasive positive pressure ventilation *Respir Care.* 1997;42:432–442.

76. Hill N, Lin D, Levy M, et al. Noninvasive positive pressure ventilation (NPPV) to facilitate extubation after acute respiratory failure: a feasibility study [abstract]. *Am J Respir Crit Care Med.* 2000;161:A263

77. Holm BA, Notter RH, Siegle J, et al. Pulmonary physiological and surfactant changes during injury and recovery from hyperoxia. *J Appl Physiol.* 1985;59: 1402–1409.

78. Hudson LD, Hurlow RS, Craig KC, Pierson DJ. Does intermittent mandatory ventilation correct respiratory alkalosis in patients receiving assisted mechanical ventilation? *Am Rev Respir Dis.* 1985;132: 1071–1074.

79. Hurst JM, Branson RD, Davis K, Barnette RR. Cardiopulmonary effects of pressure support ventilation. *Arch Surg.* 1989;124:1067–1070.

80. International Consensus Conferences in Intensive Care Medicine. Noninvasive positive pressure ventilation in acute respiratory failure. *Am J Respir Crit Care Med.* 2001;163:283–291.

81. Jackson RM. Molecular, pharmacologic, and clinical aspects of oxygen-induced lung injury. *Clin Chest Med.* 1990;11:73–86.

82. Jardin F, Genevray B, Brun-Ney D, et al. Influence of lung and chest wall compliance on transmission of airway pressure to the pleural space in critically ill patients. *Chest.* 1985;88:653–665.

83. Jiang JS, Kao SJ, Wang SN. Effect of early application of biphasic positive airway pressure on the outcome of extubation in ventilator weaning. *Respirology.* 1999;4:161–165.

84. Jubran A. Monitoring patient mechanics during mechanical ventilation. *Crit Care Clinics.* 1998;14:629–653.

85. Kacmarek RM. The role of pressure support ventilation in reducing the work of breathing. *Respir Care.* 1988;33:99–120.

86. Kiiski R, Takala J, Kari A, Milic-Emili J. Effect of tidal volume on gas exchange and oxygen transport in the adult respiratory distress syndrome. *Am Rev Respir Dis.* 1992;146:1131–1135.

87. Keenan SP, Powers C, McCormack DG, et al. Noninvasive positive-pressure ventilation for postextubation respiratory distress *JAMA.* 2002;287:3282–3244.

88. Kolobow T, Moretti MP, Fumagalli R, et al. Severe impairment in lung function induced by high peak airway pressure during mechanical ventilation. An experimental study. *Am Rev Respir Dis.* 1987;135: 312–315.

89. Kramer NR, Meyer TJ, Meharg J, et al. Randomized, prospective trial of noninvasive positive pressure ventilation in acute respiratory failure. *Am J Respir Crit Care.* 1995;151:1799–1806.

90. Kwok H, McCormack J, Cece R, et al. Controlled trial of oronasal versus nasal mask ventilation in the treatment of acute respiratory failure. *Crit Care Med.* 2003;31:468–473.

91. Lachmann B. Open up the lung and keep the lung open. *Intensive Care Med.* 1992;18:319–321.

92. Lain DC, DiBenedetto R, Morris SL, et al. Pressure control inverse ratio ventilation as a method to reduce peak inspiratory pressure and provide adequate ventilation and oxygenation. *Chest.* 1989;95:1081–1087.

93. Leatherman JW, Lari RL, Iber C, Ney AL. Tidal volume reduction in ARDS: effect on cardiac output and arterial oxygenation. *Chest.* 1991;99:1227–1231.

94. LeBourdelles G, Viires N, Boczkowski J, et al. Effects of prolonged mechanical ventilation on contractile and biochemical properties of the diaphragm in rats: comparison with immobilization of peripheral skeletal muscle [abstract]. *Am Rev Respir Dis.* 1992;145:A148.

95. Liesching T, Kwok H, Hill NS. Acute applications of noninvasive positive pressure ventilation. *Chest.* 2003;124:699–713.

96. Lin M, Yang YF, Chiang HT, et al. Reappraisal of continuous positive airway pressure therapy in acute cardiogenic pulmonary edema: short-term results and long-term follow-up. *Chest.* 1995;107:1379–1386.

97. Lofaso F, Brochard L, et al. Home vs. intensive care pressure support devices. Experimental and clinical comparison. *Am J Respir Crit Care Med.* 1996;153:151–1599.

98. Luce JM, Pierson DJ, Hudson LD. Intermittent mandatory ventilation. *Chest.* 1981;79:678–685.

99. MacIntyre N, Nishimura M, Usada Y, Tokioka H, Takezawa J, Shimada Y. The Nagoya conference on system design and patient-ventilator interactions during pressure support ventilation. *Chest.* 1990;97:1463–1466.

100. Macintyre NR. Minimizing alveolar stretch injury during mechanical ventilation. *Respir Care.* 1996;41:318–326.

101. MacIntyre, NR. Pressure support ventilation: effects on ventilatory reflexes and ventilatory muscle work load. *Resp Care.* 1987;32:447–457.

102. MacIntyre NR. Respiratory function during pressure support ventilation. *Chest.* 1988;89:677–683.

103. MacIntyre NR, Ho LI. Effects of initial flow rate and breath termination criteria on pressure support ventilation. *Chest.* 1991;99:134–138.

104. MacIntyre NR, McConnell R, Cheng KG, Sane A. Patient-ventilator flow dysynchrony: flow-limited versus pressure-limited breaths. *Crit Care Med.* 1997;25:1671–1677.

105. Marini JJ, Capps JS, Culver BH. The inspiratory work of breathing during assisted mechanical ventilation. *Chest.* 1985;87:612–618.

106. Marini JJ, Evans RW. Round table conference: acute lung injury *Intensive Care Med.* 1998;234:878–883.

107. Marini JJ, Gattinoni L. Ventilatory management of acute respiratory distress syndrome: a consensus of two. *Crit Care Med.* 2004;32:250–255.

108. Marini JJ, Ravenscraft S. Mean airway pressure: physiologic determinants and clinical importance: Part II, clinical implications. *Crit Care Med.* 1992;20:1604–1616.

109. Marini JJ, Rodriguez RM, Lamb V. The inspiratory workload of patient-initiated mechanical ventilation. *Am Rev Respir Dis.* 1986;134:902–909.

110. Marini JJ, Smith TC, Lamb VJ. External work output and force generation during synchronized intermittent mechanical ventilation: effect of machine assistance on breath effort. *Am Rev Respir Dis.* 1988;138:1169–1179.

111. Marcy TW, Marini JJ. Inverse ratio ventilation in ARDS. Rationale and implementation. *Chest.* 1991;100:494–504.

112. Martin TJ, Hovis JD, Costantino JP, et al. A randomized, prospective evaluation of noninvasive ventilation for acute respiratory failure. *Am J Respir Crit Care Med.* 2000;161;807–813.

113. Mathru M, Rao TLK, El-Etr AA, Pifarre R. Hemodynamic response to changes in ventilatory patterns in patients with normal and poor left-ventricular reserve. *Crit Care Med.* 1982;10:423–426.

114. Mathru M, Rao TLK, Venus B. Ventilator-induced barotrauma in controlled mechanical ventilation versus intermittent mandatory ventilation. *Crit Care Med.* 1983;11:359–361.

115. Maunder RJ, Shuman WP, McHugh JW, et al. Preservation of normal lung regions in the adult respiratory distress syndrome. Analysis by computed tomography. *JAMA.* 1986;255:2463–2465.

116. Meduri GU. Noninvasive positive-pressure ventilation in patients with acute respiratory failure. *Clin Chest Med.* 1996;17:185–225.

117. Meduri GU, Fox RC, Abou-Shala N, et al. Noninvasive mechanical ventilation via face mask in patients with acute respiratory failure who refused endotracheal intubation. *Crit Care Med.* 1994;22:1584–1590.

118. Meduri GU, Turner RE, Abou-Shala N, et al. Noninvasive positive pressure ventilation via face mask: first line intervention in patients with acute hypercapnic and hypoxemic respiratory failure. *Chest.* 1996;109:179–193.

119. Mehta S, Hill NS. Noninvasive ventilation. *Am J Respir Crit Care Med.* 2001;163:540–577.

120. Meyer TJ, Hill NS. Noninvasive positive pressure ventilation to treat respiratory failure. *Ann Intern Med.* 1994;120: 760–770.

121. Morgan BC, Martin WE, Hornbein TF, et al. Hemodynamic effects of intermittent positive pressure respiration. *Anesthesiology.* 1966;27:584–590.

122. Muscedere JG, Mullen JB, Gan K, Slutsky AS. Tidal ventilation at low airway pressure can augment lung injury. *Am J Respir Crit Care Med.* 1994;149: 1327–1334.

123. Nava S, Ambrosino N, Clini E, et al. Noninvasive mechanical ventilation in the weaning of patients with respiration failure due to chronic obstructive pulmonary disease: a randomized, controlled trial. *Ann Intern Med.* 1998;128:721–728.

124. Navalesi P, Fanfulla F, Frigerio P, et al. Physiologic evaluation of noninvasive mechanical ventilation delivered with three types of masks in patients with chronic hypercapnic respiratory failure. *Crit Care Med.* 2000;28:1785–1790.

125. O'Quinn RJ, Marini JJ, Culver BH, Butler J. Transmission of airway pressure to pleural space during lung edema and chest wall restriction. *J Appl Physiol.* 1985;59:1171–1177.

126. Parker JC, Hernandez LA, Longnecker GL, Peevy K, Johnson W. Lung edema caused by high peak inspiratory pressures in dogs. Role of increased microvascular filtration pressure and permeability. *Am Rev Respir Dis.* 1990;142:321–328.

127. Parker, JC, Hernandez LA, Peevy KJ. Mechanisms of ventilator-induced lung injury. *Crit Care Med.* 1993;21:131–143.

128. Pauwels RA, Buist AS, Calverley, Jenkins CR, Hurd SS. Global strategy for the diagnosis, management, and prevention of chronic obstructive pulmonary disease. NHLBI/WHO Global Initiative for Chronic Obstructive Lung Disease (GOLD) Workshop summary. *Amer J Resp Crit Care Med.* 2001;163: 1256–1276.

129. Pelosi P, Cadringher P, Bottino N, et al. Sigh in acute respiratory distress syndrome. *Am J Resp Crit Care Med.* 1999;159:872–880.

130. Pepe PE, Marini JJ. Occult positive end-expiratory pressure in mechanically ventilated patients with airflow obstruction. *Am Rev Respir Dis.* 1982;126:166–173.

131. Pilbeam SP. Selecting initial parameters and settings. In: Pilbeam SP, ed. *Mechanical Ventilation: Physiological and Clinical Applications.* St Louis, Mo: Mosby; 1998:188–219.

132. Pierce JD, Gerald K. Differences in end-tidal carbon dioxide and breathing patterns in ventilator-dependent patients using pressure support ventilation. *Am J Crit Care.* 1994;3:276–281.

133. Pierce LNB. *Guide to Mechanical Ventilation and Intensive Respiratory Care.* Philadelphia, Pa: WB Saunders Co; 1995.

134. Prakash O, Meij S. Cardiopulmonary response to inspiratory pressure support during spontaneous ventilation versus conventional ventilation. *Chest.* 1985; 88:403–408.

135. Ranieri VM, Eissa NT, Corbeil C, et al. Effects of positive end-expiratory pressure on alveolar recruitment and gas exchange in patients with the adult respiratory distress syndrome. *Am Rev Respir Dis.* 1991;144: 544–551.

136. Rasanen J, Cane RD, Downs JB, et al. Airway pressure release ventilation during acute lung injury: a prospective multicenter trial. *Crit Care Med.* 1991;19:1234.

137. Richard JC, Maggiore S, Mercat A. Where are we with recruitment maneuvers in patients with acute lung injury and acute respiratory distress syndrome? *Curr Opin Crit Care.* 2003;9:22–27.

138. Sandhar BK, Niblett DJ, Argiras EP, Dunnill MS, Sykes MK. Effects of positive end-expiratory pressure on hyaline membrane formation in a rabbit model of the neonatal respiratory distress syndrome. *Intensive Care Med.* 1988;14:538–546.

139. Sassoon CSH, Giron AE, Ely EA, Light RW. Inspiratory work of breathing on flow-by and demand-flow continuous positive airway pressure. *Crit Care Med.* 1989;17:1108–1114.

140. Sassoon CSH, Lodia R, Rheeman CH, et al. Inspiratory muscle work of breathing during flow-by, demand-flow and continuous flow systems in patients with chronic obstructive pulmonary disease. *Am Rev Respir Dis.* 1992;145:1219–1222.

141. Schonhofer B, Sorto-Leger S. Equipment needs for noninvasive mechanical ventilation. *Eur Respir J.* 2002;20:1029–1036.

142. Shah DM, Newell JC, Dutton RE, et al. Continuous positive airway pressure versus positive end-expiratory pressure in respiratory distress syndrome. *J Thorac Cardiovasc Surg.* 1977;74:557–562.

143. Simon RJ, Mawilmada S, Ivatury RR. Hypercapnia: is there a cause for concern? *J Trauma.* 1994;37:74–81.

144. Sjostrand UH, Lichtwarck-Aschoff M, Nielson JB, et al. Different ventilatory approaches to keep the lung open. *Intensive Care Med.* 1995;21:310–318.

145. Slutsky AS. Consensus conference on mechanical ventilation—January 28–30, 1993 at Northbrook, Ill. Parts 1 and 2. *Intensive Care Med.* 1994;20:64–79, 150–162. See the published erratum. *Intensive Care Med.* 1994;20:378.

146. Smurthwaite GJ, Ford P. Skin necrosis following continuous positive airway pressure with a face mask. *Anaesthesia.* 1993;48:147–148.

147. Specht NL, Yang SC, Killeen TJ, et al. Pressure support ventilation fails to provide adequate support as a primary ventilatory mode [abstract]. *Am Rev Respir Dis.* 1989;139:A362.

148. Sydow M, Burchardi H, Ephraim, et al. Long-term effects of two different ventilatory modes on oxygenation in acute lung injury: comparison of airway pressure release ventilation and volume-controlled inverse ratio ventilation. *Amer J Respir Crit Care Med.* 1994; 149:1550–1556.

149. Tasker RC, Peters MJ. Combined lung injury, meningitis and cerebral edema: how permissive can hypercapnia be? *Intensive Care Med.* 1998;24:616–619.

150. Tharratt RS, Allen RP, Albertson TE. Pressure controlled inverse ratio ventilation in severe adult respiratory failure. *Chest.* 1988;94:755–762.

151. Thorens JB, Jolliet P, Ritz M, et al. Effects of rapid permissive hypercapnia on hemodynamics, gas exchange, and oxygen transport and consumption during mechanical ventilation for the acute respiratory distress syndrome. *Intensive Care Med.* 1996;22: 182–191.

152. Tokioka H, Saito S, Kosaka F. Effect of pressure support ventilation on breathing pattern and respiratory work. *Intensive Care Med.* 1989;15:491–494.

153. Tsuno K, Prato P, Kolobow T. Acute lung injury from mechanical ventilation at moderately high airway pressures. *J Appl Physiol.* 1990;69:956–961.

154. Tuxen DV. Permissive hypercapnic ventilation. *Am J Respir Crit Care Med.* 1994;150:870–874.

155. Van de Graaff WB, Gordey K, Dornseif SE, et al. Pressure support: changes in ventilatory pattern and components of the WOB. *Chest.* 1991:100:1082–1089.

156. Venus B, Jacobs HK, Mathru M. Hemodynamic responses to different modes of mechanical ventilation in dogs with normal and acid-aspirated lungs. *Crit Care Med.* 1980;8:620–627.

157. Viale JP, Annat G, Bertrand O, et al. Additional inspiratory work in intubated patients breathing with continuous positive airway pressure systems. *Anesthesiology.* 1985;63:536–539.

158. Viale JP, Annat GJ, Bouffard, et al. Oxygen cost of breathing in postoperative patients: Pressure support ventilation versus continuous positive airway pressure. *Chest.* 1988;93:506–509.

159. Vitacca M, Rubini F, Foglio K, et al. Noninvasive modalities of positive pressure ventilation improve the outcome of acute exacerbations in COLD patients. *Intensive Care Med.* 1993;19:450–455.

160. Ward ME, Corbeil C, Gibbons W, Newman S, Macklem PT. Optimization of respiratory muscle relaxation during mechanical ventilation. *Anesthesiology.* 1988; 69:29–35.

161. Webb HH, Tierney DF. Experimental pulmonary edema due to intermittent positive pressure ventilation with high inflation pressures: protection by positive end-expiratory pressure. *Am Rev Respir Dis.* 1974;110: 556–565.

162. West JB, Tsukimoto K, Mathieu-Costello O, et al. Stress failure in pulmonary capillaries. *J Appl Physiol.* 1991;70:1731–1742.

163. Williams TJ, Tuxen DV, Scheinkestal CD, et al. Risk factors for morbidity in mechanically ventilated patients with acute severe asthma. *Am Rev Respir Dis.* 1992;146;607–615.

164. Wysocki M, Tric L, Wolff MA, et al. Noninvasive pressure support ventilation in patients with acute respiratory failure. A randomized comparison with conventional therapy. *Chest.* 1995;107:761–768.

165. Zeravik J, Borg U, Pfeiffer UJ. Efficacy of pressure support ventilation dependent on extravascular lung water. *Chest.* 1990;97:1412–1419.

166. Zhan WZ, Sieck GC. Adaptations of diaphragm and medial gastrocnemius muscles to inactivity. *J Appl Physiology.* 1992;72:1445–1453.

Weaning from Mechanical Ventilation

Suzanne M. Burns, RN, MSN, RRT, ACNP, CCRN, FAAN, FCCM, FAANP

Weaning from Mechanical Ventilation

CASE STUDY 1: SHORT-TERM MECHANICAL VENTILATION

Mrs M, a 51-year-old schoolteacher and mother of 3, was diagnosed with unstable angina after an anterior myocardial infarct. She was admitted to the cardiovascular recovery room at 11:25 AM after an aortocoronary bypass. Mrs M's blood pressure varied from 170/84 mm Hg on admission to 100/60 mm Hg 2 hours later. Her heart rate was 90 to 112 beats per minute; the electrocardiographic pattern was a normal sinus rhythm with a bundle branch block. Central venous pressure was 16 mm Hg on admission but 7 mm Hg at 2:00 PM. She received dobutamine at 5 µg/kg per minute IV infusion. Hemoglobin was 10.9 g/100 mL on admission. Mrs M's temperature was 33.9°C, so she was placed on a warming blanket. Pulse oximetry saturation was 100% on the following ventilator settings: fraction of inspired oxygen (FIO_2), 0.60; tidal volume (V_T), 600 mL; synchronized intermittent mandatory ventilation (SIMV) rate, 8/min; and pressure support, 10 cm H_2O. Her arterial blood gases (ABGs) were pH, 7.37; partial pressure of carbon dioxide (arterial) ($PaCO_2$), 38 mm Hg; partial pressure of oxygen (PaO_2), 266 mm Hg; HCO_3^-, 21 mEq/L; and base excess, –3.5.

Mrs M was given a 500-mL bolus of lactated Ringer's and 5% dextrose, after which she awoke and indicated that she was having chest pain at the sternal incision site. She was given 2 mg of morphine sulfate intravenously. Her vital signs remained stable; her temperature rose to 36.9°C, and the warming blanket was removed. At 3:00 PM the SIMV rate was reduced to 4 breaths per minute, and Mrs M supplemented SIMV with the pressure support ventilation (PSV) spontaneous breaths for a total respiratory rate of 15 breaths per minute. Although Mrs M indicated that she wanted the endotracheal tube to be removed, she was lethargic, weak,

and barely able to lift her head off the pillow. She moved her toes and ankles on command, but not her legs; her hand grasps were weak.

Over the course of the next 4 hours Mrs M required 2 more bolus fluid challenges, for a total of 1 L, and acetaminophen and cooling blanket for a temperature of 39.2°C. At 7:30 PM, she had stronger head lifts and peripheral movements. She was placed on continuous positive airway pressure (CPAP) 5 cm H_2O, with 10 cm H_2O of pressure support, and had spontaneous respiratory rates of 15 to 16 breaths per minute and ABGs as follows: pH, 7.44; $PaCO_2$, 35 mm Hg; PaO_2, 283 mm Hg; SaO_2, 99.7%; HCO_3^-, 23 mEq/L; and base excess, –0.3. After 45 minutes on CPAP Mrs M was able to sustain a head lift for more than 10 seconds, and her negative inspiratory pressure (NIP) was –40 cm H_2O. She was extubated at 8:15 PM and put on 50% oxygen via face mask. Blood gases postextubation were unchanged with the exception of PaO_2, which dropped to 153 mm Hg. The following morning Mrs M was resting comfortably. Her hemoglobin was 11.6 g/100 mL. Her chest roentgenogram showed hilar infiltrates, consistent with fluid overload, and her weight had increased 4 kg from the previous day. Central venous pressure was 14 mm Hg with diuresis in progress.

DISCUSSION OF CASE STUDY 1

Mrs M's case is consistent with the linear progress toward ventilator liberation seen in patients who require short-term mechanical ventilation (< 3 days). When Mrs M's condition was stabilized, ventilator settings were rapidly reduced to allow for increased patient-initiated breathing. In this case clinical *and* laboratory data were used to assess Mrs M's tolerance of decreased ventilatory support. When she was fully awake and no longer demonstrating weakness secondary to anesthesia, a spontaneous breathing trial (SBT) on CPAP was initiated, and she was successfully extubated. Although continued diuresis was necessary to remove excess fluid provided during the resuscitative stage, Mrs M did well and experienced no further respiratory compromise.

CASE STUDY 2: LONG-TERM MECHANICAL VENTILATION

Mr C, a 60-year-old man, was transferred to the medical ICU (MICU) for failure to wean 10 days after coronary artery bypass graft (CABG). Significant past medical history included insulin-dependent diabetes mellitus and chronic obstructive pulmonary disease. Mr C had experienced 3 unsuccessful extubation attempts, the last resulting in a respiratory arrest. In addition, Mr C sustained a pneumothorax following attempts to insert a central line during resuscitation efforts.

Mr C was transferred to the MICU on the following settings: SIMV rate, 10; VT, 600 mL/kg; PSV, 5 cm H_2O; FIO_2, 0.5; and positive end-expiratory pressure (PEEP), 5 cm H_2O. Mr C's total respiratory rate was 30 breaths per minute, and peak airway pressure was 40 cm H_2O (auto-PEEP was 8 cm H_2O). The MICU interdisciplinary team completed a full weaning assessment, which yielded the following results: Burns Wean Assessment Program (BWAP), 34% (threshold $\geq 50\%$); rapid/shallow breathing index (f/VT), 170 (threshold < 105); NIP, –35 cm H_2O (threshold $\leq$ –20 cm H_2O) (see Appendixes 3A, 3B, 3C). Major impediments to weaning were poor nutritional state (albumin 1.8 and unable to tolerate enteral feeding), poor glucose control (despite sliding scale, glucose was frequently > 200 mg/dL), generalized weakness, immobility, poor endurance, discomfort, dyspnea, anxiety, lack of sleep, and resolving pneumothorax (chest tube in place and to water seal).

The MICU employed an outcomes-management approach to the care of all long-term mechanically ventilated patients. The approach consisted of an interdisciplinary evidence-based clinical pathway; protocols for weaning trials, sedation management and glucose control; and an advanced practice nurse called an outcomes manager (OM) to manage and monitor the process. The following plan was coordinated by the MICU OM:

1. *Change ventilator settings to enhance patient ventilator synchrony, rest the respiratory muscles and eliminate auto-PEEP.* The ventilator mode was changed to PSV. Initial settings were selected to assure respiratory muscle rest. To do so the PSV level was gradually increased to a level of 15 cm H_2O while the respiratory rate and VT were observed. At 15 cm H_2O of PSV, auto-PEEP was eliminated, and the patient's breathing pattern appeared comfortable (no accessory muscle use and a spontaneous respiratory rate of 16 breaths per minute). This level, called PSV max, was the level selected to rest the respiratory muscles. Respiratory muscle rest was to be assured for the first 24 hours, between weaning trials and at night.

2. *Initiate weaning trials as soon as "wean screen" criteria are met.* Wean screen criteria included hemodynamic stability, FIO_2 requirements below 50%, and a BWAP score of $\geq 50\%$. The wean screen was assessed daily until the criteria were met. At that point, weaning trials were initiated using a protocol for CPAP.

3. *Ensure aggressive nutritional repletion.* A duodenal feeding tube was placed and enteral feedings were prescribed by a registered nutritionist. The tube feedings were increased to full rate within 24 hours. Concomitantly an insulin continuous infusion was initiated to assure tight glucose control (glucose ≤ 110 mg/dL).

4. *Control pain and reduce anxiety.* The patient was experiencing significant pain from the chest tube and was also anxious about his condition and the many untoward events that had affected his recovery. Patient-controlled analgesia with fentanyl and anxiolysis with an oral intermediate-duration benzodiazepine were initiated.

5. *Recondition and enhance physical mobility.* Progressive physical therapy, starting with sitting at the bedside and progressing to standing and ambulation twice daily was prescribed by physical therapy and initiated on day 2.

6. *Consider tracheostomy.* The team recognized that because Mr C had already sustained 10 days of mechanical ventilation via an endotracheal tube, a tracheostomy might be necessary to enhance eating, clinical conditioning, comfort, and communication. They agreed that if rapid progress did not ensue over the next few days a percutaneous tracheostomy would be scheduled.

Mr C agreed to the weaning plan and made rapid progress. Three days after transfer to the MICU Mr C met wean screen criteria, and the team agreed that he was ready to progress to active weaning trials. His chest tube was removed on MICU day 3, he rarely used his PCA any longer, and his breathing was much more comfortable. Although nutrition was still not optimal it was improving (ie, tube feeds well absorbed and glucose well controlled at 100 mg/dL). He was also walking twice daily with the help of nurses and respiratory and physical therapists, and because he was more comfortable he was sleeping well.

The team initiated the CPAP weaning protocol, which required that Mr C be placed on 5 cm H_2O CPAP for 1 hour followed by a second hour on 0 CPAP (CPAP turned off). The 2-hour trial was to be stopped and Mr C returned to PSV max settings if he developed any signs of intolerance. Mr C was also to be returned to his PSV max settings at night. Extubation would be considered if no signs of intolerance were noted for the full duration of the weaning trial.

The CPAP trials proceeded smoothly. Mr C was extubated on MICU day 4 and did not require reintubation. He was transferred to a medical floor on 2 L oxygen via nasal prongs the following morning, and he was discharged on hospital day 17.

DISCUSSION OF CASE STUDY 2

This case exemplifies the complexity of designing a weaning plan for a patient who requires prolonged mechanical ventilation. These patients are often debilitated, uncomfortable, and suffering from multiple physical impediments that make liberation from mechanical ventilation difficult. The term *chronically critically ill* (Other References: 38) is appropriate to describe patients like Mr C who, despite resolution of the underlying reason for mechanical ventilation (ie, CABG), have not returned to baseline status and have other comorbidities and conditions complicating clinical progress.

The MICU interdisciplinary weaning assessment used a number of assessment tools: the BWAP for comprehensive assessment of a wide variety of general and pulmonary factors that contribute to weaning potential (Appendix 3A), NIP and the f/VT (Appendixes 3B and 3C) to evaluate pulmonary-specific components. For example, the BWAP of 34% indicated that of the 26 BWAP factors that affect weaning potential, 18 were assessed as suboptimal (Annotated Bibliography: 2). Multiple factors such as nutrition, mobility, and comfort needed to be corrected before aggressive weaning attempts were initiated. The elevated f/VT (Annotated Bibliography: 11) was consistent with poor respiratory muscle endurance and potential ventilatory muscle fatigue. These assessment tools helped the team identify that weaning trials were unlikely to be successful and could potentially fatigue and frustrate Mr C. They therefore developed the collaborative weaning plan as described above that focused on correcting the factors underlying his debilitated state. They also selected a mode of ventilation to offset fatigue and support Mr C during aggressive rehabilitation and conditioning.

The need for a tracheostomy was considered; however, the team decided to briefly delay the procedure while they worked on improving Mr C's condition. A recent study suggests that early tracheostomy (on day 2 of mechanical ventilation) in patients likely to experience long-term ventilation results in improved outcomes (Other References: 128). Mr C's MICU team recognized that there were many readily reversible factors affecting Mr C's progress and chose to aggressively manage them prior to placing a tracheostomy. Had rapid progress not ensued, a percutaneous tracheostomy would have been scheduled immediately and performed at the bedside by the pulmonary consult team.

The importance of an interdisciplinary, systematic, and comprehensive approach to weaning, as referred to above, cannot be overemphasized. In the past, disciplines often worked separately to attain discipline-specific goals for patients. Unfortunately this *silo* approach is not collaborative; it is inefficient and it does not serve the best interests of patients and families. Communication and collaboration are essential in order that interventions are both appropriate and timely.

Although standard traditional weaning criteria such as NIP have been used for years to determine weaning potential, the criteria have not proven to be strong positive predictors (ie, a good number does not predict weaning success) for patients requiring prolonged ventilation. In Mr C's case the NIP was −35 cm H_2O, a value used successfully in the thoracic cardiovascular ICU to determine timing of extubation in postoperative CABG patients. Unfortunately for Mr C, numerous other factors were responsible for his inability to sustain spontaneous breathing. The MICU team measured NIP to evaluate respiratory muscle strength, not extubation potential. NIP is also a component of the BWAP calculation. By considering NIP from this broader perspective, the team recognized that strength (defined by the traditional threshold of −20 cm H_2O) could not adequately compensate for lack of endurance and poor pulmonary reserve.

The plan was coordinated by the OM who assured daily systematic assessment of Mr C's status. By monitoring the BWAP score and completing a daily wean screen in collaboration with the respiratory therapist, the OM was able to identify rapid improvement in the multiple factors contributing to Mr C's need for prolonged ventilation. The team was notified as soon as Mr C met weaning screen criteria. At that time, Mr C was assigned to the CPAP weaning protocol and trials were initiated.

Weaning potential results from the complex interaction of a wide variety of factors; no single factor has been identified as contributing most to success. Given Mr C's rapid progress, the team selected an aggressive spontaneous breathing weaning protocol using CPAP. The protocol was implemented, progress was tracked by the OM, and the team agreed to extubate Mr C following successful completion of the trials as defined by the protocol.

The effectiveness of well-designed protocols for weaning has been described in the literature (Annotated Bibliography: 1, 4–7). Use of the protocols decreases practice variation, assures aggressive testing of readiness, and is associated with improved outcomes such as duration of ventilation and length of stay. The protocols include a weaning screen (a set of minimally restrictive criteria that indicate stability and potential readiness for a trial), the method and duration (generally CPAP or T-piece for between 30 minutes to 2 hours), and criteria for stopping. In addition, systematic methods to monitor progress and assure timely care provision, such as the OM approach used with Mr C, are also linked to improved outcomes (Annotated Bibliography: 3). The components of protocols and interdisciplinary system initiatives are described in detail later in this protocol.

GENERAL DESCRIPTION

Weaning is the process of liberating a patient from mechanical ventilation. Though extubation is a desired goal of weaning, patients may be weaned (ie, able to sustain spontaneous breathing indefinitely) and still require an artificial airway for airway protection. Most patients who are placed on mechanical ventilation require support for the short term, defined as ≤ 3 days by the AACN 3rd National Study Group on Weaning from Mechanical Ventilation (Other References: 21, 68, 87, 88). Of those patients who are expected to require short-term mechanical ventilation, 1 in 5 have difficulty weaning; these patients fall into the category of weaning from long-term (ie, ≥ 3 days) mechanical ventilation.

Weaning may be viewed as a continuum with multiple stages. The stages include the prewean, wean, and outcome stages. Some authors also describe a fourth acute stage, which occurs as a subset of the prewean stage. This stage is included in the description below and in the protocol. (Other References: 23). There are differences in duration and characteristics of the stages between short-term and long-term mechanical ventilation patients.

Description of the Weaning Stages

The *acute stage* is that time, generally during the first 24 to 72 hours, when the patient is initially placed on a ventilator and is not stable. The main focus of interventions is the restoration of stability and reversal of the condition that necessitated mechanical ventilation. During this stage full ventilatory support and hemodynamic support are often necessary. The goals of mechanical ventilation during this stage are to protect the lung from volutrauma (see Chapter 2, Invasive and Noninvasive Modes and Methods of Mechanical Ventilation), to ensure noninjurious oxygenation, and to provide adequate ventilation and acid-base status.

The *prewean stage* is that time when the patient is stable, yet may still require numerous care interventions to restore baseline status. Ventilatory settings are selected to enhance patient interaction on modes such as PSV and lower levels of oxygen and PEEP. Weaning ability is assessed regularly, and trials may be initiated as both a means of testing readiness and to condition respiratory muscles. Again, early testing with the use of a wean screen (as described earlier) is essential to assure that patients are liberated from the ventilator as early as possible.

The *weaning stage* is generally short with rapid progress toward ventilator liberation occurring over consecutive days. Spontaneous breathing modes such as CPAP and PSV are commonly used for trials with the goal being a predetermined (generally 1–2 hours) trial without evidence of intolerance. When the patient completes the trial successfully, extubation follows. In some cases, such as when the patient has required a tracheostomy, more prolonged trials of spontaneous breathing (24–48 hours) are attempted. In addition, a variety of techniques are employed to enhance weaning the patient with a tracheostomy and include short periods of capping the tracheostomy tube, using speaking valves, and tube downsizing (see Chapter 1, Airway Management). Complete weaning, generally defined as breathing spontaneously for 24 consecutive hours, is one outcome of the weaning process but other outcomes are possible.

The *outcome stage* is the last stage of the weaning process and consists of any of the following scenarios: complete weaning with removal of the artificial airway; complete weaning with an artificial airway still necessary; incomplete weaning with partial ventilatory support required; full ventilatory support required; or death. As noted previously, weaning most commonly results in complete withdrawal of ventilatory support *and* the removal of the artificial airway. Unfortunately, some patients may require an artificial airway indefinitely for airway protection.

Studies testing the stages of weaning as described have suggested they are accurate (Other References: 23, 37). In addition, they are practical and helpful for organizing approaches to weaning. To this end they are used in this protocol.

The Weaning Process: Short- and Long-Term Mechanical Ventilation Trajectory

The weaning process with short-term mechanical ventilation is linear and clear definition of stages may not be possible. For example, a patient may have surgery and require anesthesia, but when awake the weaning trajectory is rapid, lasting only hours. The expected weaning outcome is 100% spontaneous breathing, usually followed by extubation. Readiness to wean after short-term mechanical ventilation is determined by level of consciousness, hemodynamic stability, general physiologic stability, adequacy of gas exchange, spontaneous ventilation capability, and pulmonary mechanics. Progression with the weaning process is monitored with pulse oximetry, ABG analysis , and pulmonary mechanics in addition to continued monitoring of level of consciousness, hemodynamics, general status, and spontaneous ventilation. Weaning outcome is time dependent and is determined by the degree to which the patient is able to sustain spontaneous ventilation.

In contrast, with long-term mechanical ventilation (≥ 3 days) progress is slower and is generally nonlinear. Peaks and valleys that represent progress, plateaus, and sometimes declines are common. Research supports the definition of long-term mechanical ventilation and further suggests that the risk of very prolonged stays on the ventilator (≥ 2 weeks) increases each day after 3 days of consecutive mechanical ventilation.

The long-term ventilated patient may regress from a stable stage such as the wean stage to the acute stage with a clinical condition that results in instability. Such patients frequently suffer from a wide variety of iatrogenic complications (eg, pneumothorax, ventilator-associated pneumonia, urinary tract infection, deep vein thrombosis, and pulmonary embolus) that prolong ventilator duration, ICU and hospital length of stay, and increased mortality. Care planning is complex and focuses on improving the myriad factors that impede weaning ability. In addition, extensive physical rehabilitation is often necessary. Patients, families, and healthcare workers often become frustrated and dissatisfied with the slow and unpredictable course.

Because the process of weaning from long-term mechanical ventilation is both time- and labor-intensive and unsuccessful weaning trials can be harmful to the patient and frustrating for all involved, investigators have attempted to delineate criteria that predict weaning ability. Unfortunately, no indices, predictors, or criteria exist that are superior, but weaning indices do provide important information about the factors that contribute to weaning potential. A comprehensive, interdisciplinary approach, which includes a systematic plan that decreases variability in care provision, weaning assessment, and weaning trials, is the goal.

Weaning Methods

Weaning modes and methods vary and questions on how best to wean abound. Advocates of specific ventilator modes vigorously promote their preferences despite mounting evidence that the use of spontaneous breathing protocols using CPAP or T-piece may be superior (Annotated Bibliography: 8). Unfortunately only 1 comparison trial suggests that the use of PSV is equally effective (Other References: 55). It may be that other modes such as PSV should be reserved for those who do not proceed well with CPAP trials or are poor candidates for the use of CPAP. Regardless of the mode, protocols should include distinct criteria for initiating trials (wean screen) and criteria for stopping the trials. Also, a balance between respiratory muscle rest and respiratory muscle conditioning may be important, especially for patients ventilated long term. Weaning trial protocols are covered in the protocol, and examples may be found in Appendix 3D.

Alternative therapies such as hypnosis, biofeedback, and relaxation techniques have also been proposed as methods to improve weaning outcomes, but there has been little research in this area (Other References: 1, 2, 10, 14, 15, 75, 94). Advocates believe these therapies may provide physiologic or psychologic support in difficult cases. The techniques appear to add little risk, but they are time consuming and require specialized clinical skills, so widespread application is unlikely until clear outcomes associated with their use are scientifically demonstrated. Although selected techniques are touched on briefly in the protocol, they are not emphasized. The interested reader is encouraged to access related references and other resources on the topic.

Finally, system approaches to weaning patients from prolonged ventilation have emerged that focus on decreasing variability in care and maintaining quality while reducing costs. Special care units, weaning teams, outcomes management approaches, and the use of critical pathways have been suggested, and some have demonstrated extraordinary results (Annotated Bibliography: 3, 10). It appears that these interdisciplinary approaches result in positive clinical and economic outcomes and are to be encouraged. They are discussed further in the protocol.

Implementation

Despite the importance of the systematic approaches discussed above, few resources exist to help clinicians with implementation of the protocols, assessment tools, and other evidence-based interventions. Protocols and care plans do not progress on their own, and it is essential that the process be deliberately defined and monitored over time. As described by Ely et al and Burns et al (Other References: 53; Annotated Bibliography: 3), this complex, vulnerable patient population requires rigorous planning and follow-up.

ACCURACY

As already noted, no specific weaning predictor has emerged as superior. However, methods to identify weaning readiness (ie, wean screens and assessment tools), and weaning protocols are essential for both short-term and long-term ventilated patients if outcomes are to be positive. Accuracy then is dependent on the education and training of the clinicians involved in the process. Competency of the clinician is directly linked to the accuracy of the assessments and the use of the protocols (discussed below).

COMPETENCY

Competencies related to weaning patients from short-term or long-term mechanical ventilation are best organized under the categories of assessment (weaning screen criteria, indices) and planning (application of protocols, modes, and methods). For example, the use of weaning indices requires that the person measuring the index perform the measurement correctly. Unfortunately, studies indicate that poor reproducibility of standard weaning criteria make reliance on the measurements questionable. Recommendations are discussed in specific sections of the protocol.

Perhaps most important is the nurse's ability to assess the patient's tolerance of mechanical ventilation and subsequently, weaning. To do so, it is essential that an in-depth understanding of mechanical ventilation exists. Although respiratory care practitioners are available in most units that manage ventilated patients, they are at the bedside of the patient intermittently and cannot be solely responsible for the respiratory care of the ventilated patient. Given the fact that mechanical ventilation is ubiquitous to critical care it is essential that nurses not only understand the therapy but be able to respond accurately and quickly when necessary.

Clinicians can become familiar with the various modes used for weaning by reviewing the concepts underlying each mode (see Chapter 2, Invasive and Noninvasive Modes and Methods of Mechanical Ventilation). Technical competence may be achieved by practice and demonstration–return demonstration under the tutelage of an expert. Periodic, frequent monitoring of peak inspiratory pressure, plateau pressure, respiratory rate, tidal volume, and minute ventilation using the ventilator gauges or displays is mandatory. Therefore, clinicians must be familiar with how to obtain these data from the specific ventilator model in use.

For patients being weaned with spontaneous breathing modes or methods (ie, T-piece, CPAP, or PSV), measurement of respiratory rate and tidal volume is a required competency. Practice and demonstration–return demonstration are appropriate to validate competency. Whatever the weaning mode used, competency with assessment of vital signs, respiratory pattern, breath sounds, hemodynamics, mentation, airway patency, and gas exchange is required. Clinicians can become familiar with measurement of standard weaning criteria (pulmonary mechanics) by reviewing the concepts (see Appendix 3B) and by demonstration–return demonstration. In many institutions, these measurements are done by respiratory therapists. Regardless, the nurse must understand the tests and the meaning of the results.

ETHICAL CONSIDERATIONS

Concerns related to the prolonged ventilation of the elderly and those with terminal illnesses focus on the futility of using such a high-cost form of life support as well as on discomfort and inherent loss of dignity. Mortality rates of 30% to 40% are associated with prolonged ventilation. Additionally, 1-year survival rates in patients who require weaning from long-term ventilation are reportedly lower than 50% (Other References: 44), making many question the practice, especially in select populations such as the elderly.

Although these concerns are reasonable and important to consider with respect to each patient, the US healthcare system does not restrict or ration healthcare of this type. Also, it is the experience of many institutions that few patients committed to mechanical ventilation have written living wills or documents assuring a durable power of attorney for healthcare to help guide decision making. It is important to keep the patient and family accurately informed and to discuss health care options fully in order to avoid overly burdensome treatments in terminal cases. It may also be that teams of health care professionals who are specially trained in humane, end-of-life decision making and care should be used to help the critical care teams. Campbell and Frank (Other References: 24) report on a hands-on approach to the care of dying patients by a palliative care team that offers patients, families, and clinicians the support needed for satisfactory end-of-life care while realizing substantial cost savings.

The use of survival prediction models with critically ill ventilated patients is increasingly an area of ethical concern. Although it is likely that survival prediction will increase with the use of the Acute Physiology and Chronic Health Evaluation (APACHE) system (APACHE Medical Systems: Cerner Corporation, Kansas City, Mo), it is doubtful that such predictions will dominate decisions related to care options. Instead, as in the use of weaning predictors, they should be used as one, but not the only, source of information.

OCCUPATIONAL HAZARDS

Occupational hazards are the same as those associated with day-to-day care of any intubated or mechanically ventilated patient, particularly exposure to pathogens, blood, and improperly grounded electrical equipment.

Exposure risk from pathogens and blood are substantially decreased with the appropriate use of universal blood, body, and respiratory precautions; ventilator filters; and in-line suctioning catheters.

Although electrical equipment used in hospitals is routinely tested for safety purposes, equipment from outside the hospital (especially with patients ventilated at home) should never be used until checked by the electrical engineering department of the hospital. An emergency electrical backup must be assured. Generally, electrical outlets that are supplied with emergency electrical backup in the case of a sudden failure are clearly marked as such.

FUTURE RESEARCH

Studies in patients ventilated *short-term* should continue to determine the optimal timing for extubation (ie, "fast track"). Much of this may relate to drugs used for anesthesia and amnesia and the rapidity with which they are eliminated. Additionally, studies that explore methods of assessing weaning readiness and which predictors are best in this population would be very helpful.

Weaning patients from *long-term* mechanical ventilation is costly and involves much time and effort. Identification of factors responsible for delayed ventilator liberation and how best to correct them would be useful and assure improved clinical outcomes. Unfortunately, definitive answers continue to elude investigators.

Research focusing on weaning predictors that can accurately forecast outcomes are needed so that clinicians can determine when to proceed and when to stop, thereby preventing fatigue and unsuccessful trials. There is evidence that commonly used weaning criteria that have been tested at extubation do not change reliably over time (Annotated Bibliography: 2, 4). Therefore, it will be important to test weaning predictors over the course of the weaning continuum so that clinicians can use them appropriately.

Studies comparing the ventilator duration associated with the different modes appear contradictory (Annotated Bibliography: 1, 6). It is important that studies to compare weaning modes develop entry criteria that include stages of weaning and adequately address the definition and application of respiratory muscle work and rest. To date, the protocols used in such studies have attempted to balance distinct weaning trial intervals with resting levels of ventilatory support. Unfortunately, the work of breathing associated with the trials and the resting modes has not been identified, making comparisons difficult.

The use of protocols for SBTs decrease variation and are to be encouraged (Annotated Bibliography: 5, 7). However, to be effective the components of the protocols must be clear to all who use them. The components include a wean screen, the protocol (mode and method), criteria for stopping a trial (signs of intolerance), and how to rest the patient. To date most of the SBTs have used CPAP or T-piece as the method, and they appear to result in better outcomes. However research on each of the components of the protocols and different modes will help determine the best combinations for weaning.

The assessment of weaning trial tolerance consists of subjective and objective data. Objective data (eg, increased heart rate, respiratory rate, lung sounds, breathing pattern) have a physiologic basis and are linked to tolerance or intolerance. Unfortunately, subjective symptoms such as dyspnea, discomfort, or anxiety are less well understood. They are assumed to affect weaning trials negatively, and interventions are often aimed at improving them. Studies are needed to test the validity of these assumptions so that the efficacy of interventions designed to control symptoms can be explored.

Studies in the area of adjunctive and alternative therapies will be difficult. However, given the widespread use of weaning protocols that identify entry criteria (wean screen criteria) and distinct SBT duration, studies comparing the efficacy of alternative therapies during trials may be more readily accomplished than in the past.

Lastly, care delivery systems that focus on systematic, comprehensive, and collaborative care for the patient requiring prolonged ventilation are likely to continue to be a major focus of future work in the area. These initiatives combine numerous elements of evidence-based care in order to assure consistency in care provision. It will be difficult to determine which of the elements of the initiatives (protocols, pathways, prophylaxis standards, etc) are responsible for the resultant clinical and economic outcomes. Because of their popularity and success to date, it is unlikely that randomized controlled trials will be accomplished. However, the initiatives will need to continue to demonstrate patient, staff, and economic outcomes if they are to continue.

SUGGESTED READINGS/RESOURCES

Evidence-Based Recommendations on Weaning

Cook D, Meade M, Guyatt G, Griffith L, Booker L. *Evidence Report on Criteria for Weaning from Mechanical Ventilation.* Rockville, Md: Agency for Health Care Policy and Research; 1999. Contract No. 290–97–0017. *(This article appears in the Annotated Bibliography.)*

MacIntyre NR, Cook DJ, Ely EW Jr, et al. Evidence-based guidelines for weaning and discontinuing ventilatory support: a collective task force facilitated by the American College of Chest Physicians; the American Association for Respiratory Care; and the American College of Critical Care Medicine. *Chest.* 2001;120(Suppl 6):375S-395S. *(This article appears in the Annotated Bibliography.)*

Ely EW, Meade MO, Haponik EF, et al. Mechanical ventilator weaning protocols driven by nonphysician healthcare professionals: evidence-based clinical practice guidelines. *Chest.* 2001;120:454S–463S.

Dellinger RP, Carlet JM, Masur H, et al. Surviving Sepsis Campaign guidelines for management of severe sepsis and septic shock. *Crit Care Med.* 2004;32:858–873.

Textbooks That Discuss Weaning and Weaning Techniques

Hess DR, Kacmarek RM. *Essentials of Mechanical Ventilation.* New York, NY: McGraw Hill; 2003.

Lynn-McHale Wiegand DJ, Carlson KK. *AACN Procedure Manual for Critical Care.* 5th ed. Philadelphia, Pa: Elsevier Saunders; 2005. (See specifically the chapters on mechanical ventilation and weaning.)

Tobin MJ. *Principles and Practice of Mechanical Ventilation.* New York, NY: McGraw Hill Inc; 1994.

Pierce LNB. *Guide to Mechanical Ventilation and Intensive Respiratory Care.* 2nd ed. Philadelphia, Pa: Elsevier Saunders. In press.

Internet Resources

Critical care tutorials: www.ccmtutorials.com/rs/mv

Vent World: www.ventworld.com

CLINICAL RECOMMENDATIONS

The rating scales for the Level of Recommendation range from I to IV, with levels indicated as follows: I, manufactuer's recommendations only; II, theory based, no research data to support recommendations; recommendations from expert consensus group may exist; III, laboratory data only, no clinical data to support recommendations; IV, limited clinical studies to support recommendations; V, clinical studies in more than 1 or 2 different populations and situations to support recommendations; VI, clinical studies in a variety of patient populations and situations to support recommendations.

Period of Use	Recommendation	Rationale for Recommendation	Level of Recommendation	Supporting References	Comments
Selection of patients: short- and long-term mechanical ventilation (MV)	Patients who require MV for ≤ 3 days generally have conditions that rapidly improve. For example, many patients are intubated for surgery and when fully awake from general anesthesia are quickly extubated.	Approximately 80% of patients on MV for ≤ 3 days will wean completely and without difficulty. Note that 20%, however, will move into the long-term category.	VI: Clinical studies in a variety of patient populations and situations to support recommendations	See Other References: 26, 32, 43–45, 86, 136–139, 151	Considerable research exists on duration of MV in some patient populations (eg, adult respiratory distress syndrome, neuromuscular diseases) that typically require long-term MV. In general, however, duration of MV appears to be dictated more by patients' pre-existing conditions and complications, rather than by diagnosis per se.
	Patients who require MV for ≥ 3 days are appropriately categorized as long-term mechanically ventilated.	Correctly identifying patients who require prolonged MV results in earlier interventions that may decrease total ventilator duration. While 3 days seems a relatively short ventilator duration, patients who extend beyond 3 days often continue to require support for weeks and sometimes months.	V: Clinical studies in more than 1 or 2 patient populations and situations to support recommendations	See Annotated Bibliography: 1, 3, 6, 8 See Other References: 21, 45, 68	
	Patients may be suffering from a wide variety of conditions that result in prolonged ventilator dependence.	The debilitated, immuno-compromised, and elderly are at especially at risk, as are those with COPD and other chronic ventilatory conditions: neurological diseases (eg, Guillain-Barré) or trauma (spinal cord injury, head trauma), congestive heart failure, multiple organ dysfunction, acute respiratory distress syndrome (ARDS), sepsis, and pneumonia (including ventilator-associated pneumonia [VAP]).	VI: Clinical studies in a variety of patient populations and situations to support recommendations	See Annotated Bibliography: 1, 3, 6, 8 See Other References: 36, 46, 47, 52, 54, 58, 63, 84, 86, 96, 115, 118	Patient management during the acute stage affects ventilator duration and other clinical and economic outcomes. For example, the patient with ARDS is at risk for volutrauma if lung protective strategies (eg, low-volume ventilation) are not used (See Other References: 150). Refer to protocol on MV for more on lung protective strategies (See Other References: 122).

Period of Use	Recommendation	Rationale for Recommendation	Level of Recommendation	Supporting References	Comments
Selection of patients: short- and long-term mechanical ventilation (MV) *(cont.)*	Identify patients at risk and assure interventions to prevent complications and improve outcomes.				The longer the patient is on the ventilator, the greater the chance that the patient will suffer a complication such as VAP, deep vein thrombosis (DVT), gastrointestinal bleeding (GIB), urinary tract infection (UTI), and sinusitis.
Application and initial use	**The stages of the weaning continuum** Identify the weaning stage.	It is helpful to identify the stages of weaning so that care planning and interventions may be appropriately initiated. Multiple aspects of care affect weaning outcomes.	IV: Limited clinical studies to support recommendations	See Other References: 21, 23, 37, 68, 87, 88	Examples of interventions that may be included in the acute stage include protective lung strategies and prophylaxis for VAP, DVT, urinary track infection, gastrointestinal bleeding, and sinusitis. During the preweaning stage, more attention may be focused on such interventions as nutrition, glucose control, and activity. Finally, during the weaning stage, protocols for weaning may be implemented. Some patients improve rapidly through the stages and are extubated while others progress slowly, irregularly, or not at all. Some may die or have MV withdrawn
	• The *acute stage* is that time, generally the first 24–72 hours, when the patient is initially placed on a ventilator and is unstable.	The *acute stage* is marked by the use of a high level of ventilatory support and often hemodynamic support as well. Weaning is not anticipated and ventilator adjustments are required to protect the lung (eg, low Vₜs), provide adequate oxygenation and ventilation, and assure a reasonable acid-base status.		See Other References: 21, 23, 37, 68, 87, 88	
	• The *prewean stage* is that stage where the patient is stable, yet may still have numerous factors impeding weaning readiness.	During this stage ventilatory settings are selected to enhance patient interaction on modes such as pressure support ventilation (PSV) and lower levels of oxygen and PEEP. Interventions are focused on restoring or improving baseline status.	V: Clinical studies in more than 1 or 2 different patient populations and situations to support recommendations		The prewean stage may be very short (ie, hours) in the short-term ventilated patient. In the long-term ventilated patient this stage may last for days, weeks, or months.

Period of Use	Recommendation	Rationale for Recommendation	Level of Recommendation	Supporting References	Comments
Application and initial use *(cont.)*	• The *weaning stage* is short with rapid progress over consecutive days. It is marked by physiologic stability and attempts to liberate the patient from MV. Complete weaning is generally defined as breathing spontaneously for 24 consecutive hours. Other outcomes are possible such as ventilator dependence, incomplete weaning (ventilator support required for a portion of a day), and/or death.	Spontaneous breathing trials (SBT) with modes such as continuous positive airway pressure (CPAP) and PSV are commonly used. The goal of an SBT is spontaneous breathing for a predetermined period of time without the emergence of signs of intolerance. When the predetermined trial criteria are met, a decision is made to extubate, or in the case of a tracheostomy, to attempt prolonged trials of spontaneous breathing (> 24 hours, etc).		See Annotated Bibliography: 5, 7, 9 See Other References: 23	Only complete weaning is discussed here. Refer to Chapter 4, Management of Ventilated Patients Beyond the ICU: Home Care Management, and other references on this topic.
	Assessment of weaning readiness Early, accurate assessment of weaning readiness may result in improved weaning outcomes. It is important to assess weaning readiness and to address weaning impediments before initiating weaning trials.	The risk of iatrogenic complications increases with prolonged MV further promoting ventilator dependence. However, attempting to wean short- or long-term ventilated patients prematurely (eg, when the patient is not fully recovered from anesthesia or weak, malnourished, tired, or febrile) may have negative physiological and psychological outcomes.	VI: Clinical studies in a variety of patient populations and situations to support recommendations	See Annotated Bibliography: 3, 8 See Other References: 54, 55, 84, 148	Studies demonstrate that unplanned or premature extubations that result in reintubation increase the chances of aspiration pneumonia, lengthen ICU and hospital LOS, and increase mortality.
	In the patient ventilated ≤ 3 days, the assessment is directed at level of consciousness, hemodynamic stability, oxygenation, ventilation, and respiratory mechanics.	Details related to the assessment factors follow later in this protocol.			
	Assessment in the patient ventilated ≥ 3 days is more comprehensive because changes in physiologic status occur over time. These include factors such as hydration and nutrition. Additionally, iatrogenic complications such as pneumothorax, VAP, and DVT are common and contribute to an overall debilitated state.	Details related to the assessment factors follow later in this protocol. For positive outcomes to result, systematic attention to factors that impede weaning progress is essential. Many interventions that ultimately affect ventilator dependence and other clinical and economic outcome are initiated during specific weaning stages.		See Annotated Bibliography: 3, 8 See Other References: 54, 55, 84, 148	

Period of Use	Recommendation	Rationale for Recommendation	Level of Recommendation	Supporting References	Comments
Application and initial use *(cont.)*	*Wean assessment criteria* The reason for MV is resolved or improved before the start of weaning.	It is important to recognize that patients can have multiple reasons for MV and that the reasons may change over time. This is common in patients ventilated long-term.	VI: Clinical studies in a variety of patient populations and situations to support recommendations	See Annotated Bibliography: 1, 3, 6, 8 See Other References: 36, 47, 48, 52, 54, 58, 63, 84, 86, 96, 115, 118, 131	For example, a patient may initially require ventilation for a drug overdose; however, aspiration and subsequent pneumonia may require that weaning be deferred even though the patient has recovered from the overdose. (In this example, the patient may move from the weaning stage back to the acute stage.)
	The patient's physiological status should be stable before the start of weaning.	Weaning trials are considered when the patient is stable, the underlying reason for MV is resolved, and additional pulmonary and nonpulmonary factors are improved. The stage is called the *weaning stage,* and spontaneous breathing trials are commonly used to test the patient's ability to be liberated from the ventilator.	VI: Clinical studies in a variety of patient populations and situations to support recommendations	See Annotated Bibliography: 1, 3, 5–9 See Other References: 21, 68	
	Having a wean screen, or checklist of factors to assess weaning readiness, is an essential first step prior to initiating weaning trials.	Wean screen criteria are the first step in the determination of whether or not to activate a weaning protocol. The criteria vary depending on whether the patient is ventilated short or long term.	VI: Clinical studies in a variety of patient populations and situations to support recommendations	See Annotated Bibliography: 1, 3, 5, 6, 8, 9, 10 See Other References: 6, 67, 68	An example of a weaning protocol with wean screen criteria is found in Appendix 3D.
	Patients ventilated ≤ 3 days Criteria generally focus on cardio-pulmonary stability, minute ventilation, breathing pattern (rate and V_T), oxygenation, and strength. If extubation is desired, the ability to protect the airway is essential. The criteria are selected to assure stability but not to be overly restrictive.	Specific factors that impact weaning in the patient ventilated < 3 days are delineated below.			

Period of Use	Recommendation	Rationale for Recommendation	Level of Recommendation	Supporting References	Comments
Application and initial use *(cont.)*	***Patients ventilated ≥ 3 days*** Systematically assess and correct pulmonary and nonpulmonary impediments to weaning.	Though many factors have been associated with weaning outcomes in patients ventilated ≥ 3 days, no single factor has yet been identified as the most important. It may be that a combination of factors is responsible for ventilator dependence.	V: Clinical studies in more than 1 or 2 different patient populations and situations to support recommendations	See Annotated Bibliography: 2, 8 See Other References: 38	As Daly et al (See Other References: 38) note, chronically critically ill patients are often weak and debilitated. Even if the underlying reason for MV is resolved, overall status may not be at the level necessary to progress to weaning trials. Unfortunately, progress in those who require prolonged ventilation is often slow, which may frustrate and demoralize the patient, family, and staff.
	Use a checklist (or other process tool) of factors to assure regular assessment of weaning impediments. Such a method decreases variability and assures that care provision is consistent and timely	Studies by Burns et al and Morgenroth et al demonstrate the contribution of nonpulmonary factors to weaning readiness in long-term mechanically ventilated patients. Both show the great variability in weaning progress associated with changes in physical status, and that improvement in pulmonary status alone (and the attainment of pulmonary parameter thresholds) was not sufficient to predict weaning readiness. Processes of care that decrease variability result in improved outcomes.		See Annotated Bibliography: 2, 3 See Other References: 112	Few tools exist for bedside assessment of the long-term MV patient. See Appendix 3A for the BWAP, a comprehensive tool designed to track physiological progress over time.
	Assess *pulmonary and nonpulmonary* factors in order to ***identify and correct*** impediments to weaning.	As noted earlier, weaning readiness in the patient ventilated short term is often focused on level of consciousness and specific pulmonary factors. In contrast, the long-term ventilated patient has many more impediments that may require correction.	V: Clinical studies in more than 1 or 2 different patient populations and situations to support recommendations	See Annotated Bibliography: 3, 8 See Other References: 21 22, 27, 29, 33, 34, 67, 74, 107, 108, 115,117, 136, 137, 140, 157	

Period of Use	Recommendation	Rationale for Recommendation	Level of Recommendation	Supporting References	Comments
Application and initial use (*cont.*)	Use of a checklist (or other systematic process) assures consistency in assessment and management.				The BWAP was designed for patients requiring long-term MV. It assesses 26 pulmonary and nonpulmonary factors associated with weaning. The importance of the factors may vary depending on whether the patient has been ventilated for ≤ 3 days or ≥ 3 days. Many of the BWAP factors are described below.
	1. Neurological status (eg, alert, awake, protective reflexes, spinal integrity)	Change in level of consciousness may indicate underlying problems such as a neurological condition or oversedation. The etiology of the decreased mental status should be investigated prior to weaning. Weaning is possible, but tracheostomy for airway protection may be required.	IV: Limited clinical studies to support recommendations	See Other References: 34, 115, 155	Coma, by itself, is not an indicator of inability to wean. The importance of mental status to weaning outcome was addressed in studies by Coplin and colleagues and Namen et al. Conclusions differed. Coplin suggests that waiting for an improvement in mental status in brain-injured patients is not warranted and needlessly lengthens ventilator time and associated outcomes. In contrast, Namen et al note the importance of the Glasgow Coma Scale score to weaning outcome.
	The use of sedatives provided by infusion is linked to delayed weaning and longer ICU and hospital LOS. Use of sedation management protocols and algorithms are associated with improved outcomes and are encouraged. Daily sedation interruption is recommended, when possible, to assure that patients are not overly sedated.	Randomized controlled trials by Brooks et al and Kress et al demonstrated that the use of a nurse-managed sedation algorithm and once-daily interruptions of sedation infusions respectively resulted in shorter ventilator duration and ICU lengths of stay. Once-daily interruptions of sedation infusions do not adversely affect psychologic well-being. Kress et al demonstrated that patients assigned to the method actually had lower post-traumatic stress scores than those not assigned.	VI: Clinical studies in a variety of patient populations and situations to support recommendations	See Other References: 18, 89, 90, 97	If sedation for continued anxiolysis is necessary during the weaning stage, it is important to try to transition from sedation by infusion to a steady state via an oral route (ie, via gastric tube). The use of sedation infusions is linked to prolonged ventilator duration. Refer to Chapter 6, Sedation and Neuromuscular Blockade.

Period of Use	Recommendation	Rationale for Recommendation	Level of Recommendation	Supporting References	Comments
Application and initial use *(cont.)*	2. Hemodynamic (eg, heart rate, rhythm) and metabolic stability	Patient response to MV varies according to myocardial function and reserve capacity. Cardiac failure can be exacerbated by weaning.	VI: Clinical studies in a variety of patient populations and situations to support recommendations	See Annotated Bibliography: 8 See Other References: 6, 30, 96, 104, 140	Hemodynamic instability results in compromised oxygen transport. Signs of hemodynamic instability include acute or gradual fall in arterial blood pressure, tachycardia, bradycardia, dysrhythmias, weak peripheral pulses, decreased pulse pressure, acute or gradual increase in pulmonary capillary wedge pressure, decreased cardiac output, and decreased mixed venous oxygen saturation.
		Patients experiencing sepsis, bacteremia, fever, or seizures have a greatly increased metabolic rate. By controlling or normalizing these factors, oxygen consumption and CO_2 production will decrease. For example, metabolic rate is adversely affected by thyroid status; hypothyroidism blunts the response to hypoxia and hypercarbia.	IV: Limited clinical studies to support recommendations	See Other References: 12, 107, 117	
	3. Hemoglobin/ hematocrit	Low hemoglobin and hematocrit, especially those that are the result of acute hemorrhage, affect oxygen-carrying capacity. An imbalance between supply and demand is created. Oxygen consumption secondary to the work of breathing (WOB) during weaning can further magnify this imbalance. Decreased oxygen delivery to vital organs such as the heart increases the risk of ischemic injury and complications that will further impede weaning. Transfusions should be cautiously yet appropriately provided.	IV: Limited clinical studies to support recommendations	See Other References: 35, 78	The exact level of hemoglobin required varies with the condition. Although more conservative transfusion recommendations have been published for critically ill patients, a recent study suggests that they are not followed. Herbert et al noted that a restrictive strategy (transfuse only when hemoglobin < 7 g/dL) was as effective and possibly superior to a liberal strategy (transfused to keep hemoglobin 10–12 g/dL). Corwin et al found that few followed such a strategy. However, they noted that a level < 9 g/dL was a predictor of increased mortality and LOS. Those with acute bleeding, acute myocardial infarction, and unstable angina generally require more liberal transfusion.

Period of Use	Recommendation	Rationale for Recommendation	Level of Recommendation	Supporting References	Comments
Application and initial use *(cont.)*	4. Fluids, electrolytes, nutrition	• Fluctuations in intravascular volume may result in compromised pulmonary, cardiac, renal, and cerebral function.	IV: Limited clinical studies to support recommendations	See Other References: 12, 29, 67, 96, 104, 108, 112, 119, 136, 137	
		• Electrolyte alterations affect cardiac and respiratory muscle function and can lead to muscle fatigue, decreased muscular contractility, and dysrhythmias. Especially important are potassium, magnesium, phosphate, and calcium because they are required for adequate respiratory muscle function and overall muscular strength and endurance.			
		• Malnutrition results in a diminished immune response, respiratory muscle fatigue, electrolyte disturbances, inefficient gas transport, and weakness. Metabolic requirements often exceed available energy stores in debilitated patients. Low albumin stores also result in low intravascular oncotic pressures and third spacing of fluid. Glucose control is necessary for many reasons, including improved substrate utilization, decreased infections, and the prevention of gastroparesis and ileus. Recent data suggests that glucose must be tightly controlled for best effect.			Refer to Chapter 5, Nutritional Support in Mechanically Ventilated Patients.
	An important element of nutrition in the critically ill patient is the maintenance of *tight glucose control* (80–110 mg/dL). Glucose should be monitored and controlled to assure good outcomes.	In a randomized controlled trial, Van den Berghe et al demonstrated the importance of tight glucose control using insulin infusions in critically ill ventilated surgical patients. Those assigned to tight glucose control demonstrated statistically significant improvement in mortality rates, wound infections, time on the ventilator, and ICU and hospital LOS.		See Other References: 157	

Period of Use	Recommendation	Rationale for Recommendation	Level of Recommendation	Supporting References	Comments
Application and initial use *(cont.)*	5. Anxiety, pain, and rest/sleep	These 3 subjective symptoms are important to assess in weaning patients. The critical care environment can be frightening and uncomfortable, and patients often are anxious and uncomfortable. In addition, patients' sleep cycles are often disrupted by care providers, extraneous noise, etc. The restorative stages of sleep are difficult to attain. Further, the need for information is great in these patients.	V: Limited clinical studies to support recommendations	See Other References: 61, 62, 125, 142, 143	Management of these subjective symptoms is essential. All may benefit from specific pharmacologic interventions but other nonpharmacologic interventions are also helpful such as the use of massage, music therapy, and other nontraditional forms of therapy. Perhaps most important, the nurse's use of a comforting presence may go a long way toward alleviating these symptoms. Also, it is important to provide regular, supportive, and easily understood updates to the patient and the family. Studies on patient experiences of MV are old but still applicable.
	6. Bowel problems	Bowel elimination problems (diarrhea, constipation, ileus) result in inadequate enteral alimentation, discomfort, and inefficient respiratory muscle function (diaphragm may be displaced) making weaning difficult.	IV: Limited clinical studies to support recommendations	See Other References: 28, 113 See Other References: 119	• Assess the causes of diarrhea and treat accordingly. *Clostridium difficile*, a potential cause of diarrhea, is a medical emergency and should be treated prior to proceeding with weaning. • Bowel routines should be established early and maintained throughout hospitalization. • Investigate the etiology of ileus. Early mobilization and turning may help improve or decrease ileus.
	7. Mobility, conditioning, and exercise	Deconditioning occurs rapidly with negative results. It is known that within 2–3 days of recumbency skeletal muscle atrophies and balance difficulties emerge. Rehabilitation takes longer and weaning is more difficult when the patient is weak.	IV: Limited clinical studies to support recommendations	See Other References: 106, 145	• Recruitment of muscle happens with weight bearing activities. Sitting on the side of the bed, standing, and other such activities help regain proprioception and balance and are to be encouraged. • Remember that while actively conditioning, increased ventilatory support may be necessary. Shortness of breath during exercise is a deterrent to patient acceptance and effort. (See Other References: 14)

Period of Use	Recommendation	Rationale for Recommendation	Level of Recommendation	Supporting References	Comments
Application and initial use *(cont.)*		Prolonged neuromuscular weakness (ie, critical illness myoneuropathy) has been associated with neuromuscular blockade and the use of steroids. Ventilator duration is longer as are ICU and hospital LOS. Refer to Chapter 6, Sedation and Neuromuscular Blockade in Mechanically Ventilated Patients		See Other References: 40–42	
	8. Respiratory rate and pattern	Rapid, shallow breathing patterns herald an increased WOB and potential fatigue. (Refer to section on fatigue for more details.)	VI: Clinical studies in a variety of patient populations and situations to support recommendations	See Other References: 30, 65, 123, 126, 152, 153	
	9. Secretions	Secretions increase the resistive workload of the patient. In very weak patients, thick or copious secretions will make airway clearance difficult.	V: Clinical studies in more than 1 or 2 different patient populations and situations to support recommendations	See Other References: 85, 103	While secretions may not impede weaning, they may be a deterrent to extubation. If extubation is to be considered despite the presence of copious or thick secretions, cough is assessed prior to doing so. A strong cough should be present to assure airway clearance. Positive expiratory pressure (PEP) is a good correlate of cough. (See Other References: 103)
	10. Neuromuscular disease or deformities	WOB is increased in patients with neuromuscular diseases and/or deformities (eg, myopathies, severe kyphoscoliosis).	IV: Limited clinical studies to support recommendations	See Other References: 40–42	Weaning modes and methods that gently and gradually build endurance and strength are helpful interventions.
	11. Abdominal size	Full excursion of the diaphragm is impeded with obesity, distention, and ascites. Patients with large abdomens have a decreased functional residual volume and thus an increased WOB.	V: Clinical studies in more than 1 or 2 different patient populations and situations to support recommendations	See Other References: 141, 164	Higher levels of PEEP and/or PS may be necessary to offset the work associated with the mass loading of a large abdomen.
		The position of the patient with a large abdomen is important during weaning trials. A study of weaning patients with large abdomens suggests that RR and VT are adversely affected in the 90° and 0° positions.		See Other References: 20	WOB may be decreased in the patient with a large abdomen by using a reverse Trendelenburg position during trials.

Period of Use	Recommendation	Rationale for Recommendation	Level of Recommendation	Supporting References	Comments
Application and initial use *(cont.)*	12. Airway size (ie, tube diameter and length)	As diameter decreases, resistance increases. Nasally placed tubes are generally smaller, plus the nasal passages impinge on the tube diameter. And, because nasotracheal tubes also increase the risk of sinusitis and VAP, they are to be avoided.	VI: Clinical studies in a variety of patient populations and situations to support recommendations	See Other References: 58, 59, 148	Nasally placed tubes of any variety increase the risk of sinusitis and VAP. They are to be avoided.
	13. Airway clearance	For extubation to be successful, the patient must be able to protect his or her airway. This means an effective swallow and cough are necessary. Weaning from MV (ie, off ventilatory support for > 24 hours) is possible; however, an artificial airway may still be required.	VI: Clinical studies in a variety of patient populations and situations to support recommendations	See Annotated Bibliography: 8	
	14. Gas exchange (eg, oxygenation, ventilation, and minute ventilation) and pH	ABGs are the gold standard for evaluating acid-base status.	V: Clinical studies in more than 1 or 2 different patient populations or situations to support recommendations	See Other References: 110, 160–162	While ABGs are the *gold standard* for evaluating acid-base status and gas exchange, frequent blood sampling during weaning may not be necessary and in fact may result in anemia. The judicious use of other noninvasive monitoring tools such as pulse oximetry and capnography are encouraged. Refer to *Noninvasive Monitoring* and protocols on $ETCO_2$ monitoring and pulse oximetry. (See Other References: 70, 146)
		Most important to monitor are pH and PaO_2 because critical values may result in death. In the weaning patient a pH below normal requires compensation. Generally this means an increase in minute ventilation and an increase in the WOB.		See Other References: 39, 110, 160–162	
		High FIO_2 requirements (ie, greater than 50% with or without PEEP) suggest shunt, VQ mismatch, or diffusion block.		See Other References: 115, 161, 162	
		Minute ventilation, viewed in relation to $PaCO_2$ is important to monitor. For example a minute ventilation of 20 L/min to main-		See Other References: 161, 162	$MV = RR \times V_T$ A minute ventilation of 5–10 L/min is normal but rare in the mechanically ventilated patient.

Period of Use	Recommendation	Rationale for Recommendation	Level of Recommendation	Supporting References	Comments
Application and initial use *(cont.)*		tain a $Paco_2$ of 40 mm Hg demonstrates that gas exchange is inefficient.			
		It is important to consider concomitant physical signs and symptoms of decreased reserve when evaluating oxygenation and ventilation.		See Annotated Bibliography: 11 See Other References: 30, 82, 152, 153, 156	Rapid, shallow breathing demonstrates increased WOB and is especially noteworthy if the rapid shallow breathing pattern is not consistent with a chronic condition.
		Occasionally minute ventilation is high secondary to a neurologic cause. In these cases, the $Paco_2$ will be low (reflective of the high MV). This is in contrast to a normal or high $Paco_2$ and a high MV that indicate a dead space abnormality or increased CO_2 production.		See Other References: 34, 161, 162.	
	15. Measures of respiratory muscle strength and endurance are referred to as traditional (or standard) weaning predictors (or criteria). They include: negative inspiratory pressure (NIP), PEP, spontaneous tidal volume (VT sp) and vital capacity (VC).	Respiratory muscle strength and endurance are important measures of the ability to sustain spontaneous breathing trials. A full description follows in the section on weaning predictors. (See weaning predictors below.)	IV: Limited clinical studies to support recommendations	See Annotated Bibliography: 4, 8 See Other References: 4, 129, 130	These standard criteria are commonly measured prior to weaning. They provide information about strength and endurance of the respiratory muscles but may not be predictive, especially in the long-term ventilated patient. Standard weaning predictors and others are described below.
	Weaning predictors				
	Most weaning predictors do not predict wean ability in patients ventilated > 3 days. However, their use is encouraged in order to evaluate factors important to weaning and to track progress over time.	Though many more indices exist, only those that have been adapted for clinical use, and are commonly seen in clinical practice, are described. The concepts related to the use of the indices may be helpful to consider.	VI: Clinical studies in a variety of patient populations and situations to support recommendations	See Annotated Bibliography: 2, 4, 8	Standard weaning predictors have not proven to be strong positive predictors. However, evaluation of the components is helpful in order to direct interventions.
	Weaning predictors generally focus on pulmonary factors to the exclusion of nonpulmonary factors.				Two studies (see Annotated Bibliography: 2; Other References: 112) monitored comprehensive weaning predictor scores (both general and pulmonary factors) over the course of weaning. Both described the wide variability and fluctuations of the scores and showed a progressive, if not dramatic, upward trend until weaning was accom-

Period of Use	Recommendation	Rationale for Recommendation	Level of Recommendation	Supporting References	Comments
Application and initial use *(cont.)*					plished. Thus it is unlikely that a predictor that does not change over time is predictive.
	Methods are needed that systematically track overall status (and thus weaning ability) in order to prevent unsuccessful trials that may be counterproductive (eg, result in fatigue or other sequelae).	There have been multiple attempts to develop weaning predictors that indicate when the patient is ready to wean. Unfortunately, most predictors have been tested at the end of the process (extubation). Clinicians interested in determining when trials of gradual ventilator withdrawal may begin are therefore unable to rely on the predictors to determine weaning readiness.			
	1. Pulmonary-specific weaning indices (traditional or standard weaning criteria)	These criteria are useful for assessing respiratory muscle strength and may be especially helpful in the assessment of weaning readiness in the patient ventilated < 3 days.	V: Clinical studies in more than 1 or 2 different patient populations or situations to support recommendations	See Other References: 60, 109, 129, 130	See Appendix 3B for a description of the measurement and thresholds for standard weaning criteria.
	a. Negative inspiratory pressure (NIP) is considered the most reliable as it is an effort-independent measurement.	Providing the patient's central drive is intact, this measurement may be measured regardless of the patient's level of consciousness.	V: Clinical studies in more than 1 or 2 different patient populations or situations to support recommendations	See Other References: 109, 129, 130 See Other References: 82, 102, 163	The reliability of NIP has been questioned in a number of studies. Investigators have noted that measurements of NIP vary among those performing the test. Others have also noted the test's poor reproducibility and reliability in elderly patients. (See Other References: 91, 92) Cautious evaluation of measurements obtained daily is important for comparison because results can vary greatly with different clinician techniques, changes in the patient's physical status, the use of sedation, cuff inflation, and even the time of day.
	• Measured with attention to technique and timing, NIP can provide evidence of improved respiratory muscle strength over time. NIP can also measure loss of strength (or fatigue) during or following a weaning trial.	Respiratory muscle strength is greatly affected by fatigue, so NIP values will decrease. This kind of evidence, in addition to other signs of respiratory muscle fatigue such as dyspnea, tachypnea, chest abdominal asynchrony, and hypercarbia (late sign), indicate the need to abort the weaning trial.	V: Clinical studies in more than 1 or 2 different patient populations or situations to support recommendations	See Annotated Bibliography: 11 See Other References: 4, 39, 60, 66, 109, 123, 129, 130, 147, 152, 153	

Period of Use	Recommendation	Rationale for Recommendation	Level of Recommendation	Supporting References	Comments
Application and initial use *(cont.)*	• NIP is best used as a negative predictor.	NIP has been shown to have poor positive predictive power in patients on long-term MV but good negative predictability—meaning an NIP exceeding the threshold value (in this case, more negative than -20 cm H_2O) does not indicate that the patient will wean. However, a number that does not meet the threshold (ie, more positive than -20 cm H_2O) indicates profound weakness and the probability of unsuccessful weaning trials.	V: Clinical studies in more than 1 or 2 different patient populations or situations to support recommendations	See Annotated Bibliography: 2 See Other References: 21, 67, 68, 112, 149, 154	
	b. Positive expiratory pressure (PEP) is more effort-dependent than the NIP. It is best used to evaluate the strength of the expiratory muscles and cough effectiveness, but the result must be evaluated in context with the patient's effort.		IV: Limited clinical studies to support recommendations	See Other References: 85, 103	
	c. Spontaneous tidal volume (VTsp) and vital capacity (VC): Measure volumes rather than pressures and tell more about endurance than strength of respiratory muscles.	When respiratory muscles are approaching a fatigued state, VT decreases and respiratory rate (RR) increases. This rapid, shallow breathing pattern indicates a need for respiratory muscle rest. In the patient with little reserve, a reasonable VT may be sustained for some time; however, the VC may be greatly reduced. The normal VT:VC ratio is 1:3.	V: Clinical studies in more than 1 or 2 different patient populations or situations to support recommendations	See Annotated Bibliography: 11 See Other References: 152, 153	
	d. Vital capacity (VC)	Although measuring VC is difficult in the intubated patient, some investigators have found it to be useful in select patient populations (eg, Guillain-Barré syndrome).	IV: Limited clinical studies to support recommendations	See Other References: 27	In the Chevrolet and Deleamont study, VC accurately determined the need for intubation as well as the time to begin weaning trials in patients with Guillain-Barré syndrome.
	e. Minute ventilation (VE) is a good indicator of efficiency of gas exchange; however, it must always be evaluated in conjunction with $PaCO_2$ to determine significance.	An increased VE is a normal response to pain or exercise; it may also indicate increased dead space (from disease or iatrogenic causes such as auto-PEEP) or high CO_2 production.	V: Clinical studies in more than 1 or 2 different patient populations and situations to support recommendations	See Other References: 109, 123	

Period of Use	Recommendation	Rationale for Recommendation	Level of Recommendation	Supporting References	Comments
Application and initial use *(cont.)*	2. Additional pulmonary indices (nontraditional)				
	a. Work of breathing (WOB) and central drive (CD)				
	Airway occlusion pressure (P0.1): Few clinically adapted measures of WOB and central drive exist, but P0.1 measured 1 sec after onset of inspiration has potential use as a bedside clinical weaning index. Unfortunately, its application has not been well demonstrated for routine clinical use despite numerous studies advocating its usefulness.	Studies using P0.1 in weaning patients found it increases in respiratory failure and decreases with recovery. Higher levels of P0.1 correlate with increased ventilatory muscle demand, potential fatigue, and respiratory failure.	V: Clinical studies in more than 1 or 2 different patient populations or situations to support recommendations	See Annotated Bibliography: 4 See Other References: 64, 111, 114, 134, 135	No single value of P0.1 has distinguished between weaning success and failure. Measurement at the bedside is difficult, making widespread use unlikely. Some bedside monitoring systems calculate P0.1 but to date, none correlate with weaning potential. Thresholds for when to stop or when to proceed with weaning trials do not exist.
	b. Breathing pattern Rapid/shallow breathing index (f/VT): based on the premise that a rapid, shallow breathing pattern reflects an increased respiratory load that may result in fatigue and failure. The index may best be used to indicate extubation potential rather than as an index to determine weaning readiness.	Studies that have used the f/VT suggest it is predictive of extubation success. However when used during the weaning process the index does not reliably change over time and does not predict well. f/VT has been found to have good negative but poor positive predictability. In elderly patients the cited threshold of the index is not reliable.	V: Clinical studies in more than 1 or 2 different patient populations or situations to support recommendations	See Annotated Bibliography: 2, 4, 11 See Other References: 3, 92, 152, 153	See Appendix 3C for f/VT index measurement and thresholds.
	3. Comprehensive (combined pulmonary and nonpulmonary) indices				
	The Burns Wean Assessment Program (BWAP) is a 26-item assessment tool that combines 12 general and 14 respiratory factors in a single score. The total score may be used to track the progress of the patient and as a negative weaning predictor.	The BWAP was designed for the systematic assessment of factors important to weaning (described earlier in the protocol). Investigators noted wide fluctuations in the patient's physical status (and thus BWAP score) during the prewean phase. The BWAP score changed reliably over the duration of weaning and was shown to have strong negative predictive ability.	IV: Limited clinical studies to support recommendations	See Annotated Bibliography: 2, 3 See Other References: 23	See Appendix 3A for BWAP tool and thresholds. The BWAP has been used in more than 1 patient population and a score of ~50% appears to herald the weaning stage.

Period of Use	Recommendation	Rationale for Recommendation	Level of Recommendation	Supporting References	Comments
Application and initial use *(cont.)*	**The weaning process** For ventilator liberation to occur, ventilator support must be withdrawn. The process may be gradual or abrupt, and decisions related to the selection of the mode or method may depend on whether the patient has been ventilated short- or long-term. Regardless, the weaning process consists of selecting an effective, safe, and efficient mode or method. The use of protocols is encouraged.		VI: Clinical studies in a variety of patient populations and situations to support recommendations	See Annotated Bibliography: 8	
	A mode or method for weaning is selected when the patient is assessed to be ready. Readiness requires that the reason for MV has resolved or is stable, and additional factors impeding weaning (as described previously) have improved. Please refer to "Assessment of Weaning Readiness" above for discussions on the importance of assessing and correcting different factors.	As noted earlier, patients who require prolonged MV often have many coexistent conditions that make weaning difficult. Some are comorbid conditions such as renal disease, or there may be complications such as VAP or deep vein thrombosis. Refer to prevention of complications at the end of this protocol for more on these topics.			
	Concepts of respiratory muscle work, rest, conditioning, and fatigue are important to incorporate into the design of a weaning plan and the selection of a mode or method. Also important is the determination of when a tracheostomy should be performed. A discussion of these concepts follows.				

Period of Use	Recommendation	Rationale for Recommendation	Level of Recommendation	Supporting References	Comments
Application and initial use *(cont.)*	1. Respiratory muscle work, rest, fatigue, and conditioning				
	a. Select a mode of ventilation and apply carefully in order to prevent respiratory muscle fatigue.	Respiratory muscle fatigue is difficult to quantify clinically. Instead, signs and symptoms of potential respiratory muscle fatigue (eg, dyspnea, tachypnea, chest abdominal asynchrony, and finally increased $PaCO_2$—a late sign) must be recognized. Tobin and colleagues demonstrated that rapid shallow breathing and chest abdominal asynchrony were demonstrative of compensation for an increased WOB. If the workload continues, fatigue follows.

A fatigued patient may take 12 to 24 hours to recover. | V: Clinical studies in more than 1 or 2 different patient populations or situations to support recommendations | See Other References: 9, 30, 82, 126, 152, 153 | When the patient is fatigued, MV is used to offset the fatigue. However the method varies with volume and pressure modes of ventilation. |
| | b. Design weaning trials to include defined periods of rest. | Because it is not known how much work is too much, it is prudent to recognize that all patients are at risk for respiratory muscle fatigue, especially those who are debilitated, malnourished, and hypermetabolic. Providing periods of respiratory muscle rest is prudent, especially in the long-term ventilated patient. | V: Clinical studies in more than 1 or 2 different patient populations or situations to support recommendations | See Annotated Bibliography: 1, 3, 5, 6, 8, 9

See Other References: 7, 16, 22 | During the weaning process, it is prudent to provide respiratory muscle rest periods. In the long-term ventilated patient this is easily accomplished at night. |
| | c. Respiratory muscle work may continue during ventilatory support. To assure rest and respiratory muscle recovery, adjust the volume or pressure modes to offset WOB. | To allow respiratory muscles to rest and recover, work must be greatly reduced or eliminated. | V: Clinical studies in more than 1 or 2 different patient populations or situations to support recommendations | See Other References: 16, 17, 105 | |
| | | *Volume modes*

It used to be thought that respiratory muscles were rested when volume delivered ventilator breaths were delivered, such as with assist-control (A/C). Marini and colleagues demonstrated that if the patient initiates a breath such as with A/C, patient work continues throughout the volume delivered ventilator breath. This means that simply increasing the | | See Other References: 105 | This is an important clinical concept. For example, with volume modes of ventilation, the rate may need to be increased until the patient is *not initiating breaths* in order to assure muscle rest. A practical way to assure rest is to increase the level of support at night and when signs and symptoms of fatigue emerge. |

Period of Use	Recommendation	Rationale for Recommendation	Level of Recommendation	Supporting References	Comments
Application and initial use *(cont.)*		ventilator rate with A/C may not result in decreased workload—unless the patient is not initiating any breaths at all.			
		Pressure modes			
		In the pressure support (PS) mode, muscle "unloading" may be accomplished (despite spontaneous respiratory effort), providing PS level is high enough.	V: Clinical studies in more than 1 or 2 different patient populations or situations to support recommendations	See Other References: 16, 17, 59, 83, 99, 100, 132	To accomplish unloading with PS, increase the PS level to attain RR < 20/min and a eupneic respiratory pattern. Pressure support max (PS max) describes the level of PS that results in RR, < 20/min; V_T, 8 to 12 mL/kg; and the absence of accessory muscle activity.
	2. The quality of work depends on the mode and method of ventilation used during weaning. Respiratory muscle conditioning consists of endurance and strengthening work.	The use of 2 classifications may help with practical clinical applications of specific weaning modes and methods: high-pressure, low-volume work; low-pressure, high-volume work.			
	a. High pressure, low volume work: Associated with the use of T piece, CPAP, low intermittent mandatory ventilation (IMV) rates, and some inspiratory resistive training devices. Generally, any mode or method that requires that the patient breathe spontaneously without support results in high-pressure, low-volume work.	The concept of strengthening as it relates to high-pressure, low-volume work is adapted from exercise physiology where muscle recruitment and strengthening occurs when a great or maximum force is required to move a given weight a small distance. When applied to the respiratory muscles, it is similar to the negative pressure required to attain a relatively small volume in many spontaneous breathing modes (PS excepted; see below) or methods of weaning. Similar to any strength training, with optimal loading of the muscles, full rest must be assured to assure optimal training affect. This allows for muscle repair and unloading of lactic acid.	IV: Limited clinical studies to support recommendations	See Annotated Bibliography: 6 See Other References: 55, 57, 99, 100	Although these distinctions appear to relate well to specific modes and methods of weaning, studies are needed that clearly elucidate the associated quality and quantity of work. The quality and quantity of work necessary to assure respiratory muscle conditioning is unclear. In studies by Esteban, short duration trials of high-pressure, low-volume work appeared to result in optimal training effect. Between trials, the patients were rested on high-level ventilatory support. Very short spontaneous breathing trials employing high-pressure, low-volume work (ie, ½ hour) appear to be as effective as 2-hour trials.
	b. Low pressure, high volume work: Associated with the use of PS where inspiration is aug-	Low-pressure, high-volume work is often referred to as *endurance conditioning* as a relatively small pressure is required to attain a given	IV: Limited clinical studies to support recommendations	See Annotated Bibliography: 1 See Other References: 99, 100	As with high-pressure, low-volume work, the optimal duration of a trial is unknown. However, drawing from

Period of Use	Recommendation	Rationale for Recommendation	Level of Recommendation	Supporting References	Comments
Application and initial use *(cont.)*	mented. For any given PS level the volume is larger than if the patient were to breathe spontaneously without PS. At high levels of PS, little work occurs, but as the level is reduced, muscle workload increases.	volume: muscles are not worked to maximum effort; training focuses on maintaining a specific level of work for progressively longer intervals.			exercise physiology concepts, endurance training, if done correctly, may be of longer duration.
	With both endurance and strengthening conditioning, rest periods are essential. With strengthening conditioning, trials are shorter than with endurance conditioning.	Because strengthening conditioning requires high-pressure, low-volume work and the recruitment of fast-twitch muscle fibers, fatigue ensues more quickly than with endurance conditioning, which uses slow-twitch muscle fibers (the dominant fibers of the respiratory muscles).	IV: Limited clinical studies to support recommendations	See Annotated Bibliography: 1 See Other References: 5, 99, 100	With weight training, athletes are encouraged to work out every other day rather than daily to assure muscle recovery and muscle recruitment (muscle mass). A work/rest ratio appears to be necessary for an optimal training effect to be realized. Weaning protocols using these concepts will tend to use shorter conditioning episodes (ie, 30 minutes to 2 hours) than with endurance conditioning. (Refer to sample protocols in Appendix 3D.)
	Work associated with ventilator breathing circuits: All modes and methods of weaning require that a source gas be delivered to the patient via a circuit. Ventilator response time, sensitivity setting, and patient requirements all affect the adequacy of gas flow delivery.	Most ventilator modes require that a negative pressure be sensed (pressure-triggered flow) in the ventilator before a flow of gas is delivered to the patient during spontaneous breathing. This can result in an increased workload if sensitivity is not adequately adjusted. Additionally, the ventilator response time (lag time) may be magnified when the respiratory rate is high. Flow-triggering results in less work for the patient (if set correctly). With flow triggering, a selected flow of gas is always available at the patient wye. Flow is measured by the ventilator on the expiratory limb of the patient circuit. When the patient inspires, a drop in flow "down stream" is sensed immediately and the ventilator immediately provides additional flow to meet the patient's inspiratory demand.	VI: Clinical studies in a variety of patient populations and situations to support recommendations	See Other References: 8, 11, 65, 73, 133, 122	Refer to Chapter 2, "Invasive and Noninvasive Modes and Methods of Mechanical Ventilation" for more indepth discussion of pressure and flow triggering.

Period of Use	Recommendation	Rationale for Recommendation	Level of Recommendation	Supporting References	Comments
Application and initial use *(cont.)*	Match ventilator and patient inspiratory times carefully to ensure synchrony.	When gas flow is inadequate (does not match patient's requirement) the patient experiences air hunger. Work may be excessive and exceed patient's endurance. Patient-ventilator dyssynchrony occurs when the patient's peak inspiratory demand is not matched during the inspiratory phase of the ventilator breath.	VI: Clinical studies in a variety of patient populations and situations to support recommendations	See Other References: 8, 11, 65, 73, 133

See other References: 19

See Other References: 122 | Respiratory waveform monitoring is useful in identifying patient-ventilator asynchrony. Refer to Chapter 2, Respiratory Waveforms Monitoring in *Noninvasive Monitoring,* and Chapter 2, Invasive and Noninvasive Modes and Methods of Mechanical Ventilation. |
| | Work associated with auto-PEEP
• Monitor auto-PEEP (an iatrogenic complication) routinely.
• Apply interventions to offset auto-PEEP. | Auto-PEEP develops when expiratory time is inadequate, resulting in an elevated functional residual capacity and dead space (wasted ventilation). WOB will increase as a result.

Patients at risk: COPD, bronchospasm, high VE (> 10 L/min), rapid RR (> 25/min), small-diameter artificial airways, and long inspiratory times.

Water in the circuit can also result in auto-PEEP. | VI: Clinical studies in a variety of patient populations and situations to support recommendations | See Other References: 101, 120, 121, 123, 124 | Interventions to reduce auto-PEEP include lengthening expiratory time, decreasing respiratory rate, increasing diameter of artificial airways, and pharmacological therapies (eg, bronchodilators, sedatives). Increasing set-PEEP is effective in conditions such as COPD where the addition of set-PEEP maintains airway patency throughout exhalation, thereby preventing early airway closure and gas trapping. |
| | 3. Weaning modes and methods
a. Assist control (A/C) ventilation: Delivers volume breaths at a clinician selected rate. Between the control breaths, spontaneous effort results in the delivery of a full volume breath.

Unfortunately, this makes weaning difficult. A/C is generally used as a support or resting mode. Patients are placed on T-piece, CPAP, or a different ventilation mode for weaning trials. They are covered below. | | VI: Clinical studies in a variety of patient populations and situations to support recommendations | Refer to Chapter 2, Invasive and Noninvasive Modes and Methods of Mechanical Ventiltation.

See Other References: 122 | Remember that full ventilatory rest may not be accomplished if the patient is initiating breaths. If A/C is used to rest the patient, it may not accomplish this goal. |

Period of Use	Recommendation	Rationale for Recommendation	Level of Recommendation	Supporting References	Comments
Application and initial use *(cont.)*	A common application of A/C is to intersperse T piece or CPAP trials (or other spontaneous methods or modes) with rest on A/C. If used in this manner it is important to remember to assure adequate rest periods.	Spontaneous breathing trials require high-pressure, low-volume muscle work. Rest is essential for full recovery.		See Annotated Bibliography: 5, 6, 7, 9 See Other References: 55, 57, 122	In those studies using high-pressure, low-volume work via T-piece or CPAP respiratory muscle rest was assured between trials. The trials lasted for 2 hours only. In the Esteban study the best results were demonstrated in those patients assigned to only 1 spontaneous breathing trial.
	b. T-piece or CPAP trials: These spontaneous breathing trial (SBT) methods require that the patient breathe entirely on his or her own.			Refer to Chapter 2, Invasive and Noninvasive Modes and Methods of Mechanical Ventilation See Other References: 122	
	Recent research in the area suggests that protocol-driven weaning using distinct SBTs with CPAP or T-piece results in shorter ventilator duration and may be a superior method of weaning.	Studies using T-piece or CPAP used 2-hour trials to test ability. Subsequently, evaluation of length of trial duration suggests that one-half to 1 hour may be adequate.	VI: Clinical studies in a variety of patient populations and situations to support recommendations		Other methods of weaning such as the use of PS or IMV and/or the combined use of PS and IMV continue to be used but little data exists to suggest the modes are better than trials of CPAP or T-piece. In fact, in a survey of hospitals to determine the most prevalent weaning modes and methods, the ventilator duration was longest in those who were assigned to the combined IMV/PSV mode (see Other References: 56). However, PS may be a better choice for those who fail trials of spontaneous breathing on CPAP or T-piece, those who are very weak or debilitated, and those with poor cardiac reserve. A discussion of these and other related concepts follows.
	Assure adequate gas flow when using T-piece or CPAP for weaning or conditioning trials.	For example, if the T-piece or trach collar method is used, make sure that a high flow of gas is delivered to the patient by observing flow during inspiration.	VI: Clinical studies in a variety of patient populations and situations to support recommendations	See Other References: 8, 133	

Period of Use	Recommendation	Rationale for Recommendation	Level of Recommendation	Supporting References	Comments
Application and initial use (*cont.*)	Adjust the flow so that the mist is never entirely absent at peak inspiration.			.	
	• A reservoir with a T-piece can also help ensure adequate source gas during inspiration. • With CPAP, ensure that sensitivity is set so that the patient can easily trigger flow from the ventilator. Flow triggering is a superior method.	See discussion of flow vs pressure triggering above and refer to Chapter 2, Modes and Methods of Invasive and Noninvasive Mechanical Ventilation.			
	c. Intermittent mandatory ventilation (IMV) requires that the clinician select a mandatory rate for the volume breaths. Between breaths, the patient is able to breathe at own rate and volume.			Refer to Chapter 2, Invasive and Noninvasive Modes and Methods of Mechanical Ventilation. See Other Reference: 122	
	1) Do not require long weaning trials on low levels of IMV. IMV rates below 4/min may result in a high level of work.	Traditionally, weaning with IMV occurs by gradually reducing the ventilator (mandatory) breaths until the patient is breathing entirely spontaneously. This amount of work may be too much for some, resulting in fatigue.			
	2) When low IMV rates are used, rest should be assured to prevent fatigue.	Remember that WOB is increased with low IMV rates.	IV: Limited clinical studies to support recommendations	See Other References: 11, 65, 73, 133	
	3) IMV plus PS may be used to decrease WOB associated with spontaneous breaths. During weaning, however, the combined modes may result in prolonged weaning duration. Consider switching to PSV alone for weaning trials (see below).	Since the advent of PS, application of IMV+PS is widespread. PS can reduce the work associated with spontaneous breathing through circuits and small endotracheal tubes and may be used with IMV to accomplish this goal.	IV: Limited clinical studies to support recommendations	See Other References: 56, 59, 116, 133	

Period of Use	Recommendation	Rationale for Recommendation	Level of Recommendation	Supporting References	Comments
Application and initial use (*cont.*)		At least 1 study that looked at weaning duration with the use of IMV+PS noted longer weaning times with the combined method than with any other mode or method. The reasons are unclear, but the following have been hypothesized: • The mixing of volume and pressure breaths is not physiological. Patients may not adjust well. • The process of weaning with the mixed modes is cumbersome and potentially variable. Delays result.	IV: Limited clinical studies to support recommendations	See Other References: 56	This multisite study used a survey designed to describe weaning practices. The authors proposed the listed hypotheses; other explanations may also account for the differences. Studies are needed to evaluate this relationship further.
	d. Pressure support ventilation (PSV) requires that the clinician select a pressure level. When the patient initiates a breath, the ventilator senses the negative pressure and delivers a high flow of gas; the selected pressure level is reached early in inspiration. The pressure level is maintained throughout the inspiratory phase.	With PSV the patient controls the parameters of RR, inspiratory time, and V_T.	VI: Clinical studies in a variety of patient populations and situations to support recommendations	Refer to Chapter 2, Invasive and Noninvasive Modes and Methods of Mechanical Ventilation. See Other References: 122	PSV is a spontaneous breathing mode and may be used for weaning trials. However, PSV at any level provides more support than do the CPAP or T-piece methods. The trials are less aggressive. Thus, PSV may be especially well suited for those patients who do not do well with CPAP or T-piece trials, are extremely deconditioned and weak, and in those whose cardiac reserve is such that abrupt intrathoracic pressure fluctuations are poorly tolerated. An example of this is the patient with congestive heart failure who benefits from positive pressure ventilation (ie, decreased venous return). In this patient the increased preload during CPAP or T-piece trials overwhelms the hearts ability to compensate.
	1) Weaning may be accomplished gradually by reducing the PS level. PS is associated with less WOB than with the volume	PS provides low-pressure, high-volume work, which may be tolerated for longer intervals than high-pressure, low-volume work.		See Other References: 17, 116	

Period of Use	Recommendation	Rationale for Recommendation	Level of Recommendation	Supporting References	Comments
Application and initial use *(cont.)*	modes, so longer weaning trials may be well tolerated. Lower VTs and higher RRs are expected during trials.				
	2) To ensure respiratory muscle rest increase PS level to attain RR, < 20; no accessory muscle use; and V_I, 8 to 10 mL/kg (PSV max).	Respiratory muscle unloading is possible during PS breathing, provided the level is adjusted to attain these goals.	V: Clinical studies in more than 1 or 2 different patient populations or situations to support recommendations	See Other References: 16, 17, 116, 132	To assure adequate rest, some clinicians prefer switching to a volume mode (or mixing PS with IMV) at night or at rest. In some cases (eg, patients with secretions) the combination of secretions and a decreased ventilatory drive during sleep may prevent attainment of target V_T and RR. Volume is assured with volume ventilation, so switching to a volume mode may be more protective.
	4. Weaning protocols These are guidelines or algorithms for systematic progression of ventilator weaning. Commonly identified protocol components consist of a weaning screen, identification of a mode and method, criteria for when to stop a trial (signs of intolerance), and how to provide respiratory muscle rest.	Protocols are designed to give clinicians the authority to move the patient through the different steps ordered by the physician. Protocols and algorithms are becoming more common in units. Their use decreases variation in care practices that may prolong ventilator duration.		See Annotated Bibliography: 1, 3–10 See Other References: 71, 158	Weaning protocols use a wide range of vital signs, symptoms, laboratory data, assessment findings, and noninvasive techniques to monitor progress. (See "Ongoing Monitoring" below and sample protocols in Appendix 3D.) The evidence strongly supports the use of protocols for weaning.
		In addition to protocols for weaning, other protocols designed to manage sedation and glucose have resulted in improved clinical and financial outcomes in weaning patients (discussed in assessment section).			

Period of Use	Recommendation	Rationale for Recommendation	Level of Recommendation	Supporting References	Comments
Application and initial use *(cont.)*	a. The use of weaning trial protocols is linked to improved outcomes in ventilated patients. Protocols should be used to ensure timely, efficient, and safe weaning trials in both short- and long-term ventilated patient populations.	A number of randomized controlled studies suggest that the use of protocols to test ability and progress weaning shortens weaning duration.	VI: Clinical studies in a variety of patient populations and situations to support recommendations	See Annotated Bibliography: 1, 5, 6, 7, 8, 9	One major advantage of a weaning protocol is that progress is not impeded by common system problems such as waiting until rounds are completed to obtain weaning trial orders. Unlike other studies, Krishnan et al, found no difference between protocol-directed trials and intensivist-driven trials (see Other References: 93). This finding may have been a result of the physicians' awareness of studies demonstrating the effectiveness of aggressive application of spontaneous breathing trials on outcomes.
	• Although studies on protocols to date have predominately used spontaneous breathing trials (SBT) using CPAP or T-piece that clearly demonstrate their positive impact on outcomes, the efficacy of other potential modes or methods has not been clarified. • Use of protocols (regardless of the mode or method) have been linked to better outcomes. • An essential aspect of protocols may be the attention paid to the amount of work provided. Rest intervals are also important to prevent respiratory muscle fatigue and to attain the greatest conditioning effect.	In studies by Brochard et al and Esteban et al, weaning methods were compared to determine which resulted in the shortest weaning duration. Although the results appear contradictory as to which method was superior, the findings may be a result of the application of the modes (eg, adequacy of rest/work ratio) rather than the modes themselves. Vitacca et al compared different protocolized methods of weaning patients with COPD to determine the best method for this patient population. No mode or method emerged as superior; however, all patients assigned to a protocol did better than those with no protocol.	V: Clinical studies in more than 1 or 2 different patient populations or situations to support recommendations	See Annotated Bibliography: 1, 6 See Other References: 158	In the sample protocols in Appendix 3D it is important to note the shorter weaning trial durations suggested for use with CPAP. This is because CPAP (T-piece, etc) provides higher workloads. Training intervals are necessarily shorter than with PSV, which provides for lower workloads. While the studies cited suggest that these applications may result in shorter weaning times, more studies are needed with better control of the work/rest ratios and using different modes and methods before the concept can be fully endorsed.
	b. Use a weaning screen to identify those ready to attempt a weaning trial. Generally the screens include such criteria as: resolution of the reason for mechanical ventila-	Long-term ventilation patients assigned to a protocol that assured daily testing of ability to breathe spontaneously were weaned more quickly than were the control groups.	VI: Clinical studies in a variety of patient populations and situations to support recommendations	See Annotated Bibliography: 1, 5, 6, 9	Results suggest that aggressive, well-monitored testing of ability shortens ventilator duration without harming the patient. An example of a wean screen is found in the Appendix 3D.

Period of Use	Recommendation	Rationale for Recommendation	Level of Recommendation	Supporting References	Comments
Application and initial use *(cont.)*	tion, patient stability, identification of threshold levels of FIO$_2$, and PEEP to name just a few. The screen is designed to assure that physiologic stability is present and that the patient is improving. It is important that the criteria not be overly restrictive. Protocols that encourage prompt recognition of weaning trial readiness may result in earlier ventilator discontinuance. Entry criteria (wean screen criteria) help identify attainment of the weaning stage.				
	c. Identify a mode or method for weaning trials. Trial duration should be defined and adherence monitored.	Numerous randomized trials using protocols for SBTs with CPAP or a T-piece have been accomplished. The methods result in shorter ventilator duration and other clinical outcomes. These methods are highly recommended as having the highest scientific merit and should be used in practice. PS has also been used successfully in a few studies. See comments on the use of PSV for weaning trials in the section on modes and methods.	VI: Clinical studies in a variety of patient populations and situations to support recommendations	See Annotated Bibliography: 5, 7, 8, 9 See Other References: 55	Generally the trials with CPAP or T-piece last only 1–2 hours. Data from Esteban et al suggest that 1 hour (or less) may be sufficient to determine successful weaning in the majority of patients and that PSV may be equally effective. Signs of intolerance generally emerge early in these trials.
		Trial duration may be different, depending on the mode or method. (Please refer to discussion of respiratory muscle work earlier in this table.)		See Annotated Bibliography: 8 See Other References: 29, 40, 41, 68, 96, 104, 136, 137, 155	

Period of Use	Recommendation	Rationale for Recommendation	Level of Recommendation	Supporting References	Comments
Application and initial use *(cont.)*	d. Identify when to stop a trial, ie, signs of intolerance	Decisions related to the choice of mode or method for trials should incorporate consideration of individual characteristics of the patient.	VI: Clinical studies in a variety of patient populations and situations to support recommendations	See Annotated Bibliography: 1, 3, 5–9	For example, a patient with limited cardiac reserve may not tolerate abrupt changes in positive pressure. Venous return may be increased substantially during spontaneous breathing trials with CPAP or T-piece and overwhelm the patient's ability to compensate. In this example PS may be a gentler, better tolerated mode. Patients with severe myopathies may also do better with a PS wean trial.
	e. If signs of intolerance emerge, the trial should be stopped and the patient supported (and rested) on the ventilator.	Weaning trial intolerance may be assessed with a combination of noninvasive signs and symptoms. Included are V_T (if using CPAP this is easily measured by observing the ventilator digital readout display), RR, change in BP or HR, dyspnea, diaphoresis, and other signs of distress. ABGs are helpful but often not required. When these signs and symptoms occur, little is gained by continuing the trials. Fatigue and failure are likely.	VI: Clinical studies in a variety of patient populations and situations to support recommendations	See Annotated Bibliography: 1, 3, 5–9	
	5. Tracheostomy: Timing and weaning trials				
	Until recently no randomized controlled trials had been done to determine the importance of tracheostomy, and timing of tracheostomy, in patients requiring prolonged MV. Recently however, data has emerged suggesting that early tracheostomy in those likely to require ventilation for > 14 days, improves outcomes.	In a study by Rumback et al, 120 patients projected to require MV for > 14 days were randomly assigned to percutaneous tracheostomy within 48 hours. Mortality, incidence of pneumonia, and accidental extubations were all statistically significantly improved in the early tracheostomy group compared to the controls. They also had shorter ICU lengths of stay, shorter ventilator duration, and less damage to the mouth and larynx.	V: Clinical studies in more than 1 or 2 different patient populations or situations to support recommendations	See Other References: 128	These findings are intriguing but must be cautiously interpreted. Weaning trials with tracheostomy tubes in place may be more aggressively implemented than with an endotracheal tube. Because extubation is not required to determine ability to spontaneously breath for > 24 hours it is likely that this may account for the improved outcomes noted in this study. It is also likely that the requirement for sedation is less than what may be required to assure patient comfort and safety when endotracheal tubes are used.

Period of Use	Recommendation	Rationale for Recommendation	Level of Recommendation	Supporting References	Comments
Application and initial use *(cont.)*	Although we have learned much about the superiority of weaning trials using aggressive weaning screens and protocols, this new data suggest that additional benefits may be realized with early tracheostomy in those likely to require ventilation for > 14 days. At a minimum, tracheostomy should be considered earlier in the course of MV than has traditionally been the case.	With the exception of those conditions where the need for a tracheostomy was obvious (eg, spinal cord injury), prior to this study tracheostomy was commonly considered only after 10–12 days of MV. Other reasons included a history of unsuccessful weaning trials, patient comfort, and patients who could not protect their airway. This study suggests that the major determinant for the need of tracheostomy should be the judgment of clinicians that the patient may require ventilation longer than 14 days.			
	The presence of a tracheostomy tube does allow for more aggressive weaning trials as the end point is not extubation but spontaneous breathing for at least 24 hours. In difficult-to-wean cases, trials should be progressed gradually. A plan incorporating daytime trials, with nighttime rest on the ventilator, often works well. Progression to spontaneous breathing during the night is accomplished when daytime goals are attained. Concepts of respiratory muscle rest, work, and fatigue apply, as does the need for systematic assessment of impediments and correction of same.	Currently no studies exist that demonstrate a superior method for weaning tracheostomy patients who require extremely prolonged stays on the ventilator (ie, weeks to months).			
	Care delivery systems (systematic, comprehensive approaches)				
	Systematic approaches are to be encouraged as they decrease variation in care and are associated with improved clinical and economic outcomes in patients ventilated both short term and long term.	System models vary in scope and design, but the common focus is a systematic, progressive approach to weaning. Generally these models include numerous process components designed to assure evidence-based care. To	V: Clinical studies in more than 1 or 2 different patient populations or situations to support recommendations	See Annotated Bibliography: 3, 10 See Other References: 22, 76, 77	Institutional buy-in for these initiatives is essential for success. Further, due to the complexity of some of the models of care, responsibility for the management, monitoring, and updating of the process is essential.

Period of Use	Recommendation	Rationale for Recommendation	Level of Recommendation	Supporting References	Comments
Application and initial use (*cont.*)		that end they often include a clinical pathway and protocols for weaning trials and the management of other aspects of care (ie, glucose control and sedation management). Importantly, clinicians (often advanced practice nurses) are identified to manage and monitor the approaches.			
	Care delivery models vary in complexity and scope and examples are described below.				
	1. Weaning teams: a. May promote systematic, comprehensive care and positive outcomes.	Few studies exist that focus on the use of collaborative weaning teams. While at least 1 study using a weaning team (physician, nurse, and respiratory care practitioner) did demonstrate improved outcomes in those managed by the team versus the in-house physician staff, the study used a retrospective-prospective design and has not been replicated.	IV: Limited clinical studies to support recommendations	See Other References: 31	While the use of such a team inherently makes sense and is likely to be helpful, the development and sustained support of such a team is difficult to assure. In addition the complexity of these patients may require a more comprehensive approach as seen with more comprehensive system initiatives (described below).
	b. Weaning teams are composed of caregivers most involved in the weaning process. For a weaning team to be effective, the members must be knowledgeable, able to clearly articulate the plan to caregivers, and agree to a common philosophy of weaning.	In traditional models of care, weaning is often considered the work of respiratory therapists. The physician writes the orders and the therapist is the sole consultant to the physician regarding weaning plans. This approach does not serve this complex patient population well as it is neither collaborative nor coordinated. For weaning teams to be effective, all essential caregivers should be represented. Team members must agree on some philosophical premises that guide the weaning process and have institutional buy-in to ensure weaning plans and recommendations are followed.	IV: Limited clinical studies to support recommendations		To be efficient, weaning teams must not be too large, but they must incorporate the professionals most involved in the patient's care. Further, it is important that the team members regularly seek additional information from other professionals whose input is supportive to the process. Follow-up is essential and includes note writing and communication with bedside caregivers, MDs, family, and the patient.

Period of Use	Recommendation	Rationale for Recommendation	Level of Recommendation	Supporting References	Comments
Application and initial use *(cont.)*	2. Comprehensive system initiatives (outcomes management, case management, etc): These programs incorporate institutional buy-in and the inclusion of multidisciplinary input. A well-designed program contributes to positive outcomes for ventilated patients.	To date only 2 large system initiatives have been published.	V: Clinical studies in more than 1 or 2 different patient populations or situations to support recommendations	See Annotated Bibliography: 3, 10	
	The systematic focus of the models ensures streamlined, efficient, and cost effective care and are recommended.	However, other systematic approaches with more limited scope (ie, based in only a single unit), also demonstrate positive results. Programs that decrease variability in care are linked to positive outcomes.		See Annotated Bibliography: 5, 7, 9 See Other References: 71, 76, 77	Henneman et al used a grease board in a MICU to assure that a collaborative weaning plan was developed, implemented, and followed.
		In a study by Burns et al patients ventilated > 3 days were managed and monitored using outcomes managers (advanced practice nurses) in 5 adult critical care units. The program incorporated the use of a multidisciplinary, evidence-based clinical pathway, protocols for weaning trials, and the management of sedation. Significant improvements were noted in all variables of interest (ventilator duration, ICU and hospital LOS, and mortality).		See Annotated Bibliography: 3	Both of these studies represented large numbers of patients. Importantly, the programs are unlikely to do well without consistent attention being paid to the multiple aspects of care. Further, as new evidence emerges related to best practices, it is essential that they be incorporated into the standardized plans (ie, pathway or algorithm).
		Smyrinos et al, using a similar comprehensive approach (weaning algorithm, multidisciplinary evidence-based plan of care, and a nurse to manage the process) in 3 critical care units, demonstrated significant positive gains in ventilator duration and ICU and hospital LOS.		See Annotated Bibliography: 10	

Period of Use	Recommendation	Rationale for Recommendation	Level of Recommendation	Supporting References	Comments
Application and initial use *(cont.)*	Unlike some surgical populations of patients assigned to a clinical pathway, it is difficult to predict when certain elements of care should be initiated in the patient ventilated long-term. For example, critical pathways designed for the long-term ventilated patient cannot be designed in time increments. Instead, stages of the weaning process may be a more reasonable approach.	The value of a critical pathway is as a tool to help focus and advance care. This systematic approach may help reduce the lapses in care delivery that traditionally have resulted in complications and, thus, longer hospitalizations.	II: Theory based, no research data to support recommendations; recommendations from expert consensus group may exist	See Annotated Bibliography: 3 See Other References: 22, 38	If a pathway is used to chart care for the patients, it is essential that appropriate progression of the pathway be assured. Pathways do not progress automatically.
	A knowledgeable clinician manager is essential to the effective use of such a system. Successful attributes and qualifications include clinical expertise (ie, advanced knowledge of pulmonary diseases and weaning), excellent communication skills, ability to lead a multidisciplinary team, and demonstrated effectiveness as a change agent.	While many institutions use less stringent criteria to select a care manager, and have designated utilization review nurses and others to fill this role, experts who work with patients requiring long-term ventilation believe that such applications will not result in positive outcomes. Appropriate and timely interventions are required to assure progressive care delivery. If the care manager is not an expert, applications are likely to be more superficial in scope, less sophisticated in reasoning, and less accepted by the multidisciplinary team.	IV: Limited clinical studies to support recommendations	See Annotated Bibliography: 3, 10 See Other References: 53	While critical pathways are helpful tools to assure systematic attention to important care elements, it is a knowledgeable clinician who can effect a reasoned and individualized application of the model. It is unlikely that any protocol or plan of care will be consistently used unless someone is charged with the authority to do so. In a study by Ely, application of a weaning protocol beyond the medical units in which it had been tested (ie, surgical units) was difficult. Though respiratory care practitioners were well trained and charged with protocol implementation, compliance with the spontaneous breathing trial portion of the protocol was poor. Reasons cited included such variables as lack of consistency of therapists in the units and lack of buy-in from the surgeons. Compliance did improve modestly with educational intervention. Use of a knowledgeable clinician, such as an outcomes manager, may provide a more efficient and effective method of assuring appropriate management, monitoring, and evaluation of such an initiative.

Period of Use	Recommendation	Rationale for Recommendation	Level of Recommendation	Supporting References	Comments
Application and initial use *(cont.)*	3. Special weaning units: may provide quality and cost effective care for patients requiring prolonged ventilation.				
	a. Specially designated weaning units are helpful.	The complex care of patients requiring prolonged ventilation focuses on rehabilitation and restoration of baseline status rather than the emergency or urgent care typically found in ICUs. The cost of care associated with stays in ICUs is very high, prompting many to look at different care models.	VI: Clinical studies in a variety of patient populations and situations to support recommendations	See Other References: 13, 24, 29, 49–51, 69, 81, 136–139, 159 Refer to Chapter 4, Management of Ventilated Patients Beyond the ICU: Home Care Management (Other Reference: 48)	
		Institutions frequently lose money on costly DRGs (eg, DRGs for tracheostomy 541 and 542 [previously 483]). Because each DRG is associated with a specific reimbursement linked to LOS, ventilator duration beyond the DRG-designated LOS may result in a financial shortfall. Hence the interest in transferring these patients to subacute rehabilitation units or to home.		See Annotated Bibliography: 8 See Other References: 13, 24, 29, 49–51, 69, 81, 136–139, 159 See Other References: 48	Unfortunately, the prevalence of *weaning centers* is decreasing and many hospitals are developing programs (such as those described and others) to care for patients requiring very long stays on the ventilator (ie, weeks to months and even years). Increasingly, home care of the ventilated patient is being considered as an option. Refer to Chapter 4, Beyond the ICU: Home Care Management of Patients Receiving Mechanical Ventilation.
	b. Weaning units have in many cases demonstrated that difficult-to-wean patients can be successfully weaned and that care is also cost effective.	Recent work suggests that outcomes of these very long-term ventilated patients are the same regardless of whether they are cared for in traditional critical care/acute care settings or in a ventilator weaning unit.	VI: Clinical studies in a variety of patient populations and situations to support recommendations	See Other References: 38, 43–45, 51, 52, 127, 136–139	

Period of Use	Recommendation	Rationale for Recommendation	Level of Recommendation	Supporting References	Comments
Application and initial use *(cont.)*	c. Weaning units may provide an environment more conducive to the process of weaning.	Weaning units focus on long-term patients' unique rehabilitation needs. ICUs are sometimes seen as insensitive to the needs of patients and families (eg, restricted visiting hours, noisy, numerous interruptions from a wide variety of caregivers). ICU staff may be frustrated with the lack of progress associated with these patients' care and the need to prioritize care planning based on the emergency needs of more critically ill patients.	II: Theory based, no research data to support recommendations; recommendations from expert consensus group may exist	See Other References: 38, 69, 136–139	Although it seems obvious that care in ICUs is not conducive to optimizing the weaning process, much can be done there to improve the care of MV patients (eg, open visiting hours, encouraging families to participate in the patient's care). Schedules to keep care planning on target are important. Protocols can be developed that empower team members such as nursing, physical therapy, and respiratory care to advance weaning and rehabilitation as needed.
Ongoing monitoring	Monitoring patient tolerance during weaning can be accomplished with a wide variety of clinical assessment techniques and invasive and noninvasive technology. Given the longer duration of hospitalization associated with these patients, noninvasive monitoring is more comfortable for the patient, less expensive than the frequent use of arterial blood gases (ABGs), and effective when used by knowledgeable caregivers. 1. Invasive monitoring: ABGs and arterial lines	Although the gold standard for assessing oxygenation and ventilation status in weaning patients is the measurement of ABGs, noninvasive technology (eg, pulse oximetry, ETCO$_2$ monitoring and respiratory waveforms) can be effectively used to decrease the frequency of ABG analysis. Assessment findings such as breathing pattern, RR, and V$_T$ can be safely used as criteria to start or stop trials.	VI: Clinical studies in a variety of patient populations and situations to support recommendations	Refer to *AACN Protocols for Practice: Noninvasive Monitoring,* 2nd ed. See Other References 19, 70, 146	See sample weaning protocols in Appendix 3D for examples of noninvasive criteria for starting and stopping weaning trials.
	a. Frequent use of arterial lines or ABGs in patients on prolonged ventilation is often unnecessary during weaning.	In the studies noted, the presence of knowledgeable caregivers (the use of a weaning team and advanced nurse clinicians) resulted in fewer tests, shorter ventilator duration, and increased cost savings.	VI: Clinical studies in a variety of patient populations and situations to support recommendations	See Annotated Bibliography: 3, 5, 8, 10 See Other References: 31, 71	Technology is only as good as the person using it. It is important to use a thoughtful, knowledgeable approach to assessment in the weaning patient to avoid excessively invasive and costly care. The use of experts to systematically guide the weaning process is key in any care delivery model.

Period of Use	Recommendation	Rationale for Recommendation	Level of Recommendation	Supporting References	Comments
Ongoing monitoring *(cont.)*	b. ABGs are necessary periodically to confirm the adequacy of oxygenation and ventilation.	While noninvasive technology allows for fewer ABGs, there is no better measurement to assess tolerance. ABGs may not be required with each ventilator parameter change but should be considered with any acute changes or when noninvasive techniques provide insufficient assessment information.	VI: Clinical studies in a variety of patient populations and situations to support recommendations		
	2. Noninvasive monitoring should be used when available to help with weaning trials.	Detailed descriptions of noninvasive technologies is beyond the scope of this protocol. Therefore, for detailed descriptions and evidence-based recommendations *Noninvasive Monitoring*. The technologies, pulse oximetry, capnography, and respiratory waveforms are briefly described below.	VI: Clinical studies in a variety of patient populations and situations to support recommendations	See Other References: 19, 70, 146	
	a. Use pulse oximetry to monitor patients in whom oxygenation status is of concern.	Patients requiring MV are at risk for oxygenation problems. Continuous monitoring of oxygenation is expected because the technology is simple, accurate, and available.	VI: Clinical studies in a variety of patient populations and situations to support recommendations	See Other References: 70	Remember that while oxygenation status can be assessed with pulse oximetry, ventilation status cannot. If there are concerns related to adequacy of ventilation, obtain an ABG analysis.
	Pulse oximetry (SpO_2) is a noninvasive method of continually monitoring arterial oxygen saturation. The SpO_2 probe detects pulsatile flow and calculates the absorption of light by functional hemoglobin, which is then translated into an SpO_2.				
	b. End-tidal carbon dioxide ($ETCO_2$) monitoring may be useful for monitoring patients during weaning trials. End-tidal carbon dioxide monitoring ($ETCO_2$) (also called capnometry or capnography): Uses a sampling/sensor connection at the patient	The technology may be especially helpful to evaluate weaning trial tolerance and efficiency of ventilation; however, $ETCO_2$ is most useful to trend changes in CO_2. An ABG analysis may still be required to assess actual $PaCO_2$.	IV: Limited clinical studies to support recommendations	See Other References: 146	Concerns about $ETCO_2$ monitoring are frequently cited. The equipment may be cumbersome and heavy, and "trending" is not always accurate—especially when the spontaneous breathing pattern is rapid and shallow. With rapid, shallow breathing, an increase in dead space ventilation makes $ETCO_2$ readings

Period of Use	Recommendation	Rationale for Recommendation	Level of Recommendation	Supporting References	Comments
Ongoing monitoring *(cont.)*	wye. Exhaled CO_2 is continually measured breath to breath. $ETCO_2$ waveforms can be used to evaluate breathing patterns during weaning.				difficult to interpret (often the $ETCO_2$ will be markedly lower than that attained with an ABG). With mechanical breaths, there is less dead space ventilation and trends in $ETCO_2/PaCO_2$ will be more consistent and accurate. Trends may also be affected by whether a sidestream or main-stream sensor is used. To use $ETCO_2$ effectively in assessing weaning tolerance, clinicians must understand these concepts.
	c. Respiratory waveform monitoring Waveform displays are currently available on most new ventilators. Pressure, volume, flow, and loop waveform configurations are displayed on the ventilators and are helpful to monitor patient-ventilator synchrony, auto-PEEP, and tolerance.	The respiratory waveforms can provide important information to clinicians. Unfortunately, they are often not understood.	II: Theory based, no research data to support recommendations; recommendations from expert consensus group may exist	See Other References: 19	The use of respiratory waveforms is an effective way to teach concepts related to MV, flow, and WOB. The waveforms, which may be graphed, clearly document patient tolerance. Often such graphic evidence is adequate to make decisions related to the need for increased ventilatory support or other interventions. This may, in part, eliminate the need for frequent ABGs and, importantly, excessively long and fatiguing weaning trials.
	Signs and symptoms of intolerance 1. Breathing patterns a. Chest abdominal asynchrony may herald impending fatigue and respiratory failure. 1) Assess the etiology immediately and initiate appropriate interventions. As noted earlier, patients (except quadriplegic patients) should have eupneic breathing patterns.	See "Work of Breathing" above.	VI: Clinical studies in a variety of patient populations and situations to support recommendations	See Annotated Bibliography: 11 See Other References: 152, 153	

Period of Use	Recommendation	Rationale for Recommendation	Level of Recommendation	Supporting References	Comments
Ongoing monitoring (*cont.*)	2) Return patient to a support mode or level of ventilation.	Continued work will result in respiratory fatigue and failure.			
	b. Rapid/shallow breathing pattern: A respiratory rate above 25/min is rarely normal; explore the etiology and initiate appropriate interventions. A rapid/shallow breathing pattern may occur immediately following extubation but should not persist. Patients who fail extubation frequently evidence additional signs of intolerance such as diaphoresis, hypertension, tachycardia, and decreased oxygen saturation within 5 minutes of extubation.	As noted earlier, studies have demonstrated that this breathing pattern generally heralds fatigue.	VI: Clinical studies in a variety of patient populations and situations to support recommendations		Patients who are stressed physiologically do not have adequate pulmonary reserve; their breathing pattern may be rapid and shallow as a result. Too often, clinicians who care for these patients explain the pattern away. ("He always breathes like that.") Rapid/shallow breathing patterns are rarely normal.
	c. Cheyne Stokes respirations often present with congestive heart failure (CHF) and neurologic events. If seen in the weaning patient, defer weaning trials until the etiology is determined and treated.	CHF is the most common cause of Cheyne-Stokes breathing. This is important as the emergence of Cheyne-Stokes breathing may herald the need for aggressive preload and afterload reduction before attempting spontaneous breathing trials. When patients are switched from positive pressure ventilation to spontaneous (negative pressure ventilation), the increased venous return may overwhelm the heart's ability to compensate. Pulmonary edema and unsuccessful weaning trials may result.	IV: Limited studies to support recommendations	See Other References: 96, 140	
	2. Symptoms	Symptoms, by definition, are what the patient experiences.			
	a. Thresholds for tolerance of symptoms vary between patients. Visual analog scales are a useful way to monitor individual patient symptoms.		IV: Limited clinical studies to support recommendations	See Other References: 25, 98	

Period of Use	Recommendation	Rationale for Recommendation	Level of Recommendation	Supporting References	Comments
Ongoing monitoring *(cont.)*	b. Symptoms such as dyspnea, anxiety, discomfort, fear, and panic are assumed to affect weaning trial outcomes negatively. Interventions to offset the symptoms (eg, sedating agents, relaxation techniques, biofeedback) are considered appropriate.	Patient perceptions of the ventilation experience have been described as uncomfortable and anxiety-producing. Complicating the issue is the finding in a number of studies that patient symptoms may not correlate with the caregiver perceptions of symptoms. In addition, 1 study suggests that much of the communication between caregiver and patient may be inaccurately interpreted making the accurate application of symptom assessments very difficult. Much work in the area of symptom management (specifically dyspnea) has been done in COPD patients, where commonly tracked outcome measures include quality-of-life and functional measures. In the weaning patient other measures are necessary. In 1 study in which biofeedback was used to enhance relaxation, decrease anxiety, and maintain V_T during weaning, the result was increased V_T and reduced mean ventilator days in the biofeedback group versus the control group. While this study suggests that controlling symptoms may result in positive outcomes, more work needs to be done to define the relationship. Though many of the studies in the area of symptoms were done in the late 1980s and early 1990s, the work is still applicable.	V: Clinical studies in more than 1 or 2 different patient populations or situations to support recommendations	See Other References: 1, 2, 10, 15, 25, 72, 75, 79, 94, 98	Often clinicians respond to symptoms with interventions designed to decrease the symptom severity (eg, suctioning, repositioning, medicating, and comforting measures). These commonsense, humane responses should be encouraged. Too often dyspnea is assumed to have a psychological origin and physiological reasons are inadequately explored.
	c. Dyspnea: Etiologies vary. Though anxiety may be associated with dyspnea it is often difficult to determine if the dyspnea has a psychological or physiologic etiology. Therefore, eliminate the physiological reasons for dyspnea before determining	Physiological causes include states that result in hypoxemia and/or pain. Examples include but are not limited to: • Ventilator malfunction or inappropriate settings (eg, inadequate flow adjustment) • Excessive secretions • Bronchospasm • Auto-PEEP	V: Clinical studies in more than 1 or 2 different patient populations or situations to support recommendations	See Other References: 25	Inaccurate assessments of the etiology of dyspnea can result in needlessly prolonged ventilator duration. Use of a scale (eg, 0–10) to rate dyspnea is helpful to assess the degree of dyspnea and the efficacy of interventions.

Period of Use	Recommendation	Rationale for Recommendation	Level of Recommendation	Supporting References	Comments
Ongoing monitoring *(cont.)*	that the symptom is of psychological origin.	• Respiratory muscle fatigue • Left ventricular failure or overload • Atelectasis • Pleural effusion • Pneumothorax • Pulmonary embolus • Inappropriate use of narcotics or sedatives			
Prevention of complications	Clinicians caring for weaning patients must be competent and knowledgeable to ensure accurate risk assessment and appropriate and timely interventions.	Numerous complications are associated with MV, especially prolonged ventilation, and include barotrauma, patient-ventilator asynchrony, aspiration pneumonia, infections, and death. Complications related to MV are briefly discussed below as they are inexorably linked to weaning. However, extensive discussion is beyond the scope of this protocol.	VI: Clinical studies in a variety of patient populations and situations to support recommendations	See Other References: 122	
	Quality control measures must be in place (see below).				
	1. Identify the potential for barotrauma.	Frequently associated with the use of high pressures and large V_Ts in patients with ARDS and status asthmaticus.		Refer to Chapter 2, Invasive and Noninvasive Modes and Methods of Mechanical Ventilation (Other References: 122, 150)	
	a. During the acute stage identify patients at risk. Use protective ventilatory strategies (ie, low V_T ventilation, optimal PEEP levels, and permissive hypercarbia) as appropriate.	High distending pressures (plateau pressures > 30 cm H_2O) are associated with volutrauma and alveolar fractures. As a result, ventilatory strategies are employed. Refer to mechanical ventilation protocol.		Refer to Chapter 2, Invasive and Noninvasive Modes and Methods of Mechanical Ventilation.	While these strategies are necessary in the acute stage versus the weaning stage, they greatly affect outcomes such as duration of ventilation, ICU and hospital LOS, and mortality and should be part of the continuum of care provided for the ventilated patient. Other modes of ventilation such as bi-phasic ventilation, airway pressure release ventilation (APRV) and high-frequency oscillation may offer attractive characteristics for the ventilation of the stiff lung. For

Period of Use	Recommendation	Rationale for Recommendation	Level of Recommendation	Supporting References	Comments
Prevention of complications *(cont.)*					example, bi-phasic ventilation and APRV allow for high levels of PEEP to be used to "open the lung" in conjunction with patient initiated spontaneous breathing.
	b. Monitor for auto-PEEP (inadequate expiratory time), especially in those at risk (ie, asthmatics, patients with high minute ventilations, COPD).	Interventions to offset auto-PEEP include decreasing respiratory rate, shortening inspiratory time, lengthening expiratory time, and using bronchodilators.			
	c. Monitor changes in airway pressure when on volume modes of ventilation and VT in those on pressure modes. Evaluate the etiology of the changes and intervene quickly.	Changes in compliance may be secondary to a pneumothorax. Early detection may prevent cardiac tamponade and death.			
	2. Ensure patient ventilator synchrony. a. Asynchrony most often results from inadequate flow delivery during inspiration.	See "Ongoing Monitoring" and section on "Work of Breathing" above in addition to mechanical ventilation protocol.			
	b. With rapid respiratory rates, asynchrony can be magnified by the inability of the ventilator to provide adequate flow to meet the patient's inspiratory demand.	Often called *bucking the vent* or *out-of phase,* patient-ventilator asynchrony is common yet poorly managed in many cases. Often it is a result of inadequate flow delivery. See "Work of Breathing."			Because the concept is often misunderstood, interventions may inappropriately focus on sedating the patient instead of adjusting ventilator flow. The assessment of respiratory waveforms is an extremely useful noninvasive technique to assess patient-ventilator asynchrony or intolerance. (See Other References: 19)
	3. Nosocomial or hospital-acquired pneumonias: VAP is described as a pneumonia developing after 3–5 days of MV.	VAP is associated with poor outcomes (eg, increased ventilator duration, LOS, and mortality).		See Other References: 36, 58, 84, 148	

Period of Use	Recommendation	Rationale for Recommendation	Level of Recommendation	Supporting References	Comments
Prevention of complications *(cont.)*	Use interventions to prevent this common complication of prolonged ventilation. Some are noted.	CDC guidelines for the prevention of "healthcare-associated pneumonia" have been published. The reader is encouraged to refer to the guideline for detailed recommendations. The recommendations include: • Scrupulous hand washing and preventing the backflow of secretions and fluid into the lungs • Maintaining the head of the bed at 30° or higher • Avoiding unnecessary circuit changes (Dreyfuss et al noted that pneumonia risk was not higher when circuits were not changed for the duration of patient use than when changed every 48 hours.) • The use of continuous aspiration of subglottic secretions (CASS) tubes • Prevention of reintubation (unsuccessful extubation) • The use of noninvasive ventilation when possible • Avoiding unnecessary nasally placed tubes	VI: Clinical studies in a variety of patient populations and situations to support recommendations	See Other Reference: 148 See Other References: 46	Some unresolved issues relate to the use of oral decontamination methods (chlorhexidine, etc), the selective use of GI prophylaxis agents, and gastric feeding-free intervals. The use of gastric feeding-free intervals, thought to decrease pH and thus prevent bacterial overgrowth, is less likely to be explored as an option given the current common use of insulin infusions (for tight glucose control). The gastric feeding-free intervals in this case may potentiate severe swings in glucose levels. (See Other References: 95, 144, 157)
Quality control	Weaning criteria	Using weaning criteria requires that the person measuring the criteria be adequately trained and the equipment be accurate.			For issues related to accurate measurement of weaning parameters, see related sections in this protocol and Appendixes 3A, 3B, 3C, 3D.
	Institutional outcomes measures: Care delivery models (eg, protocols, care paths) must be monitored in order to evaluate effectiveness.	Measuring care outcomes provides patients, payers, and institutions with quantifiable data on system interventions.		See Annotated Bibliography: 3, 10 Other Reference: 22	Outcomes measures depend on the system initiative. For the patient requiring prolonged ventilation, measures may include (but are not limited to) individual, aggregate, and long-term outcomes, including: • Complications (VAP, aspirations, pneumothorax, etc.) • Extubation, reintubation, weaning, and mortality rates • Ventilator duration • Tracheostomy (when placed, type of tra-

Period of Use	Recommendation	Rationale for Recommendation	Level of Recommendation	Supporting References	Comments
Quality control *(cont.)*					cheostomy, time to wean, etc.) • LOS (in critical care, step-down, institution, etc.) • Quality of life • Functional state, transfer, or disposition • Mortality (in the hospital and following hospitalization).

ANNOTATED BIBLIOGRAPHY

1. Brochard L, Rauss A, Benito S, et al. Comparison of three methods of gradual withdrawal from ventilatory support during weaning from mechanical ventilation. *Am J Respir Crit Care Med.* 1994;150:896–903.

Study Sample

Researchers tested 456 mechanically ventilated patients from 3 ICUs with standard weaning criteria and assigned them to a 2-hour trial of spontaneous breathing. Of this sample, 109 who were not able to sustain the spontaneous breathing trial were included in the randomized study.

Comparison Studied

Patients were assigned to 1 of 3 weaning techniques: T-piece, synchronized intermittent mandatory ventilation (SIMV), or pressure support ventilation (PSV). Criteria for stopping trials and extubation were standardized among methods.

Study Procedures

T-piece: Patients were placed on multiple trials of T-piece for up to 2 hours (providing signs of intolerance did not occur) with 1-hour rest periods on the assist-control (A/C) mode (with a high backup rate) between trials. When a 2-hour trial was accomplished without signs of intolerance, the decision was made to extubate.

SIMV: SIMV rate for trials was set at half that of controlled or A/C mode rate. Twice daily the ventilator rate was decreased by 2 to 4 breaths if no signs of intolerance were demonstrated, in which case ventilator rate was increased to the preceding level. When the patient was able to tolerate an SIMV rate of ≤ 4 for 24 hours, extubation was considered.

PSV: PSV level was adjusted to attain a respiratory rate of 20 to 30 per minute. Twice each day PSV was decreased by 2 to 4 cm H_2O. If signs of intolerance evolved the PSV level was increased back to the preceding level. When the patient was able to tolerate PSV of ≤ 8 cm H_2O for 24 hours, extubation was considered.

Key Results

With PSV both weaning duration and total length of stay in the ICU were significantly shorter.

Study Strengths and Weaknesses

Study strengths are the large sample; the clear, replicable entry and exit criteria for the different methods; and the well-designed study methods. Of major concern is the lack of control related to the work associated with each of the methods. For example, breathing spontaneously through a ventilator circuit on an SIMV of ≤ 4 for more than 24 hours

is considered excessive. The protocols may not have provided comparable respiratory muscle rest, making the results difficult to interpret.

Clinical Implications

Weaning outcomes may be influenced by the ventilatory strategy chosen. Weaning protocols are helpful tools to guide weaning trials regardless of the mode or method.

2. Burns SM, Burns JE, Truwit JD. Comparison of five clinical weaning indices. *Am J Crit Care.* 1994;3:342–352.

Study Sample

The prospective convenience sample consisted of 37 adult critical care patients requiring mechanical ventilation for at least 7 days and identified as stable and ready to wean.

Comparison Studied

The Burns Wean Assessment Program (BWAP); weaning index (WI); respiratory frequency to tidal volume (f/V_T) ratio; compliance, rate, oxygenation, and pressure (CROP) index; and negative inspiratory pressure (NIP) were measured in order to test the efficacy of the 5 indices and establish a threshold for the BWAP.

Study Procedures

Indices were measured every other day until the patient weaned.

Key Results

With the exception of the BWAP, none of the indices changed significantly from preweaning scores. All indices had good negative predictive power but weak positive predictive power.

Study Strengths and Weaknesses

This is one of the first studies to test weaning criteria over the course of the weaning continuum rather than at the end (ie, extubation). The study describes the weaning process as gradual, with many peaks and valleys until weaning occurs, and clearly demonstrated the importance of nonpulmonary factors in weaning. However, the sample size (n = 37) was small and the prospective, noninterventional design lacks control over duration of weaning. In other words, patients may have been able to wean earlier, so the established BWAP threshold may actually be lower.

Clinical Implications

Systematic approaches using comprehensive weaning indices such as the BWAP may be useful to track trends in progress, keep care planning on target, and prevent unsuccessful weaning trials.

3. **Burns SM, Earven D, Fisher C, et al. Implementation of an institutional program to improve clinical and financial outcomes of patients requiring mechanical ventilation: one year outcomes and lessons learned. Crit Care Med. 2003;31:2752–2763.**

Study Sample

Patients from 5 adult critical care units (coronary, medical, neurological, surgical-trauma, thoracic-cardiovascular) who had been mechanically ventilated for greater than 3 consecutive days were monitored prospectively before the application of an outcomes managed (OM) approach (n = 595) and then following the institution of the model (n = 510). The OM model of care included an evidence-based clinical pathway, protocols for weaning and sedation use, and the selection of 4 advanced practice nurses (called *outcomes managers*) to manage and monitor the program.

Comparison Studied

Clinical and financial data were compared between pre-OM (control group) and post-OM groups.

Study Procedures

The OM approach was applied to all patients requiring mechanical ventilation longer than 3 consecutive days in the 5 units.

Key Results

Statistically significant differences in all clinical outcomes were demonstrated in the OM managed patients as compared to the control patients. Improved outcomes included: ventilator duration, intensive care length of stay, hospital length of stay, and mortality. Cost savings were over $3,000,000 in the OM group.

Study Strengths and Weaknesses

The strength of the study is the number of patients followed and the prospective rigorous study design. The major weakness of the study is that it is not a randomized controlled trial.

Clinical Implications

Few similar initiatives have been published. The OM approach assures that systematic assessment, management, and evaluation of this complex patient population occurs. By decreasing variation, outcomes improved. The approach and lessons learned in this process improvement project may be helpful to other institutions.

4. **Cook D, Meade M, Guyatt G, Griffith L, Booker L. *Evidence Report on Criteria for Weaning from Mechanical Ventilation.* Rockville, Md: Agency for Health Care Policy and Research; 1999. Contract No. 290-97-0017.**

Study Sample

This project, the McMaster University Evidence-Based Review of Weaning from Mechanical Ventilation, was sponsored by the US Agency for Health Care Policy and Research (AHCPR). Over 5,000 weaning citations were reviewed and 154 studies further analyzed for this evidence-based report. The report consists of 15 comprehensive data tables and 15 appendices.

Key Results

This comprehensive review determined the scientific merit of existing weaning criteria (eg, predictors). The report concluded that published weaning criteria fell short; indeed, they were not strong positive predictors. The report also suggested that multidisciplinary approaches to weaning and protocols did improve weaning outcomes.

5. **Ely EW, Baker AM, Dunagan DP, et al. Effect on the duration of mechanical ventilation of identifying patients capable of breathing spontaneously. *N Engl J Med.* 1996;335: 1864–1869.**

Study Sample

A randomized control trial of 300 adult patients receiving mechanical ventilation in medical and coronary ICUs formed the study sample.

Comparison Studied

Researchers sought to determine if daily screening of patients to identify those who were able to breathe spontaneously (and notifying their physicians of same) would promote earlier ventilator discontinuance as compared to those not screened.

Study Procedures

In the intervention group respiratory function was tested by physicians, nurses, and respiratory therapists to identify those who met criteria for "spontaneous breathing." Those identified were then assigned to a 2-hour trial of spontaneous breathing (SB) (T-piece or flow-by). If the trial was successful, a printed message was left in the chart noting that the patient had successfully completed a 2-hour trial and had an 85% chance of successfully staying off the ventilator for 48 hours. Decisions related to extubation were made by the attending physician, not the researchers. The control group was screened but received no other interventions.

Key Results

Patients randomly assigned to the intervention group had significantly shorter ventilator durations (median 4.5 vs 6 days) than those in the control group with a reintubation rate of 4%.

Study Strengths and Weaknesses

Strengths were the large sample size, clear entry and exit criteria, and spontaneous breathing methods that were more comparable (T-piece and flow-by) for work of breathing than other similar studies using spontaneous breathing trials (eg, CPAP, T-piece). Weaknesses were no control of resting levels of support, and decisions related to extubation were made by attending physician rather than the research team.

Clinical Implications

Daily screening and testing of weaning potential using SBTs appear to result in shorter ventilator duration. Weaning protocols are safe and effective.

6. Esteban A, Frutos F, Tobin M, et al. A comparison of four methods of weaning patients from mechanical ventilation. *N Engl J Med.* 1995;332:345–350.

Study Sample

The study sample consisted of 546 patients who had received mechanical ventilation for more than 7 days and were considered ready for weaning by their physicians. Of this sample 130 patients "failed" a 2-hour trial of spontaneous breathing and were randomly assigned to 1 of 4 weaning techniques. Criteria for "intolerance" were standardized for all techniques.

Comparison Studied

In this prospective, randomized, multicenter study, 4 weaning techniques were compared to determine duration of weaning.

Study Procedures

Subjects were randomly assigned to (1) intermittent mandatory ventilation (IMV) of 10, then decreased if tolerated twice daily by 2 to 4 breaths per minute; (2) PSV, which was initially set at 18 cm H_2O and reduced, if tolerated, by 2 to 4 cm H_2O twice daily; (3) intermittent trials of spontaneous breathing conducted at least twice daily; or (4) a once-daily trial of spontaneous breathing.

Key Results

Once-daily trials of spontaneous breathing led to statistically significantly quicker extubations (3 times quicker) than the other techniques.

Study Strengths and Weaknesses

This study had a large sample, well-designed study methods, and clear and replicable entry and exit criteria. As with the Brochard study (Annotated Bibliography: 1), concerns center around the level of rest provided by the different protocols. For example, with the spontaneous breathing method a high A/C level of 20 was used to rest compared to IMV where the resting level was 10.

Clinical Implications

Weaning outcomes may be influenced by the ventilatory technique used and by the type of respiratory muscle rest provided. Weaning protocols are helpful tools to direct weaning trials.

7. Kollef MH, Shapiro SD, Silver P, et al. A randomized, controlled trial of protocol-directed versus physician-directed weaning from mechanical ventilation. *Crit Care Med.* 1997;25:567–574.

Study Sample

Medical and surgical patients requiring mechanical ventilation in 2 university-affiliated teaching hospitals were studied.

Comparison Studied

Patients were randomly assigned to either a protocol-directed (n = 179) or physician-directed (n = 178) weaning.

Study Procedures

Protocol-directed weaning was carried out by trained nursing and respiratory care staff. The protocols defined entry criteria, definitions of intolerance (when to stop) and rest, and how to progress the trials. Physician-directed weaning consisted of a plan of care directed by the in-house critical care staff.

Key Results

The primary outcome variable, ventilator duration, was significantly better in the protocol-directed group. No difference in hospital length of stay or hospital mortality was demonstrated, but cost savings were realized in the protocol-directed group.

Study Strengths and Weaknesses

Weaknesses included the fact that the patients were drawn from short-term and long-term ventilated patients. A clearer definition of these categories would have made interpretation of the findings more helpful. An additional weakness is that medical and surgical housestaff were used for the physician-directed groups, and these physicians in training may not have had the experience to make good decisions about weaning. Additionally, the attending physicians could intervene with the weaning protocols potentially changing their effectiveness. Also, nurses and therapists may have wanted the protocol-directed weaning group to do better thus introducing a strong bias. The strength of the study is that it is a randomized controlled trial with a large sample size.

Clinical Implications

Protocol-directed weaning provided by nurses and therapists is both safe and effective. The protocols decrease practice variability.

8. **MacIntyre NR, Cook DJ, Ely EW Jr, et al. Evidence-based guidelines for weaning and discontinuing ventilatory support: a collective task force facilitated by the American College of Chest Physicians; the American Association for Respiratory Care; and the American College of Critical Care Medicine.** *Chest.* **2001;120(6 Suppl):375S–395S.**

Study Sample

This project sought to create a set of evidence-based clinical practice guidelines for ventilator weaning and discontinuation. The report did use the McMaster report (described above) in addition to additional evidence. A consensus process, based on the evidence (when available), was used to make recommendations.

Clinical Implications

This comprehensive report used both evidence and, when not available, expert opinion and consensus to make recommendations for the discontinuation of mechanical ventilation. The guidelines are extremely helpful for clinicians who work with this patient population.

9. **Marelich GP, Murin S, Battistella F, Inciardi J, Vierra T, Roby M. Protocol weaning of mechanical ventilation in medical and surgical patients by respiratory care practitioners and nurses: effect on weaning time and incidence of ventilator associated pneumonia.** *Chest.* **2000; 118:459–467.**

Study Sample

A group of 385 medical and surgical mechanically ventilated patients was studied. However, only 253 were evaluated from study entry to ventilator discontinuance.

Comparison Studied

A respiratory care practitioner and nurse-driven ventilator management protocol (VMP) for weaning was compared to standard (physician-directed) weaning.

Study Procedures

After enrollment, patients were randomly assigned to either VMP weaning or standard weaning. Ventilator duration and the incidence of ventilator-associated pneumonia (VAP) were compared between the study groups.

Key Results

VMP weaning demonstrated statistically significantly improved ventilator duration as compared to the control group, and VAP was lower in trauma patients but not significant.

Study Strengths and Weaknesses

The study was not (and could not be) blinded to the nurses and therapists. Thus the clinicians may have been biased in favor of the VAP and resulted in positive outcomes. VAP was defined with a clinical definition versus a pathologic definition.

Clinical Implications

These results, similar to others that report on the use of weaning protocols suggest that VMPs are effective and safe in the hands of nurses and therapists and superior to traditional physician weaning.

10. **Smyrnios NA, Connolly A, Wilson MM, et al. Effects of a multifaceted, multidisciplinary, hospital-wide quality improvement program on weaning from mechanical ventilation.** *Crit Care Med.* **2002;30:1224–1230.**

Study Sample

Patients deemed ventilator dependent in diagnosis-related groups (DRG) 475 (mechanical ventilation) and 483 (tracheostomy without head and neck surgery) admitted to adult medical, surgical and cardiac intensive care units were studied.

Comparison Studied

Baseline year data (n = 220) was compared to data from the intervention group in the first year (n = 246) and second year (n = 267).

Study Procedures

A weaning management program was implemented in the 3 ICUs. The program included the use of a standardized weaning protocol and multitiered system of caring for all ventilator dependent patients. Common medical barriers to weaning were managed with a standardized approach, and the process was managed and monitored by a pulmonary and critical care specialist and 2 pulmonary nurses.

Key Results

Significantly improved outcomes in the managed group included ventilator duration and ICU and hospital lengths of stay. Mortality improved but not significantly so.

Study Strengths and Weaknesses

The authors' definition of ventilator dependence is confusing and thus difficult to compare to other programs. Regardless, the strength of the study is its prospective design and the use of relatively rigorous methodology for such a large-scale institutional quality initiative.

Clinical Implications

This study, which uses a systematic approach to the care and management of mechanically ventilated patients, may be helpful to those who wish to implement a similar process improvement initiative.

11. Yang KL, Tobin MJ. A prospective study of indexes predicting the outcome of trials of weaning from mechanical ventilation. *N Engl J Med.* 1991;324:1445–1450.

Study Sample

Researchers selected 100 medical ICU patients who had received 8 days of ventilator support and who were clinically stable and considered ready to wean by their physician.

Comparison Studied

The threshold values for 2 indices were determined between successful and unsuccessful weaning trials in 36 patients, and the predictive accuracy of the values were tested prospectively on an additional 64 patients.

Study Procedures

Two indices, the index of rapid/shallow breathing (fx/VT) and the integrated CROP index, were calculated on the first 36 patients who were weaned (n = 24) or failed weaning (n = 12) to establish threshold values. The predictive power of the threshold values for each index were then assessed in the remaining 64 patients.

Key Results

The fx/VT ratio was the best predictor of successful weaning and failure but both the fx/VT and the CROP index were significantly associated with weaning outcome.

Study Strengths and Weaknesses

This was a well-designed study with a reasonable sample size. But testing was done at the end of the process (extubation), and the decision to extubate was made by the attending physician. Thus, it is difficult to determine the effect of individual clinician practices on the threshold level.

Clinical Implications

Both CROP and fx/VT are designed for clinical use and are relatively easy to calculate at the bedside. They do provide important information about the specific components important to weaning.

OTHER REFERENCES

1. Acosta F. Biofeedback and progressive relaxation in weaning the anxious patient from the ventilator: a brief report. *Heart Lung.* 1988;17:299–301.

2. Acosta F. Weaning the anxious ventilator patient using hypnotic relaxation: case reports. *Am J Clin Hypn.* 1987;29:273–280.

3. Afessa B, Hogans L, Murphy R. Predicting 3-day and 7-day outcomes of weaning from mechanical ventilation. *Chest* 1999;116:456–461.

4. Aldrich TK, Prezant DJ, Karpel JP, Multz AS, Hendler JM. Maximal inspiratory pressure in respiratory failure. *Chest.* 1990;97:975.

5. Anzueto A, Andrade FH, Maxwell LC, et al. Resistive breathing activates the glutathione redox cycle and impairs performance of rat diaphragm. *J Appl Physiol.* 1992;72:529–534.

6. Arom K, Emery R, Petersen R, et al. *Ann Thorac Surg.* 1995;60:127–132.

7. Arora KS, Rochester DF. Respiratory muscle strength and maximal voluntary ventilation in undernourished patients. *Am Rev Resp Dis.* 1982;126:5–8.

8. Banner MJ, Blanch PB, Kirby RR. Imposed work of breathing and methods of triggering a demand-flow continuous positive airway system. *Crit Care Med.* 1993;21:183–190.

9. Bellemare F, Grassino A. Evaluation of human diaphragm fatigue. *J Appl Physiol.* 1982;53:1196–1206.

10. Bergbom-Engberg I, Haljamae H. Assessment of patients' experience of discomforts during respirator therapy. *Crit Care Med.* 1989;17:1068–1072.

11. Beydon L, Chasse M, Harf A, Lemaire F. Inspiratory work of breathing during spontaneous ventilation using demand values and continuous flow systems. *Am Rev Respir Dis.* 1988;138:300–304.

12. Bolton CF, Young GB, Zochodne DW. The neurological complications of sepsis. *Ann Neurol.* 1993;33:94–100.

13. Bone RC, Balk RA. Noninvasive respiratory care unit. A cost effective solution for the future. *Chest.* 1988;93:390–394.

14. Bouley GH, Froman R, Shah H. The experience of dyspnea during weaning. *Heart Lung.* 1992;21:471–476.

15. Bowen DE. Ventilator weaning through hypnosis. *Psychosomatics.* 1989;30:449–450.

16. Brochard L, Harf A, Lorino H, Lemaire F. Inspiratory pressure support prevents diaphragmatic fatigue during weaning from mechanical ventilation. *Am Rev Respir Dis.* 1989;139:513–521.

17. Brochard L, Pluskwa F, Lemaire F. Improved efficacy of spontaneous breathing with inspiratory pressure support. *Am Rev Respir Dis.* 1987;136:411–415.

18. Brook AD, Ahrens TS, Schaff R, et al. Effect of a nursing-implemented sedation protocol on the duration of mechanical ventilation. *Crit Care Med.* 1999; 27:2609–2615.

19. Burns SM. Respiratory waveforms monitoring. In: *AACN Protocols for Practice: Noninvasive Monitoring.* 2nd ed. Sudbury, Mass: Jones and Bartlett; 2005: 31–55.

20. Burns SM, Egloff MB, Ryan B, Carpenter R, Burns JE. Effect of body position on spontaneous respiratory rate and tidal volume in patients with obesity, abdominal distention and ascites. *Am J Crit Care.* 1994;3: 102–106.

21. Burns SM, Clochesy JM, Goodnough-Hanneman SK, Ingersoll GL, Knebel AR, Shekleton ME. Weaning from long-term mechanical ventilation. *Am J Crit Care.* 1995;4:4–22.

22. Burns SM, Marshall M, Burns JE, et al. Design, testing, and results of an outcomes-managed approach to patients requiring prolonged mechanical ventilation. *Am J Crit Care.* 1998;7:45–57.

23. Burns SM, Ryan B, Burns JE. The weaning continuum: use of Apache III, BWAP, TISS, and WI scores to establish stages of weaning. *Crit Care Med.* 2000;28:2259–2267.

24. Campbell M, Frank RR. Experience with an end-of-life practice at a university hospital. *Crit Care Med.* 1997;25:197–202.

25. Carrieri-Kohlman V. Dyspnea in the weaning patient: assessment and intervention. *AACN Clin Issues.* 1991; 2:462–471.

26. Carson SS, Bach PB, Brzozowski L, Leff A. Outcomes after long-term acute care: an analysis of 133 mechanically ventilated patients. *Am J Respir Crit Care Med.* 1999;159:1568–1573.

27. Chevrolet J, Deleamont P. Repeated vital capacity measurements as predictive parameters for mechanical ventilation need and weaning success in the Guillain-Barré syndrome. *Am Rev Resp Dis.* 1991;144:814–818.

28. Cleary RK. Clostridium difficile-associated diarrhea and colitis: clinical manifestations, diagnosis, and treatment. *Dis Colon Rectum.* 1998;41:1435–1449.

29. Clochesy JM, Daly BJ, Montenegro HD. Weaning chronically critically ill adults for mechanical ventilation: a descriptive study. *Am J Crit Care.* 1995;4:93–99.

30. Cohen CA, Zagelbaum G, Gross D, Roussos CH, Macklem PT. Clinical manifestations of inspiratory muscle fatigue. *Am J Med.* 1982;73:308–316.

31. Cohen IL, Bari N, Strosberg MA, et al. Reduction of duration and cost of mechanical ventilation in an intensive care unit by use of a ventilatory management team. *Crit Care Med.* 1991;19:1278–1284.

32. Combes A, Costa M, Trouillet J, et al. Morbidity, mortality, and quality-of-life outcomes of patients requiring ≥ 14 days of mechanical ventilation. *Crit Care Med.* 2003;31:1373–1381.

33. Conti G, DeBlasti R, Pelaia P, et al. Early prediction of successful weaning during pressure support ventilation in chronic obstructive pulmonary disease patients. *Crit Care Med* 1992;20:366–371.

34. Coplin WM, Pierson DJ, Cooley KD, Newell DW, Rubenfeld GD. Implications of extubation delay in brain-injured patients meeting standard weaning criteria. *Am J Respir Crit Care Med.* 2000;161:1530–1536.

35. Corwin HL, Gettinger A, Pearl RG, et al. The CRIT Study: anemia and blood transfusion in the critically ill—current clinical practice in the United States. *Crit Care Med.* 2004;32:290–291.

36. Craven D, Kunches LM, Killinsky V, et al. Risk factors for pneumonia and fatality in patients receiving mechanical ventilation. *Am Rev Respir Dis.* 1986; 133:792–796.

37. Curley, MAQ, Fackler JC. Weaning from Mechanical Ventilation: Patterns in young children recovering from acute hypoxemic respiratory failure. *Am J Crit Care.* 1998; 7: 335–345.

38. Daly BJ, Rudy EB, Thompson KS, Happ MB. Development of a special care unit for chronically critically ill patients. *Heart Lung.* 1991; 20:45–52.

39. DeHaven CB, Hurst JM, Branson RD. Evaluation of two different extubation criteria: attributes contributing to success. *Crit Care Med.* 1986;14:92–94.

40. De Jonghe B, Bastuji-Garin S, Sharshar T, Outin H, Brochard L. Does ICU-acquired paresis lengthen weaning from mechanical ventilation? *Intensive Care Med.* 2004;30:1117–1121.

41. De Jonghe B, Sharshar T, Hopkinson N, Outin H. Paresis following mechanical ventilation. *Curr Opin Crit Care.* 2004;10:47–52.

42. De Jonghe B, Cook D, Sharshar T, Lefaucher JP, Carlet J, Outin H. Acquired neuromuscular disorders in critically ill patients: a systematic review. *Intensive Care Med.* 1998;24:1242–1250.

43. Douglas SL, Daly BJ, Brennan PF, Gordon NH, Uthis P. Hospital readmission among long-term ventilator patients. *Chest* 2001;120:1278–1286.

44. Douglas SL, Daly BD, Brennan PF, Harris S, Nochomovitz M, Dyer MA. Outcomes of long-term ventilator patients: a descriptive study. *Am J Crit Care.* 1997;6:99–105.

45. Douglas SL, Daly BJ, Gordon N, Brennan PF. Survival and quality of life: short-term versus long-term ventilator patients. *Crit Care Med.* 2002;30:2655–2662.

46. Dreyfuss D, Djedaini K, Weber P, et al. Prospective study of nosocomial pneumonia and of patient and circuit colonization during mechanical ventilation with circuit changes every 48 hours vs no change. *Am Rev Resp Dis.* 1991;143:738–743.

47. Dreyfuss D, Soler P, Basset G, Saumon G. High inflation pressure pulmonary edema: respective effects of high airway pressure, high tidal volume, and positive end-expiratory pressure. *Am Rev Resp Dis.* 1988;137: 1159–1164.

48. Ecklund M. Beyond the ICU: Home Care Management of Patients Receiving Mechanical Ventilation. In: Burns S, ed. *AACN Protocols for Practice: Care of Mechanically Ventilated Patients.* Sudbury, Mass: Jones and Bartlett; 2006: 161–190.

49. Elpern EH. Prolonged ventilator dependence: economic and ethical considerations. *Crit Care Nurs Clin North Am.* 1991;3:601–608.

50. Elpern EH, Larson R, Douglass P, Rosen RL, Bone RC. Long-term outcomes for elderly survivors of prolonged ventilator assistance. *Chest.* 1989;96:1120–1124.

51. Elpern EH, Silver MR, Bone RL, et al. The noninvasive respiratory care unit: patterns of use and financial implications. *Chest.* 1991;99;205–208.

52. Ely EW, Baker AM, Evans GW, Haponik EF. The distribution of costs of care in mechanically ventilated patients with chronic obstructive pulmonary disease. *Crit Care Med.* 2000;28:408–413.

53. Ely EW, Bennett PA, Bowton DL, Murphy SM, Florence AM, Haponick EF. Large scale implementation of a respiratory therapist-driven protocol for ventilator weaning. *Am J Respir Crit Care Med.* 1999;159:439–446.

54. Epstein SK, Nevins ML, Chung J. Effect of unplanned extubation on outcome of mechanical ventilation. *Am J Respir Crit Care Med.* 2000;161:1912–1916.

55. Esteban A, Alia I, Gordo F, et al. Extubation outcomes after spontaneous breathing trials with T-tube or pressure support ventilation. *Am J Respir Crit Care Med.* 1997;156:459–465.

56. Esteban A, Alia I, Ibanez J, Benito S, Tobin MJ, and the Spanish Lung Failure Collaborative Group. Modes of mechanical ventilation and weaning: a national survey of Spanish hospitals. *Chest.* 1994;106:1188–1193.

57. Esteban A, Alia I, Tobin MJ, et al. Effect of spontaneous breathing trial duration on outcome of attempts to discontinue mechanical ventilation. *Am J Respir Crit Care Med.* 1999;159:512–518.

58. Fagon J, Chastre J, Domart Y, et al. Nosocomial pneumonia in patients receiving continuous mechanical ventilation. *Am Rev Respir Dis.* 1989;139:877–884.

59. Fiastro JF, Habib MP, Quan SF. Pressure support compensation for inspiratory work due to endotracheal tubes and demand continuous positive airway pressure. *Chest.* 1988;93:499–505.

60. Fiastro JF, Habib MP, Shon BY, Campbell SC. Comparison of standard weaning parameters and the work of breathing in mechanically ventilated patients. *Chest.* 1988;94:232–238.

61. Freedman NS, Kotzer N, Schwab RJ. Patient perception of sleep quality and etiology of sleep disruption in the intensive care unit. *Am J Respir Crit Care Med.* 1999;159:1155–1162.

62. Frisk U, Nordstrom G. Patients' sleep in an intensive care unit patients' and nurses' perception. *Intensive Crit Care Nurs.* 2003;19:342–349.

63. Fu Z, Costello ML, Tsukimoto K., et al. High lung volume increases stress failure in pulmonary capillaries. *J Appl Physiol.* 1992;73:123–133.

64. Gandia F, Blanco J. Evaluation of indexes predicting the outcome of ventilator weaning and value of adding supplemental inspiratory load. *Intensive Care Med.* 1992;18:327–333.

65. Gibney NRT, Wilson RS, Pontoppidan H. Comparison of work of breathing on high gas flow and demand valve continuous positive airway pressure systems. *Chest.* 1982;82:692–695.

66. Gilbert R, Auchincloss JH, Peppi D, Ashutosh K. The first few hours off a respirator. *Chest.* 1974;65:152–157.

67. Goodnough-Hanneman SK. Multidimensional predictors of success or failure with early weaning from mechanical ventilation after cardiac surgery. *Nurs Res.* 1994;43: 4–10.

68. Goodnough-Hanneman SK, Ingersoll GL, Knebel AR, Shekleton ME, Burns SM, Clochesy JM. Weaning from short-term mechanical ventilation: a review. *Am J Crit Care.* 1994;3:421–443.

69. Gracey DR, Viggrano RW, Naessens JM, Hubmayr RD, Silverstein MD, Koenig GE. Outcomes of patients admitted to a chronic ventilator-dependent unit in an acute care hospital. *Mayo Clin Proc.* 1992;67:131–136.

70. Grap MJ. Pulse oximetry monitoring. In: Burns S, ed. *AACN Protocols for Practice: Noninvasive Monitoring,* 2nd ed. Sudbury, Mass: Jones and Bartlett; 2005:99–113.

71. Grap MJ, Strickland D, Tormey L, et al. Collaborative practice: development, implementation and evaluation of a weaning protocol for patients receiving mechanical ventilation. *Am J Crit Care.* 2003;12:454–460.

72. Gries ML, Fernsler L. Patient perceptions of the mechanical ventilation experience. *Focus Crit Care.* 1988;15:52–59.

73. Gurevitch MJ, Gelmont D. Importance of trigger sensitivity to ventilator response delay in advanced chronic obstructive pulmonary disease with respiratory failure. *Crit Care Med.* 1989;17:354–359.

74. Hansen-Flaschen J, Cowen J, Raps EC. Neuromuscular blockade in the intensive care unit: more than we bargained for. *Am Rev Resp Dis.* 1993;147:234–236.

75. Henneman EA. Effect of nursing contact on the stress response of patients being weaned from mechanical ventilation. *Heart Lung.* 1989;18:483–489.

76. Henneman E, Dracup K, Ganz T, Molayeme O, Cooper C. Effect of a collaborative weaning plan on patient outcome in the critical care setting. *Crit Care Med.* 2001;29:297–303.

77. Henneman E, Dracup K, Ganz T, Molayeme O, Cooper CB. Using a collaborative weaning plan to decrease duration of mechanical ventilation and length of stay in the intensive care unit for patients receiving long-term mechanical ventilation. *Am J Crit Care.* 2002;11:32–140.

78. Hebert PC, Wells G, Blajchman MA, et al. A multicenter, randomized, controlled clinical trial of transfusion requirements in critical care. *N Eng Jour Med.* 1999;340:409–417.

79. Holliday JE, Hyers TM. The reduction of weaning time from mechanical ventilation using tidal volume and relaxation biofeedback. *Am Rev Respir Dis.* 1990;141:1214–1220.

80. Hoo GWS, Park L. Variations in the measurement of weaning parameters: a survey of respiratory therapists. *Chest.* 2002;121:1947–1955.

81. Inchhar FJ. A ten year report of patients in a prolonged respiratory care unit. *Minn Med.* 1991;74:23–27.

82. Jubran A, Tobin MJ. Pathophysiologic basis of acute respiratory distress in patients who fail a trial of weaning from mechanical ventilation. *Am J Respir Crit Care Med.* 1997;155:906–915.

83. Kanak R, Fahey PJ, Vanderwarf C. Oxygen cost of breathing: changes dependent on mode of mechanical ventilation. *Chest.* 1985;87:126–127.

84. Kappstein I, Schulgen G, Beyer U, Geiger K, Schumacher M, Daschner FD. Prolongation of hospital stay and extra costs due to ventilator-associated pneumonia in an intensive care unit. *Eur J Clin Microbiol Infect Dis.* 1992;11:504–508.

85. Khamiees M, Raju P, DeGirolamo A, Amoateng-Adjepong Y, Manthous CA. Predictors of extubation outcome in patients who have successfully completed a spontaneous breathing trial. *Chest.* 2001;120:1262–1270.

86. Knaus W. Prognosis with mechanical ventilation: the influence of disease, severity of disease, age, and chronic health status on survival from an acute illness. *Am Rev Respir Dis.* 1989;140:S8–S13.

87. Knebel AR, Shekleton ME, Burns SM, Clochesy JM, Hanneman SK, Ingersoll GL. Weaning from mechanical ventilation: concept development. *Am J Crit Care.* 1994;3:416–420.

88. Knebel A, Shekleton MD, Burns S, Clochesy JM, Hanneman SK. Weaning from mechanical ventilatory support: refinement of a model. *Am J Crit Care.* 1998;7:149–152.

89. Kress JP, Gehlbach B, Lacy M, Pliskin N, Pohlman AS, Hall JB. The long-term psychological effects of daily sedative interruption on critically ill patients. *Am J Respir Crit Care Med.* 2003;168:1457–1461.

90. Kress JP, Pohlman AS, O'Connor MF, Hall JB. Daily interruption of sedative infusions in critically ill patients undergoing mechanical ventilation. *N Engl J Med.* 2000;342:1471–1477.

91. Kreiger BP, Ershowsky PF, Becker DA, Gazeroglu HB. Evaluation of conventional criteria for predicting successful weaning from mechanical ventilatory support in elderly patients. *Crit Care Med.* 1989;17:858–861.

92. Krieger BP, Isber J, Breitenbucher A, Throop G, Ershowsky P. Serial measurements of the rapid-shallow-breathing index as a predictor of weaning outcome in elderly medical patients. *Chest.* 1997;112:1029–1034.

93. Krishnan JA, Moore D, Robeson C, Rand CS, Fessler HE. A prospective, controlled trial of a protocol-based strategy to discontinue mechanical ventilation. *Am J Respir Crit Care Med.* 2004;169:673–678.

94. LaRicca PJ, Katz RH, Peters JW, Atkinson GW, Weiss T. Biofeedback and hypnosis in weaning from mechanical ventilators. *Chest.* 1985;87:267–269.

95. Lee B, Chang RWS, Jacobs S. Intermittent nasogastric feeding: a simple and effective method to reduce pneumonia among ventilated ICU patients. *Clin Int Care.* 1990;1:100–102.

96. Lemaire F, Teboul J, Cinotti L, et al. Acute left ventricular dysfunction during unsuccessful weaning from mechanical ventilation. *Anesthesiology.* 1988;69:171–179.

97. Luer J. Sedation and neuromuscular blockade in mechanically ventilated patients. In: Burns S, ed. *AACN Protocols for Practice: Care of Mechanically Ventilated Patients.* 2nd ed. Sudbury, Mass: Jones and Bartlett; 2006:253-284.

98. Lush MT, Janson-Bjerklie S, Carrieri VK, Lovejoy N. Dyspnea in the ventilator-assisted patient. *Heart Lung.* 1988;17:528–535.

99. MacIntyre NR. Respiratory function during pressure support ventilation. *Chest.* 1986;89:677–683.

100. MacIntyre NR. Weaning from mechanical ventilatory support. Volume-assisting intermittent breaths versus pressure assisting every breath. *Respir Care.* 1988;33:121–125.

101. MacIntyre NR, Cheng K-CG, McConnell R. Applied PEEP during pressure support reduces the inspiratory threshold load of intrinsic PEEP. *Chest.* 1997;111:188–193.

102. Mador MJ. Weaning parameters: are they clinically useful? *Chest.* 1992;102:1642.

103. Man WD-C, Kyroussis D, Fleming TA, et al. Cough gastric pressure and maximum expiratory mouth pressure in humans. *Am J Respir Crit Care.* 2003;168:714–717.

104. Mathru M, Rao TL, El-Etr AA, Pifarre R. Hemodynamic response to changes in ventilatory patterns in patients with normal and poor left ventricular reserve. *Crit Care Med.* 1982;10:423–426.

105. Marini JJ, Rodriguez M, Lamb V. The inspiratory workload of patient-initiated mechanical ventilation. *Am Rev Respir Dis.* 1986;134:902–909.

106. Martin UJ. Whole-body rehabilitation in long-term ventilation. *Respir Care Clin N Am.* 2002;8:593–609.

107. Massumi RA, Winnacker JL. Severe depression of the respiratory center in myxedema. *Am J Med.* 1964;36:876–882.

108. Menzies R, Gibbons W, Goldberg P. Determinants of weaning and survival among patients with COPD who require mechanical ventilation for acute respiratory failure. *Chest.* 1989;95:398–405.

109. Millbern SM, Downs JB, Jumper LC, Modell JH. Evaluation of criteria for discontinuing mechanical ventilatory support. *Arch Surg.* 1978;113:1441–1443.

110. Miwa K, Mitsuoka M, Takamori S, Hayashi A, Shirouzu K. Continuous monitoring of oxygen consumption in patients undergoing weaning from mechanical ventilation. *Respiration.* 2003;70:623–630.

111. Montgomery AB, Holle RHO, Neagley SR, Pierson DJ, Schoene RB. Prediction of successful ventilator weaning using airway occlusion pressure and hypercapnic challenge. *Chest.* 1987;91:496–499.

112. Morganroth ML, Morganroth JL, Nett LM, Petty TL. Criteria for weaning from prolonged mechanical ventilation. *Arch Intern Med.* 1984;144:1012–1016.

113. Mostafa SM, Bhandari S, Ritchie G, Gratton N, Wenstone R. Constipation and its implications in the critically ill patient. *Br J Anaesth.* 2003;91:815–819.

114. Murciano D, Boczkowski J, Lecocquic Y, Milic-Emili J, Pariente R, Aubier M. Tracheal occlusion pressure: a simple index to monitor respiratory muscle fatigue during acute respiratory failure in patients with chronic obstructive pulmonary disease. *Ann Intern Med.* 1988;108:800–805.

115. Namen AM, Ely EW, Tatter SB, et al. Predictors of successful extubation in neurosurgical patients. *Am J Respir Crit Care Med.* 2001;163:658–664.

116. Nathan SD, Ishaaya AM, Koerner SK, Belman MJ. Prediction of minimal pressure support during weaning from mechanical ventilation. *Chest.* 1993;103:1215–1219.

117. Pandya K, Lal C, Scheinhorn D, Day K, Sharma OP. Hypothyroidism and ventilator dependency. *Arch Intern Med.* 1989;149:2115–2116.

118. Parker JC, Hernandez LA, Peevy KJ. Mechanisms of ventilator-induced lung injury. *Crit Care Med.* 1993;21:131–143.

119. Parrish C, Krenitsky J, Willcutts K. Nutritional support in mechanically ventilated patients. In: Burns S, ed. *AACN Protocols for Practice: Care of Mechanically Ventilated Patients.* Sudbury, Mass: Jones and Bartlett; 2006:191-252.

120. Pepe PE, Marini JJ. Occult positive end-expiratory pressure in mechanically ventilated patients with airflow obstruction. *Am Rev Respir Dis.* 1982;126: 166–170.

121. Petrof BJ, Legare M, Goldberg P, et al. Continuous positive airway pressure reduces work of breathing and dyspnea during weaning from mechanical ventilation in severe chronic obstructive pulmonary disease. *Am Rev Respir Dis.* 1990;141:281–289.

122. Pierce L. Invasive and noninvasive modes and methods of mechanical ventilation. In: Burns S, ed. *AACN Protocols for Practice: Care of Mechanically Ventilated Patients.* Sudbury, Mass: Jones and Bartlett; 2006:59–94.

123. Pourriat JL, Lamberto CH, Hoang PH, Fournier JL, Vasseur B. Diaphragmatic fatigue and breathing pattern during weaning from mechanical ventilation in COPD patients. *Chest.* 1986;90:703–707.

124. Ranieri VM, Giuliani R, Cinnella G, et al. Physiologic effects of positive end-expiratory pressure in patients with chronic obstructive pulmonary disease during acute ventilatory failure and controlled mechanical ventilation. *Am Rev Respir Dis.* 1993;147:5–13.

125. Richards KC, O'Sullivan PS, Phillips RL. Measurement of sleep in critically ill patients. *J Nurs Meas.* 2000;8:131–144.

126. Roussos C, Fixley M, Gross D, Macklem PT. Fatigue of inspiratory muscles and their synergic behavior. *J Appl Physiol.* 1979;46:897–904.

127. Rudy EB, Daly BJ, Douglas S, Montenegro HD, Song R, Dyer MA. Patient outcomes for the chronically critically ill: special care versus intensive care unit. *Nurs Res.* 1995;44:324–331.

128. Rumbak MJ, Newton M, Truncale T, Schwartz SW, Adams JA. Hazard PB. A prospective, randomized study comparing early percutaneous dilational tracheotomy to prolonged translaryngeal intubation (delayed tracheotomy) in critically ill medical patients. *Crit Care Med.* 2004;32:1689–1694.

129. Sahn SA, Lakshminarayan S. Bedside criteria for discontinuation of mechanical ventilation. *Chest.* 1973;63:1002–1005.

130. Sahn SA, Lakshminarayan S, Petty TL. Weaning from mechanical ventilation. *JAMA.* 1976;235:2208–2212.

131. Sapijaszko MJ, Brant R, Sandham D, Berthiaume Y. Nonrespiratory predictor of mechanical ventilation dependency in intensive care unit patients. *Crit Care Med.* 1996;24:601–607.

132. Sassoon CSH, Light RW, Lodia R, Sieck GC, Mahutte CK. Pressure-time product during continuous positive airway pressure, pressure support ventilation, and T-piece during weaning from mechanical ventilation. *Am Rev Respir Dis.* 1991;143:469–475.

133. Sassoon CSH, Lodia R, Rheeman CH, Kuei JH, Light RW, Mahutte CK. Inspiratory muscle work of breathing during flow-by, demand-flow, and continuous-flow systems in patients with chronic obstructive pulmonary disease. *Am Rev Respir Dis.* 1992;145:1219–1222.

134. Sassoon CSH, Mahutte CK. Airway occlusion and breathing pattern as predictors of weaning outcome. *Am Rev Respir Dis.* 1993;143:860–866.

135. Sassoon CSH, Te TT, Mahutte CK, Light RW. Airway occlusion pressure: an important indicator for successful weaning in patients with chronic obstructive pulmonary disease. *Am Rev Respir Dis.* 1987;135:107–113.

136. Scheinhorn DJ, Artinian BM, Catlin JL. Weaning from prolonged mechanical ventilation. The experience at a regional weaning center. *Chest.* 1994;105:534–539.

137. Scheinhorn DJ, Chao DC, Stearn-Hassenpflug M, LaBree LD, Heltsley DJ. Post-ICU mechanical ventilation: treatment of 1,123 patients at a regional weaning center. *Chest.* 1997;111:1654–1649.

138. Scheinhorn DJ, Chao DC, Hassenpflug MS, Gracey DR. Post-ICU weaning from mechanical ventilation: the role of long-term facilities. *Chest.* 2001;120:482S-484S.

139. Seneff MG, Wagner D, Thompson D, Honeycutt C, Silver MR. The impact of long-term acute-care facilities on the outcome and cost of care for patients undergoing prolonged mechanical ventilation. *Crit Care Med.* 2000;28:342–350.

140. Sereika SM, Clochesy JM. Left ventricular dysfunction and duration of mechanical ventilatory support in the chronically critically ill: a survival analysis. *Heart Lung.* 1996;25:45–51.

141. Sharp J, Henry J, Sweeny S, Meadows W, Pietras R. Effects of mass loading the respiratory system in man. *J Appl Physiol.* 1964;19:959–966.

142. Simpson T, Lee ER, Cameron C. Patients' perceptions of environmental factors that disturb sleep after cardiac surgery. *Am J Crit Care.* 1996;5:173–181.

143. Simpson T, Lee ER, Cameron C. Relationships among sleep dimensions and factors that impair sleep after cardiac surgery. *Res Nurs Health.* 1996;19:213–223.

144. Spilker CA, Hinthorn DR, Pingleton SK. Intermittent enteral feeding in mechanically ventilated patients: the effect on gastric pH and gastric cultures. *Chest.* 1996;110:243–248.

145. Stiller K. Physiotherapy in intensive care: towards and evidence-based practice. *Chest.* 2000;118:1801–1813.

146. St. John RE. End-tidal carbon dioxide monitoring. In: Burns S, ed. *AACN Protocols for Practice: Noninvasive Monitoring,* 2nd ed. Sudbury, Mass: Jones and Bartlett; 2005:57–79.

147. Swartz MA, Marino PL. Diaphragmatic strength during weaning from mechanical ventilation. *Chest.* 1985;88:736–739.

148. Tablan OC, Anderson LJ, Besser R, Bridges C, Hajjeh R. Guidelines for preventing health-care–associated pneumonia, 2003. Recommendations of CDC and the Healthcare Infection Control Practices Advisory Committee. *MMWR.* 2004;53(RRO3):1–36.

149. Tahvanainen J, Salmenpera M, Nikki P. Extubation criteria after weaning from intermittent mandatory ventilation and continuous positive airway pressure. *Crit Care Med.* 1983;11:702–707.

150. The Acute Respiratory Distress Syndrome Network. Ventilation with lower tidal volumes as compared with traditional tidal volumes for acute lung injury and the acute respiratory distress syndrome. *N Eng J Med.* 2002;342:1301–1307

151. Tobin MJ. Advances in mechanical ventilation. *N Engl J Med.* 2001;344:1986–1996.

152. Tobin MJ, Guenther S, Perez W, et al. Konno-Mead analysis of ribcage-abdominal motion during successful and unsuccessful trials of weaning from mechanical ventilation. *Am Rev Respir Dis.* 1987;135:1320–1328.

153. Tobin MJ, Perez W, Guenither SM, et al. The pattern of breathing during successful and unsuccessful trials of weaning from mechanical ventilation. *Am Rev Resp Dis.* 1986;134:1111–1118.

154. Truwit JD. Rochester DF. Monitoring the respiratory system of the mechanically ventilated patient. *New Horizons.* 1994;2:94–106.

155. Vallverdu I, Calaf N, Subirana M, Net A, Benito S, Mancebo J. Clinical characteristics, respiratory functional parameters and outcome of a two-hour T-Piece trial in patients weaning form mechanical ventilation. *Am J Respir Crit Care Med.* 1998;158:1855–1862.

156. Vassilakopoulos T, Zakynthinos S, Roussos C. The tension-time index and the frequency/tidal volume ratio are the major pathophysiologic determinants of weaning failure and success. *Am J Respir Crit Care Med.* 1998;158:378–385.

157. Van den Berghe G, Wouters PJ, Bouillon R, et al. Outcome benefits of intensive insulin therapy in the critically ill: insulin dose versus glycemic control. *Crit Care Med.* 2003;31:359–366.

158. Vitacca M, Vianello A, Colombo D, et al. Comparison of two methods for weaning COPD patients requiring mechanical ventilation for more than 15 days. *Am J Respir Crit Care Med.* 2001;164:225–230.

159. Wagner DP. Economics of prolonged mechanical ventilation. *Am Rev Respir Dis.* 1989;140:S14-S18.

160. Walsh TS, Dodds S, McArdle F. Evaluation of simple criteria to predict successful weaning from mechanical ventilation in intensive care patients. *Br J Anaesth.* 2004;92:793–799.

161. West JB. *Ventilation/Bloodflow and Gas Exchange.* 5th ed. Philadelphia, Pa: Lippincott; 1990.

162. West JB. *Respiratory Physiology—The Essentials.* Baltimore, Md: Williams & Wilkins; 1990.

163. Yang KL. Reproducibility of weaning parameters. A need for standardization. *Chest.* 1992;102:1829–1832.

164. Zerah F, Harf A, Perlemuter L, et al. Effects of obesity on respiratory resistance. *Chest.* 1993;103:1470–1476.

Burns Wean Assessment Program

General Assessment

Yes	No	Not Assessed	
___	___	___	1. Hemodynamically stable? (pulse rate, cardiac output)
___	___	___	2. Free from factors that increase or decrease metabolic rate? (seizures, temperature, sepsis, bacteremia, hypo/hyperthyroid)
___	___	___	3. Hematocrit > .25 (or baseline)?
___	___	___	4. Systemically hydrated? (weight at or near baseline, balanced intake and output)
___	___	___	5. Nourished? (albumin > 2.5, parenteral/enteral feedings maximized) If albumin is low and anasarca or third spacing is present, score for hydration should be No.
___	___	___	6. Electrolytes within normal limits? (including Ca^{++}, Mg^+, PO_4) Correct Ca^{++} for albumin level.
___	___	___	7. Pain controlled? (subjective determination)
___	___	___	8. Adequate sleep/rest? (subjective determination)
___	___	___	9. Appropriate level of anxiety and nervousness? (subjective determination)
___	___	___	10. Absence of bowel problems? (diarrhea, constipation, ileus)
___	___	___	11. Improved general body strength/endurance? (ie, out of bed in chair, progressive activity program)
___	___	___	12. Chest x-ray improving or returned to baseline?

Respiratory Assessment

Yes	No	Not Assessed	*Gas flow and work of breathing*
___	___	___	13. Eupneic respiratory rate and pattern? (spontaneous respiratory rate < 25, without dyspnea, absence of accessory muscle use) This is assessed off the ventilator while measuring items 20 through 23 below.
___	___	___	14. Absence of adventitious breath sounds? (rhonchi, rales, wheezing)
___	___	___	15. Secretions thin and minimal?
___	___	___	16. Absence of neuromuscular disease/deformity?
___	___	___	17. Absence of abdominal distention/obesity/ascites?
___	___	___	18. Oral endotracheal tube ≥ #7.5 or tracheostomy tube ≥ #6.5 (inner diameter)

(Continues)

		Not	
Yes	*No*	*Assessed*	*Airway Clearance*
——	——	——	19. Cough and swallow reflexes adequate?
			Strength
——	——	——	20. Negative inspiratory pressure < –20 cm H_2O?
——	——	——	21. Positive expiratory pressure > +30 cm H_2O?
			Endurance
——	——	——	22. Spontaneous tidal volume > 5 mL/kg?
——	——	——	23. Vital capacity >10 to 15 mL/kg?
			Arterial blood gases
——	——	——	24. pH between 7.30 and 7.45?
——	——	——	25. $Paco_2$ approximately 40 mm Hg (or baseline) with minute ventilation < 10 L/min? This is evaluated while on ventilator.
——	——	——	26. Pao_2 > 60 on Fio_2 < 40%?

To score, divide the number of "yes" responses by 26.

_____

Traditional Weaning Indices

To ensure accurate measurements, make sure the endotracheal or tracheal tube cuff is inflated.

Negative Inspiratory Pressure (NIP)

Attach a 1-way valve and a pressure manometer to the patient's artificial airway, making sure the cuff is inflated. Instruct the patient to try to exhale maximally before attaching the measurement device (this is an attempt to begin at residual volume). When the measurement device is attached, instruct the patient to inhale forcefully against the closed system. The best effort (most negative number) is recorded in 20 seconds. Abort the test if the patient becomes unduly agitated or experiences dysrhythmias or desaturation.

NIP threshold: ≤ 20 cm H_2O

Positive Expiratory Pressure (PEP)

Measured as in NIP, but the measurement device is adapted to allow for the patient to inhale but not exhale. The patient is instructed to exhale forcefully against the closed system. The best effort, in this case the most positive number, is recorded in 20 seconds.

PEP threshold = ≥ 30 cm H_2O

Spontaneous Tidal Volume (VT sp)

Attach a respirometer or other volume-measuring device to the expiratory side of a 2-way valve and instruct the patient to breathe normally for 1 minute. Average VT is calculated by dividing the patient's spontaneous respiratory rate into the minute ventilation. This measurement may also be done with the patient on the ventilator on a CPAP level of zero. Observe the digital VT readout to determine the average VT.

VT sp threshold = 5 mL/kg

Vital Capacity (VC)

Obtained by using the same equipment as with VT sp (or on the ventilator as described), but the technique is markedly different and difficult to do in the intubated patient. The patient must be able to understand and follow the instructions. First, ask the patient to inhale maximally before the measurement device is attached. When the device is attached, the patient is asked to exhale maximally and forcefully. The maneuver is usually attempted more than once, and the patient is allowed to rest between attempts. Record the best effort.

VC threshold = ≥ 15 mL/kg

Minute Ventilation (VE)

Minute ventilation is obtained by multiplying respiratory rate by the VT. It may be measured manually (after a minute of spontaneous breathing) using a respirometer (as described for VT sp). More commonly, the exhaled minute ventilation (aka minute volume) may be observed on the ventilator displays.

VE threshold = 5 to 10 L/min

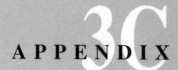
Frequency to Tidal Volume Ratio (f/VT)

f/VT Ratio

Divide spontaneous respiratory frequency (f) in 1 minute by
tidal volume (VT) in liters

Threshold: < 105 = weaning success
                    > 105 = weaning failure

Sample Weaning Protocol*

Weaning Trial Screen

The following criteria are assessed daily:

1. Hemodynamic stability (no dysrhythmias, HR ≤ 120, absence of vasopressors—low-dose dopamine and dobutamine are exceptions)
2. $FIO_2 \leq 50\%$
3. PEEP ≤ 8 cm H_2O
4. BWAP > 45% (BWAP is done only on patients ventilated ≥ 3 days)
5. If the patient meets these criteria a wean trial protocol is initiated.

Wean Trial Protocol: Continuous Positive Airway Pressure (CPAP) (1 trial—1 hour duration)

1. One trial of CPAP is attempted daily. The trial lasts for 1 hour total.
2. With any signs of intolerance (see definition below), the trial is discontinued and the patient is returned to a resting mode until the next trial.
3. When the 1-hour trial is sustained without signs of intolerance, the team is approached and extubation potential is discussed.
4. Full respiratory muscle rest is provided between trials and at night.
5. If the patient is very weak or has a cardiac condition, a more gradual wean plan (PSV) may be used for trials. See below.

OR

Wean Trial Protocol: Pressure Support Ventilation (PSV) (2 trials—4 hours duration)

1. Start at PSV max level (level to attain RR ≤ 20 with VT of 8–12 mL/kg).
2. Decrease PSV by 5 cm H_2O.
3. If no signs of intolerance are evident during the first 4-hour trial, the PSV is decreased by another 5 cm H_2O for the second trial.
4. With any signs of intolerance during trials, the patient is returned to previous level for the next 4-hour trial.
5. If unable to tolerate, the patient is fully rested until the next day when the process begins again.
6. When the patient is able to sustain 5–6 cm PSV without signs of intolerance (for 4 hours) the team is approached and extubation potential is discussed.

***Intolerance** for either the protocols is defined **as any** of the following (3–5 minutes sustained):*

1. RR ≤ 35 for 5 mins
2. O_2 sat ≤ 90% or a decrease of 4%
3. HR ≥ 140 and/or a 20% sustained change of HR in either direction
4. Systolic BP ≥ 180, ≤ 90 mm Hg
5. Excessive anxiety or agitation
6. Diaphoresis

---

*Source: Adapted from University of Virginia Health System MICU weaning protocol © 2002 by the Rector and Board of Visitors of the University of Virginia.

Rest for either protocol:

1. PSV max: PSV max is that pressure level required to attain a RR of 20 or less and a V_T of 8–10 mL/kg. Respiratory pattern should be synchronous, and there should be no accessory muscle use.
2. Other modes: With volume modes such as assist control or intermittent mandatory ventilation, respiratory muscle rest is not assured unless there is cessation of respiratory muscle activity. Therefore, rest is considered that level of support required to prevent patient-initiated breaths. When IMV is used, PSV may be added for protection (ie, as a safety). Regardless, the goal is cessation of spontaneous effort.

Beyond the ICU: Home Care Management of Patients Receiving Mechanical Ventilation

Margaret M. Ecklund, RN, MS, CCRN, APRN-BC

Beyond the ICU: Home Care Management of Patients Receiving Mechanical Ventilation

CASE STUDY 1

"Does anyone ever go home on a ventilator?" So began the process of planning Mrs F's return home, where she would undergo mechanical ventilation. Mrs F had a history of chronic obstructive pulmonary disease (COPD) and congestive heart failure and had been oxygen dependent for the last 8 years. She had spent several weeks in the medical intensive care unit prior to transfer to the progressive pulmonary care unit. After multiple unsuccessful attempts at weaning, a tracheostomy was performed and Mrs F received noninvasive positive pressure ventilation for 6 months. During this time, she had bouts of pneumonia and her dyspnea worsened, as did her functional and nutritional status. She was weak and unable to get out of bed on her own and required feeding via a small-bore feeding tube. Weaning from the ventilator was unlikely. Her husband was a committed caregiver and asked the team if he could take his wife home.

Mrs F's husband met with the team to explore options. With 2 daughters willing to help, it seemed reasonable that he might be able to care for his wife at home. Over the course of the next 2 months, preparations were made and teaching sessions were held to prepare for Mrs F's discharge. After instruction, it was clear that Mrs F's husband had an excellent understanding of the processes involved in care, and demonstrated necessary skills flawlessly. He also showed the ability to think critically and troubleshoot situations. Her daughters, though somewhat hesitant, demonstrated that they would be of help and support to their father.

Unfortunately, third-party payer financial support was inadequate to support Mrs F's care at home. Her husband realized that their retirement savings would quickly be depleted if used to care for her. It was determined that if Mrs F's income and expenses were considered separate from those of her husband, Medicaid would be an option and would make the financial burden reasonable. If Medicaid were approved, coverage would be provided for medical supplies and daily 24-hour care by licensed caregivers in the home. (This option is not available in many states since the passage of the Balanced Budget Act in 1997. In addition, availability of nurses trained in ventilator management varies.) After 6 months, when Medicaid coverage would decrease to support only 16 hours of daily care, Mrs F's husband would assume care for the remaining 8 hours.

When Mrs F left the hospital her home had been well prepared by her husband under the guidance of the home care agency. She traveled to her apartment in an advanced life support vehicle with an advanced practice nurse and a respiratory therapist. Later Mrs F's husband described the "heavy feeling" he experienced when the hospital team left the apartment and he was left with a new team to help him care for his wife.

Expectations for the success of the discharge to home were exceeded as each month passed. When Medicaid coverage was reduced to support care by licensed nurses for only 16 hours per day, Mrs F's husband assumed primary caregiving each evening. He worked through issues associated with different levels of competence of the nurses providing care, often giving the nurses pointers on ventilator troubleshooting. Organization of the home care plan was clearly in his capable hands. The advanced practice nurse from the hospital proved to be his most valuable resource when issues arose. She was in a unique position to help with technical questions over the phone or to visit periodically to review the plan of care with the primary home care nurse and the family. She also provided routine and emergency tracheostomy changes, which avoided unnecessary trips to the hospital. The advanced practice nurse's close collaboration with the attending physician was essential to provide for the expanded scope of advanced practice in the home care setting.

CASE STUDY 2

Mr C, a 40-year-old man with progressive amyotrophic lateral sclerosis, was admitted to the ICU in respiratory failure with a $PaCO_2$ of 112 mm Hg. He was somnolent but able to be aroused with verbal stimulation. Intubation and mechanical ventilation improved his arterial blood gases (ABGs) to baseline status, and he became awake and alert.

Mr C's hypoventilation was secondary to profound muscle weakness from ALS. His weakness had progressed to the point where he was unable to perform any activities of daily living. After potential care options were discussed with Mr C, his wife, and 2 daughters, he expressed the desire to pursue home mechanical ventilator therapy.

Because Mr C was not acutely ill and had made decisions related to his future care, education became the main nursing focus. A tracheostomy and percutaneous gastrostomy tube were placed, and plans were developed for teaching. For home care to be a realistic option, caregivers must be available 24 hours a day. In Mr C's case his family was supportive and capable. His parents had been caring for him while his wife worked and his daughters were in school, coming to live with him Monday to Friday and returning to their home Friday evening for the weekend. Mrs C had been responsible for her husband's care during the evenings and at weekends, with assistance from their daughters and occasionally from friends or neighbors. As a result, training progressed quickly and within 3 weeks, Mr C was discharged.

CASE STUDY 3

Ms Q, an 18-year-old female with central sleep apnea, had experienced numerous trials of nighttime continuous positive airway pressure without success. She found the therapy so uncomfortable that she could not sleep. A second method, the chest cuirass (a negative pressure ventilator), was also attempted, but this too was unsuccessful. Finally, Ms Q decided to have a tracheostomy placed so that she could learn to use nighttime home mechanical ventilation through the tracheostomy.

Ms Q was admitted to the hospital for surgery, and 2 days after the tracheostomy was learning to suction herself and perform tracheostomy care. As an active teenager who could ventilate effectively while awake, Ms Q was up and about during the day. With her tracheostomy cuff deflated, she could speak well and communication was not a problem. Also, early evaluation by a speech therapist had determined that Ms Q's swallow was effective, therefore she could continue to enjoy eating pizza and french fries as she wished.

Ms Q was eager to learn so that she could go home and continue her life. Her parents were supportive. They learned how to care for her in case she needed their help, but also encouraged her independence and self-care.

Eighteen days after admission for tracheostomy Ms Q was discharged home with her parents. Her goal was to enter college the next semester and within a year be a full-time student, living in a dorm.

About a year after her hospital admission, Ms Q returned to the hospital to share her ventilator home care management (HCM) experiences with another young woman who had begun learning to care for her own tracheostomy and intermittent mechanical ventilation needs at home. Currently, Ms Q lives independently in an apartment with a friend. She has taken some business courses and still hopes one day to attend college.

CASE STUDY 4

Recurrent chest pain after angioplasty necessitated Mr S's coronary artery bypass graft surgery. His heart recovered well but his emphysematous lungs made weaning from mechanical ventilation difficult. After 3 weeks of working to decrease ventilator support, Mr S had a tracheostomy placed. At 79 years of age, he questioned the quality of life he would have "tied to a machine"; however, after several weeks he was able to adjust to 1- to 2-hour periods without ventilator support during waking hours. A few days later he began asking how soon he could go home to enjoy his garden.

Mrs S's crippling osteoarthritis made it impossible for her to perform tracheostomy care for her husband, but she was his cheerleader as he began caring for himself. Their granddaughter lived nearby and agreed to learn Mr S's care needs and be available to help on a regular basis. Spring weather was a strong motivation to get home, and Mr S and his granddaughter quickly learned tracheostomy care, suctioning, and ventilator care. Dyspnea with any exertion was a problem, so nursing assistants to help with bathing and personal care were scheduled Monday through Friday. As soon as support systems were in place, Mr S was discharged home with his wife. Several friends from their church group scheduled visits to assist Mr S and his family during the following months. Mr S died in his sleep in late October. Home ventilation gave him time to enjoy his family and his home during the last months of his life.

GENERAL DESCRIPTION

Home mechanical ventilation is a method of supporting full or partial ventilatory needs arising from neuromuscular weakness, neurogenic hypoventilation, or ineffective gas exchange in patients who are otherwise clinically stable (see Appendix 4A). Though some needs associated with home mechanical ventilation can be partially met with noninvasive methods (eg, continuous positive airway pressure (CPAP) with nasal or face mask, bi-level ventilation, negative pressure cuirass, iron lung, or wrap), this protocol focuses on mechanical ventilation with a tracheostomy in place.

COMPETENCY

Nurses who care for ventilator-assisted patients who are planning for HCM must have a clear understanding of oxygenation, ventilation, and airway management. HCM requires a team of caregivers to organize and teach the necessary skills. Appendixes 4A and 4B show examples of assessment and responsibilities of individual team members. Each healthcare team must assess strengths and weaknesses of the plan and designate a team leader for teaching and plan coordination. The AACN Synergy Model for Patient Care[1] provides a framework that supports matching the needs of the patient with the competency and skills of the nurse.

To prepare a patient for HCM it is essential to determine clinical stability, minimum home care ventilatory parameters (fraction of inspired oxygen [FIO_2], mode, rate, and tidal volume [VT]), nutritional interventions, mobility methods and schedules, medication administration, coping strategies, and communication needs. Evaluating patient-family interaction and commitment and competency of caregivers is vital as preparation is made for discharge. Clinicians must understand the differences between ventilator support in the home and in the hospital to ensure the patient and family make an effective transition from acute care to the home without trauma or fear.

It is important that nursing staff and the healthcare team involved in preparing patients and families for HCM of ventilation have comprehensive nursing skills to promote patient and family confidence and involvement, along with strong team communication and listening skills. The healthcare team must also be able to accomplish the following:

- Teach skills at the learning level of the patient or caregivers. Consider barriers to learning and make appropriate adaptations.
- Promote structured skill development at appropriate time intervals for the selected caregivers.
- Enhance the continuity of care during the transition from hospital to home with excellent patient, family, and healthcare team collaboration in identifying and acquiring home equipment and healthcare support.
- Identify potential problems early, and solve problems as they arise.
- Evaluate caregivers' performance in order to provide support and reinforcement to achieve the level of care necessary for safe discharge of the patient.
- Differentiate home care practices (clean technique and flexible scheduling) from hospital care (sterile technique, careful charting, and strict time scheduling).

See Appendixes 4C, 4D, and 4E for checklists, sample medication administration record, and troubleshooting guides.

The following are suggested to ensure that nursing staff reach the required level of competency:

- Reference materials: Handbook for primary nurse or case manager; teaching materials for patient and family
- Educational classes: Formal classes for selected staff who serve as caregivers, primary nurses, respiratory therapists, and the case manager coordinating care. To learn teaching strategies, mentoring and coaching from senior staff members is an alternative to formal classes.
- Skills acquisition: Time for selected nurses to work with experienced staff to develop the competencies needed to care for and teach these complex patients
- Supportive interventions: Feedback from patients and families who have experienced HCM to promote continual improvement

ETHICAL AND FINANCIAL CONSIDERATIONS

Patients and families need careful and clear explanations of positive and negative aspects of both home care and long-term care in a ventilator facility so that they can properly evaluate choices. It is essential that caregivers understand the 24-hour-a-day demands of home care that make it unsuccessful for some patients. It is important to complete a financial overview with the patient, family, and home care planner to assess the financial risk of home care. Paid licensed caregivers in the home are expensive and most third-party payers supply equipment only, with no reimbursement for caregivers.

Some patients may not choose long-term ventilation therapy, and home care is not successful for some patients. Talking with other caregivers and patients may increase understanding of the ramifications of the decision to pursue home care. Problems of feeling trapped in an overwhelming, difficult, unmanageable, or intolerable situation are best prevented with a realistic practical approach. End-of-life discussions are also an option for the individual and family facing these complex choices.

OCCUPATIONAL HAZARDS

There are no specific occupational hazards associated with HCM of ventilator-dependent patients. Potential hazards are similar to those associated with any electrical device. The caregiver can be exposed to blood and body fluids with routine care. Injuries associated with lifting are also a caregiver risk.

FUTURE RESEARCH

Research focusing on the needs and outcomes of patients requiring home ventilation and on their caregivers would be helpful.

Studies that elucidate the reasons for readmission to the hospital from the home may help determine educational needs of patients and families as well as required resources for home care.

REFERENCE

1. AACN Certification Corporation. The AACN Synergy Model for Patient Care. Available at: http://www.aacn.org/certcorp/certcorp.nsf/vwdoc/SynModel?opendocument. Accessed January 5, 2006.

SUGGESTED READINGS

AARC Clinical Practice Guideline. Long-term invasive mechanical ventilation in the home. *Respir Care.* 1995;40:1313–1320.

Ecklund MM. Successful outcomes for the ventilator-dependent patient. *Crit Care Nurs Clin N Am.* 1999; 11:249–259.

Fauroux B, Howard P, Muir JF. Home treatment for chronic respiratory insufficiency: the situation in Europe in 1992. *Eur Respir J.* 1994;7:1721–1726.

International Ventilator User's Network (IVUN). 4207 Lindell Blvd #110, St Louis, Mo, 63108-2915 (314-534-0475). Available at: www.post-polio.org/ivun/. Accessed February 13, 2005.

Nellcor Puritan Bennett's Portable Ventilator User's Network. Contact Jan Nelson, 14800 28th Ave N, Plymouth, Minn, 55447 (1-800-497-4979).

Tracheostomy Tube Adult Home Care Guide. St Louis, Mo: Shiley Tracheostomy Products, Mallinckrodt Medical Inc., (888-744-1414).

CLINICAL RECOMMENDATIONS

The rating scales for the Level of Recommendation range from I to IV, with levels indicated as follows: I, manufactuer's recommendations only; II, theory based, no research data to support recommendations; recommendations from expert consensus group may exist; III, laboratory data only, no clinical data to support recommendations; IV, limited clinical studies to support recommendations; V, clinical studies in more than 1 or 2 different populations and situations to support recommendations; VI, clinical studies in a variety of patient populations and situations to support recommendations.

Period of Use	Recommendation	Rationale for Recommendation	Level of Recommendation	Supporting References	Comments
Selection of Patients	The decision to recommend HCM for ventilator-dependent patients is based on comprehensive evaluation of each patient-family situation. These are best evaluated in relation to specific conditions and the impact of these conditions on the degree of care.	Success of HCM for ventilator-dependent patients is contingent on the choice of patients. If comprehensive evaluation is overlooked, patients may do poorly or be unable to remain at home.	II: Theory based, no research data to support recommendations; recommendations from expert consensus group may exist	See Annotated Bibliography: 9, 14 See Other References: 3, 4, 12	The decision to allow HCM for ventilator-dependent patients is made individually after evaluating: • Pathophysiologic states that will benefit from HCM • Patient and family wishes, including the option of a palliative care plan for the patient to die at home • Clinical and physiologic stability • Supportive physical home environment • Available caregivers, medical and technical support • Psychosocial resources of patient and family • Financial assessment and feasibility
	1. Pathophysiologic states that often benefit from HCM: *Neuromuscular disorders* • Amyotrophic lateral sclerosis • Arnold-Chiari malformation • Guillain-Barré syndrome • Multiple sclerosis • Muscular dystrophy • Myasthenia gravis • Congenital central hypoventilation syndrome (also known as the Ondine curse,) • Poliomyelitis • Polymyositis	Neuromuscular weakness or dysfunction that results in hypoventilation can be relieved with mechanical ventilation.	IV: Limited clinical studies to support recommendations	See Annotated Bibliography: 8 See Other References: 7	

Period of Use	Recommendation	Rationale for Recommendation	Level of Recommendation	Supporting References	Comments
Selection of Patients *(cont.)*	• Spinal cord injury (above and sometimes below the 4th cranial nerve) • Surgical phrenic nerve injuries				
	2. Pathophysiologic states that may benefit from HCM: *Restrictive disorders* • Fibrothorax • Interstitial pulmonary fibrosis • Kyphoscoliosis • Obesity • Sarcoidosis	Restrictive and obstructive diseases may cause inadequate oxygenation and ventilation. Carefully selected patients with reasonably stable conditions may benefit from HCM.	IV: Limited clinical studies to support recommendations	See Other References: 12	
	Obstructive disorders • Bronchiectasis • Bronchiolitis obliterans • Bronchopulmonary dysplasia • Chronic bronchitis and emphysema • Cystic fibrosis • Sleep apnea syndrome			See Other References: 1, 11	High FIO_2 levels, inflation pressures, and respiratory rates make mechanical ventilation difficult in the home. Clinical instability because of primary pulmonary disease may decrease the benefits of HCM.
	Patient and family desire for HCM must be clearly stated after advantages and disadvantages have been presented.	A knowledgeable decision for HCM made by patient and family caregivers will help maintain commitment to the process of learning and providing care.	IV: Limited clinical studies to support recommendations	See Annotated Bibliography: 3, 4, 6, 7, 9, 12, 14 See Other References: 8, 14	In one study (Annotated Bibliography: 4) fewer than half the patients and families felt they made an informed decision for HCM. The videotape describing patient and family experiences with ventilator HCM may be useful in making the decision. A treatment plan that is effective in the hospital may be too complex for home caregivers to follow. Simplifying the plan can increase compliance and success.
	Clinical and physiologic stability are necessary before selecting HCM. • *Clinical stability:* Coexisting diseases, other organ system problems, and infections must be well controlled before patients can be sent home.	Success with HCM depends on having a simple, comprehensive plan of care that contains interventions that can be managed by the care team at home. Careful evaluation of each aspect of care enhances the probability of success.	II: Theory based, no research data to support recommendations; recommendations from expert consensus group may exist	See Annotated Bibliography: 9 See Other References: 6	

Period of Use	Recommendation	Rationale for Recommendation	Level of Recommendation	Supporting References	Comments
Selection of Patients *(cont.)*	• *Physiologic stability:* Identified when the lowest possible F$_{IO_2}$, simplest ventilatory mode, and nutritional regimen are in place and working well.				
	A supportive physical home environment is essential: • The patient must be able to receive physical care in an appropriate area and be safely evacuated in an emergency. • Adequate electrical circuits for necessary equipment, heating, and cooling; storage space for supplies and equipment; safe water supply; phone access; and a system for calling caregivers are vital. Necessary modifications of the home must be evaluated before decisions can be made about HCM.	Discharge to a safe environment is essential. Multistory homes with upper-level bedrooms may present barriers to care and socialization. Older homes and those with a history of electrical problems may present dangers to HCM. It may be necessary to evaluate well water in rural homes.	II: Theory based, no research data to support recommendations; recommendations from expert consensus group may exist	See Annotated Bibliography: 7, 9, 10	In areas with a history of electrical power outages families may need to buy a generator. The home care agency and equipment supplier can provide home care assessment.
	Available caregivers: Family members or hired caregivers are essential to successful HCM of ventilator-dependent patients. At least 2, and preferably more, people must be willing and able to be trained to provide necessary care before deciding to pursue HCM. Patients needing only nighttime ventilation may be exceptions; however they also need trained support people after discharge. A 24-hour-a-day/7-days-a-week schedule using trained family caregivers should also include coverage for relieving the caregivers. Relief for the primary caregivers is essential.	The 24-hour-a-day responsibility for giving care must be shared. If one person attempts to assume this work, success is very unlikely.	IV: Limited clinical studies to support recommendations	See Annotated Bibliography: 5, 12	Speaking with or visiting the home of a family who is experiencing ventilator HCM is often helpful.

Period of Use	Recommendation	Rationale for Recommendation	Level of Recommendation	Supporting References	Comments
Selection of Patients *(cont.)*	*Psychosocial resources of patient and family:* • Patient and family coping skills may determine feasibility of HCM, which requires motivated, optimistic people who are able to think critically.	Financial and psychological resources influence the ability of patients and families to continue HCM. Investigation of resources and evaluation of psychological strengths and weaknesses allow for systems to be put in place that will make success more likely.	IV: Limited clinical studies to support recommendations	See Annotated Bibliography: 1, 3, 7, 10	
	• A plan for comprehensive funding for HCM must be in place before discharge.	Financial resources or third party payment sources are needed to pay for equipment and supplies.			
Preparation for HCM	Once HCM has been chosen for the ventilator-dependent patient, preparation for discharge recommendations are as follows:		II: Theory based, no research data to support recommendations; recommendations from expert consensus group may exist	See Annotated Bibliography: 3, 4, 9, 14	Occasionally a patient may be evaluated at home for HCM and admission is then scheduled for tracheostomy and teaching. Before admission, a home visit by the case manager or primary nurse who will be caring for this patient may help the patient and family understand what will be expected of them. Beginning teaching before hospitalization may decrease length of stay and improve outcome. Partnership with the home health agency can help in achieving the above goals.

	The patient must be at or near the optimal functional status:
	
	• Major systems stable
	
	• Absence of acute infections
	
	• Stable metabolic status
	
	• Stable ventilator parameters with absence of sustained dyspnea or tachypnea:
	
	  – $FIO_2 \leq 0.40$
	
	  – Simplest ventilator mode possible
	
	• Secretions controlled; patient able to clear secretions either spontaneously or with tracheal suction.
		Any complications or unresolved medical problems make progress toward discharge more difficult.
		
		High FIO_2 is difficult and expensive to provide in the home. Complex ventilator modes (IMV, PEEP), although available on some ventilators, add an additional burden to the caregivers learning requirements. Generally, the least complex ventilator settings are selected prior to home discharge. Patients may need a period of adjustment to the small home ventilator because ventilation may feel different.			

Period of Use	Recommendation	Rationale for Recommendation	Level of Recommendation	Supporting References	Comments
Preparation for HCM *(cont.)*	• Review medicines; schedule time to provide periods of rest for patient and caregiver. • Simplify nutritional management; ensure adequate caloric needs met and bowel program in place. • Consider giving flu and pneumococcal vaccines before discharge.	Give only medicines that are absolutely necessary, and do so on a simplified schedule. Paid caregivers may be needed to offer family members time to sleep or get away. Discussion of the caregiver needs is important to the success of the home discharge.			
	Hold patient care conferences involving healthcare providers *and patient and family* for goal setting and evaluations of progress. • Healthcare team members vary according to the practice setting. The team may include a primary physician (often a pulmonologist), advanced practice nurse, physician assistant, primary and associate nurses, respiratory therapist, dietician, speech therapist, social worker, home care providers, care manager, and anyone else who will be involved in the patient's care (eg, physical or occupational therapy or pastoral care).	Each patient and family has different needs, so goals must be specific. Individualized plan development meets the specific needs of patient and caregivers. Clear discussion of goals and plan by all involved improves understanding and promotes progress toward discharge.	IV: Limited clinical studies to support recommendations	See Annotated Bibliography: 6	
	• Having a limited number of nurses working with the patient and family ensures consistency in teaching and increased comfort for the patient and family. Matching patient need with nurse characteristics will help with optimal patient outcomes.		II: Theory based, no research data to support recommendations; recommendations from expert consensus group may exist	See Annotated Bibliography: 4, 9 See Other References: 1	
	Identify primary and consulting physicians.	If hospital physicians will not be following the patient after discharge, it is best to involve the physician responsible for home care early.			Building a relationship with the home care company while the patient is hospitalized promotes smooth transition. Placing the patient on the home ventilator and approximating home care will increase learning and feelings of comfort.

Period of Use	Recommendation	Rationale for Recommendation	Level of Recommendation	Supporting References	Comments
Preparation for HCM (*cont.*)	Partner with home care company and providers of durable medical equipment to establish continuity of care.	Going home can be a stressful experience. Knowing who will answer questions and provide backup and emergency help relieves some of the anxiety.			
	Begin discharge teaching by defining individualized goals and instituting a teaching plan.	Begin teaching simple care as soon as caregivers are identified to allow time for them to become comfortable with the many aspects of care.	IV: Limited clinical studies to support recommendations	See Annotated Bibliography: 4, 8, 9, 11, 14	
	Give each caregiver a competency sheet to verify knowledge and accurate return demonstration of skills. Written instructions with steps provide reference information.				
	Clean (not sterile) technique with good hand washing is recommended for home care. Recommended areas of teaching, may include the following: • Tracheostomy stoma care, inner cannula cleaning or change, cuff inflation, skin care with tracheostomy tie change and tracheostomy tube change, steps to be taken in case of accidental decannulation • Airway clearance: Suctioning, hydration, signs of pulmonary infection, chest physiotherapy and augmented cough, mobility • Adequate ventilation: Use and maintenance of the home ventilator, adequate humidification, use of manual resuscitation bag and oxygen, use of SpO$_2$ monitor, home oxygen safety	Clean technique simplifies care. Infection risk at home is less than in the hospital due to limited numbers of caregivers and less exposure to drug-resistant bacteria. Begin use of home ventilator during hospitalization to allow time for teaching and for patient to adjust to a different machine.	II: Theory based, no research data to support recommendations; recommendations from expert consensus group may exist	See Other References: 5, 9, 14, 15	Cleaning and reusing suction catheters with appropriate technique may be acceptable in the home and decreases cost. Nondisposable ventilator circuits can be changed when dirty and cleaned with various cleaners, disinfected, and air dried. Cleaning by dishwasher is also possible.

Period of Use	Recommendation	Rationale for Recommendation	Level of Recommendation	Supporting References	Comments
Preparation for HCM *(cont.)*	• Maintenance of cleanliness, maximum strength, and flexibility: Bath, shampoo and shave, mouth care, bowel and bladder management, strength and flexibility exercises	Care related to activities of daily living may not need to be taught, but assessing patient or caregiver skills in this area is very important.			
	• Signs, symptoms, and prevention of irritation, infection, and skin breakdown: Turning, positioning, transfer (use of equipment such as hydraulic lift) and ambulation; percutaneous endoscopic gastrostomy (PEG) site care; Foley care; peripherally inserted central catheter (PICC) or IV line care	All teaching is patient specific.			
	• Adequate nutrition and hydration: Feeding tube care, flushing, and declogging; hydration and dehydration assessment; recognition and interventions for diarrhea and constipation	Patients able to eat may need a review of nutrition.			
	• Communication: Importance of maintaining communication techniques, including speaking valve use	During teaching, communication methods can be established with input from patient, family, nurses, and sometimes speech therapists.			
	• Effective coping skills for patient and caregivers	Identify or teach coping skills to improve responses to care after discharge.			
	• Discussion of and suggestions for social, educational, and vocational activities	Often patients need encouragement to live as normally as possible.			
	• Emergency plans: Evacuation, family or patient emergencies, available generator, backup ventilator, manual resuscitation bag, or additional batteries in case of frequent power failures	Because of decreased mobility and ventilator dependency, evacuation in case of fire or storm must be planned. Planning for emergencies before they happen increases the ability of patient and family to cope.			
	• Completion of advance directives, including clear direction for return to hospital and activation of emergency medical system.				

Period of Use	Recommendation	Rationale for Recommendation	Level of Recommendation	Supporting References	Comments
Preparation for HCM *(cont.)*	Notify community agencies (eg, electric, telephone company) and emergency medical services.	Rapid restoration of interrupted services and response to emergencies is vital.		See Annotated Bibliography: 4, 14	
	Establish a backup plan in case HCM does not succeed. Home care agencies may help and provide social worker follow-up.	Occasionally even with the best preparation, the patient is not able to be cared for at home.			
	The discharge date should be decided by the entire team with input from patient and family. Optimal time for discharge is early in the week.	Increased availability of resource staff during weekday business hours provides greater resources for troubleshooting problems before the weekend.			
Discharge	**Planning and Preparation for Discharge** Trained caregivers provide total care for 24 hours or for extended periods on consecutive days.	Learning to manage care before they arrive home decreases stress.	II: Theory based, no research data to support recommendations; recommendations from expert consensus group may exist	See Annotated Bibliography: 1, 9 See Other References: 6, 10	
	Sleep patterns of 6 to 8 hours per night are established with less frequent nighttime interventions.	Establishing this more normal home routine before discharge helps both patient and caregivers.			
	Transportation: Determine *before* discharge day how the patient will travel home and who will accompany.				Prior approval from payer may be necessary for ambulance transportation.
	Written discharge prescriptions are given to the family with appropriate instruction for medications and equipment.				
	The home care company's responsibility is to make sure all needed equipment is in the home and caregivers know how to operate all devices. If a representative does not travel with the patient he or she should be at the home to meet the patient on arrival.	Building a trusting relationship is extremely important to success in HCM.			

Period of Use	Recommendation	Rationale for Recommendation	Level of Recommendation	Supporting References	Comments
Discharge *(cont.)*	Discharging hospital staff's responsibility is to make sure caregiver has all needed equipment for the trip and phone numbers for all resource people.				
	Assess the need for the ventilator-dependent patient to have short visits at home before discharge.	Some caregivers and patients may experience less anxiety and stress if they can have short home experiences before discharge.			
	Establish a method of keeping in touch with the patient and family to ensure continuity of care (advanced practice nurse, primary nurse, or case manager may fulfill this role).	Often if things go smoothly with the home care company this is not necessary, but the safety net provided by a contact person is reassuring.			
	Identify ways to meet psychosocial needs of patient and caregiver after discharge. Counseling may be available in connection with the home care agency.	At discharge the focus is on the technical aspects of care, but as time goes on psychosocial needs may intensify, and having a system in place to meet those needs is very helpful.	IV: Limited clinical studies to support recommendations	See Annotated Bibliography: 2	
	Day of Discharge				
	At discharge it is recommended that the primary nurse or case manager accompany the patient and caregivers to the ambulance or car if possible.	Providing support as the patient leaves the secure hospital environment is meaningful.	II: Theory based, no research data to support recommendations; recommendations from expert consensus group may exist	See Annotated Bibliography: 1, 4, 9 See Annotated Bibliography: 1, 5, 9	
	Discharge instructions, medications, and teaching plan verification are given to patient and family with copies placed in the medical record and sent to the home care agency.	Organization of materials in a binder for the home helps for access of information.			
Follow-up	Home care company provides follow-up community health nurse to provide initial and ongoing assessment of need.	The stress of being responsible for care may make it hard to recall all that is taught. Caregivers need to transfer dependence to the home care company as they work on developing a measure of independence.	II: Theory based, no research data to support recommendations; recommendations from expert consensus group may exist		

Period of Use	Recommendation	Rationale for Recommendation	Level of Recommendation	Supporting References	Comments
Follow-up *(cont.)*	Advanced practice nurse, primary nurse, or care manager ensures continuity of care by following the plan for keeping in touch with the patient (this individualized plan will depend on the hospital and its resources as well as the patient's needs).	Contact with a hospital care provider during the first few days at home gives reassurance and decreases feelings of abandonment.			
	Offer family and patient the opportunity to assist others in same process they have experienced. Hospital healthcare team may keep informal contacts with HCM patients to keep in touch on progress and future networking with other patients and families.	Patients and families have much to offer; they know what their needs are and usually enjoy sharing their experiences.			
Prevention of Complications	Adequate staff education and reeducation are important as there is high complexity and risk associated with HCM of a ventilator-dependent patient.	Infrequent HCM discharge makes it important to have core staff trained or resource person available.			
	Individualize care, teaching, and planning for discharge based on specific patient needs.				
	Verify competence of each caregiver (checklists are helpful, see Appendix 4C).				
Quality Improvement Issues	Ask patient and caregivers about perceptions of the teaching and discharge process. Incorporate suggestions to improve care.	Feedback is vital to assure quality care and optimal patient satisfaction.	IV: Limited clinical studies to support recommendations	See Annotated Bibliography: 1, 5, 7, 10, 12, 14 See Other References: 12	
	Collect objective data to verify healthcare providers' observations of improved quality of life resulting from HCM. Follow up after discharge to verify adequate information provided to render care.				
	Examine readmission causes and issues.				

ANNOTATED BIBLIOGRAPHY

1. **Bertolotti G, Corone M. From mechanical ventilation to home care: the psychological approach.** *Monaldi Arch Chest Dis.* **1994;49:537–540.**

The authors discuss the life-supporting nature of mechanical ventilation giving rise to fear of death, feelings of abandonment and mutilation, and changes in self-image. At discharge the psychological needs of patients and caregivers are overshadowed by the need for technical expertise to manage the home ventilator equipment. Psychological support should be offered well before discharge. Level of communication within the family and the degree of commitment of all family members is associated with adaptation to mechanical ventilation.

2. **Criner GJ, Tzkouanakis A, Kreimer DT. Overview of improving tolerance of long-term mechanical ventilation.** *Crit Care Clin.* **1994;10:845–866.**

This article synthesizes data that define the group of patients who require long-term ventilation (≥ 6 hours per day for ≥ 30 days) and suggests ways to maximize ventilation to improve patient outcome and functional status. Noninvasive and positive pressure ventilation via tracheostomy are discussed along with problems affecting the tolerance of long-term ventilation. Optimizing ventilator settings and carefully evaluating and systematically treating psychological, medical, and physiological problems may improve patients' tolerance and maximize functional capacity.

3. **Douglas SL, Daly BJ. Caregivers of long-term ventilator patients. Physical and psychological outcomes.** *Chest.* **2003;123:1073–1081.**

Study Sample
The study sample consisted of caregivers of 135 patients who were receiving long-term ventilation (defined as patients who required more than 4 days of continuous mechanical ventilation in the hospital); were admitted to the intensive care unit of a university medical center, a Veterans Administration hospital, or a small community hospital; and resided in a home or institutional setting after discharge.

Purpose of the Study
The purpose of the study was to determine the effects on caregivers of caring for patients receiving long-term mechanical ventilation, by examining depression, burden, overload, and physical health in this caregiver population over a 6-month period after hospital discharge.

Study Procedures
Interviews of caregivers were conducted at hospital discharge and 6 months later. Established tools were used to assess caregiver depression, burden, overload, and physical health.

Key Results
Caregivers reported a drop in physical health scores from hospital discharge to 6 months after discharge. Caregivers of patient's residing in an institution reported higher depression and overload scores. Low caregiver physical health and high overload scores were significantly associated with caregiver depression.

Study Strengths and Weaknesses
The study examines a defined population of subjects who care for patients receiving long-term ventilation and provides insight into caregiver coping. This study will be helpful for clinicians who work with such caregivers in the home setting. A weakness of the study is the inexact definition of the caregiver term, which limits comparison to other studies.

Clinical Implications
Healthcare teams can better address the potential for depression and risks to physical health that may ensue as caregivers assume home care of the patient receiving long-term mechanical ventilation.

4. **Ecklund MM. Successful outcomes for the ventilator-dependent patient.** *Crit Care Nurs Clin N Am.* **1999;11:249–259.**

The author describes the model of care used in a pulmonary step-down unit. The role of the multidisciplinary team in planning for and achieving patient-focused customized care is reviewed. A case study reviews preparation for discharge to home of a ventilator-dependent patient.

5. **Glass C, Boling PA, Gammon S. Collaborative support for care givers of individuals beginning mechanical ventilation at home.** *Crit Care Nurse.* **1996;16:67–72.**

The authors conducted detailed interviews with family members responsible for the care of ventilator-dependent patients to determine caregivers' perceived needs. Questions addressed how to improve preparation for going home and the first few weeks at home and what they learned from experience that might help other caregivers. A videotape based on this information allowed caregivers and one ventilator-dependent person to share their insights and practical knowledge gained from experience. The caregivers and patient describe the advantages and disadvantages of HCM, preparation for going home, tips to help manage home care, how to create a comfortable feeling for the patient at home, and ideas for finding other caregivers for support. The videotape is available from the American Lung Association of Virginia (804-355-3295) at cost.

6. Goldstein RS, Peek JA, Gort EH. Home mechanical ventilation demographics and user perspectives. *Chest.* 1995;108:1581–1586.

Study Sample

The study population consisted of 98 (48 male, 50 female) patients undergoing home mechanical ventilation (HMV), mean age 47.4 ± 19.5 years. Diagnoses included COPD, thoracic restrictive disease, and neuromuscular disease. Subjects had received HMV a mean of 59.5 ± 58.3 months, with 53% being electively ventilated and the remainder under emergency circumstances. Users experienced continuous ventilation (18%), night only (37%), or night with occasional daytime use (45%). Twenty-eight percent of subjects were totally independent, 33% partially dependent on caregivers, and the remainder were unable to perform self-care.

Comparison Studied

The effect of diagnosis and invasive or noninvasive mechanical ventilation on the number of positive and negative comments volunteered regarding lifestyle was studied.

Study Procedures

A research assistant conducted interviews in the patient's home, during scheduled outpatient appointment, or by telephone. The research assistant followed a specific 2-part questionnaire developed with input from physicians, respiratory therapists, and members of the Committee for Independence in Living and Breathing. Section 1 gathered information on demographics, mechanical ventilator use, mobility, and living arrangements. Section 2 contained 8 open-ended questions that elicited a broad range of user responses to their experiences with HMV.

Key Results

Of the 47% of subjects who were ventilated by tracheostomy, three-fourths had a neuromuscular disease. These subjects had significantly more negative statements and fewer positive statements than those with noninvasive ventilation. Informed choice for HMV was made in only 38% of the subjects. When asked if they would choose HMV today, 89% said yes; 87% said HMV had been a positive experience overall. Aspects of the condition most difficult to deal with initially related to adjustment to equipment and ventilator, limitations in activities and dependence on others, physical symptoms, and permanence of the condition or uncertainty of prognosis. At the time the study was done, 40% indicated they had adapted almost completely to the situation; difficulties with limitations in activity, dependence, and equipment problems were considered a problem by only a few.

Study Strengths and Weaknesses

Although diagnosis is related clearly to both positive and negative statements regarding HMV experience, it is difficult to determine the effect of invasive or noninvasive HMV on the variables.

Clinical Implications

The authors concluded that in this study subjects adapted well to ongoing ventilator support in the home and would choose the therapy again if required to do so. A majority of the subjects (62%) felt that they did not make an informed choice for HMV when first starting mechanical ventilation or when the treatment became permanent. This underlines the importance of discussing HMV with patients and families without delay as the disease progresses—waiting until respiratory failure occurs or for emergency intubation means the patient cannot understand or express his or her wishes.

7. Lindahl B, Sandman P, Rasmussen BH. Meaning of living at home on a ventilator. *Nurs Inquiry.* 2003;10:19–27.

Study Sample

The study sample consisted of 9 adult patients in Sweden who were dependent on mechanical ventilation in the home for more than 2 years. Subjects required complete or partial ventilator support. Only patients able to speak were enrolled in order to allow voice recording during interviews.

Purpose of the Study

The purpose of the study was to determine perceptions of patients living at home and receiving mechanical ventilation.

Study Procedures

Interviews were conducted in person.

Key Results

The following themes related to living at home on a ventilator emerged from the analyses:

- Technology is both a burden and a relief.
- Home is a safe and comfortable space from which to reach out to others for help.
- The body is perceived as being frail, brave, and resilient.
- Strive to live in the present.
- Surrender oneself and trust others.

Study Strengths and Weaknesses

This qualitative study provides information about the perceptions of patients who receive mechanical ventilation at home. The study sample's mix of patients receiving invasive and noninvasive mechanical ventilation provides diversity;

however, the nonhomogeneous sample makes generalizing the findings difficult.

Clinical Implications

The healthcare team's knowledge and understanding of patient's perspective is important in planning care.

8. Moss AH, Oppenheimer EA, Casey P, et al. Patients with amyotrophic lateral sclerosis receiving long-term ventilation. *Chest.* 1996;110:249–255.

Study Sample

Fifty patients with amyotrophic lateral sclerosis (ALS) receiving long-term mechanical ventilation (LTMV) participated in structured interviews. Of this sample, 43 patients were ventilated via tracheostomy, 7 with noninvasive ventilation; 36 lived at home, and 14 lived in an institution.

Purpose of the Study

This study was designed to examine decision making, advance directives, and outcomes of patients with ALS receiving LTMV.

Study Procedures

Structured interviews by investigators or trained home health nurses contained open- and closed-ended questions. Separate interviews were conducted with family members or other caregivers most closely associated with the patient's treatment.

Key Results

- Decision: 42% decided in advance for LTMV, 42% decided at the time of respiratory failure crisis, 8% started LTMV without patient consent but with family consent, and 8% started LTMV without patient or family consent.
- Satisfaction with decision: 88% were glad to be alive on LTMV; 80% would choose LTMV again.
- Advance directives: 76% would stop LTMV under certain circumstances; 58% did not want cardiopulmonary resuscitation.
- Family attitudes: 42% considered care a major burden that had changed their entire life and said the situation was very stressful; 78% said insurance was "essential" to afford LTMV; 83% of the caregivers would encourage family members with ALS to choose LTMV again.
- Expenses (home versus institution): 91% of home expenses were covered by insurance; 54% had more than one insurance. Mean yearly out-of-pocket expense for home care was $10,356 (range $0 to $240,000), with home care being significantly less expensive. Annual average expense for home care was $136,560 compared to the average annual institutional expense of $366,852.

Study Strengths and Weaknesses

Of the 75 patients identified, 11 died before interview, 6 were unable to communicate well enough to be interviewed, and 8 declined to participate, decreasing the sample by one-third (13 of whom were in institutions). Patient attitudes may have been influenced by the availability of resource personnel for patients with LTMV in the study area. Interviewer bias might influence the outcome as 4 investigators interviewed, but bias was minimized by the use of standard questions with responses recorded verbatim.

Clinical Implications

Clear explanation of the progression of ALS will allow decisions about LTMV to be made in advance. Discussion about limits of LTMV should be encouraged and desires about maintaining LTMV should be clear in case institutional care is ever required.

9. O'Donohue WJ, Giovannoni RM, Keens TG, Plummer AL. Long-term mechanical ventilation guidelines for management in the home and at alternate community sites. *Chest.* 1986;90(Suppl):1S–37S.

This comprehensive article is a report of the Ad Hoc Committee, Respiratory Care Section of the American College of Chest Physicians. The consensus guidelines for patient selection and discharge criteria, which include a comprehensive plan for patient discharge, represent the opinions of adult and pediatric healthcare professionals practicing throughout the United States. There are sections on principles for respiratory care for ventilator-assisted infants, children, and adults in the home and an alternate community site.

10. Smith CE, Mayer LS, Parkhurst C, Perkins SB, Pingleton SK. Adaptation in families with a member requiring mechanical ventilation at home. *Heart Lung.* 1991;20:349–356.

Study Sample

Twenty family caregivers of patients receiving HMV were studied. Needs of the patients varied from continuous positive pressure ventilation to mask ventilation only at night. Home care ranged from full-time family care to 24-hour professional care.

Purpose of Study

The purpose of this study was to determine how family caregivers adapt to having a ventilator-dependent adult at home.

Study Procedures

In-home interviews were conducted with primary family caregivers of ventilator-dependent adults. The Family Coping Scale; Family APGAR, which measures individual satisfaction with family function; and 8 interview questions developed by the investigators followed by open-ended probes related to each subject's responses were used in the 2-hour interview session.

Key Results

Family coping scores fell within national norms if the patient required ventilation 24 hours a day or less. Family APGAR scores showed satisfaction with overall family function but decreased as ventilation time increased. Interviews related that essential knowledge and skills were taught but additional information was desired. Positive themes included satisfaction with decision to care for the family member at home and improved quality of life and confidence in ventilator care. Negative themes reflected the burden of caregiving, dependence of the patient on the caregiver, resentment, and hopelessness.

Study Strengths and Weaknesses

The small study sample with a varied patient group is of concern; however, this study is an important step toward looking at family adaptation to ventilator care in the home.

Clinical Implications

Both positive and negative feelings were expressed by the caregivers in this study. Preparing for discharge, mastery of the caregiver role, and management of equipment may overshadow the psychosocial needs of patients and caregivers. Needs for counseling and support must be assessed before discharge and followed up months and years later. As the duration of HMV increased, positive family function was perceived to decrease and caregivers expressed a need for respite care.

11. Smith CE, Mayer LS, Perkins SB, Gerald K, Pingleton SK. Caregiver learning needs and reactions to managing home mechanical ventilation. *Heart Lung.* 1994;23:157–163.

Study Sample

Twenty caregivers and ventilator-dependent adults living at home were studied.

Purpose of the Study

This study was designed to identify caregivers' learning needs and reactions to providing care for ventilator-dependent adults in the home.

Study Procedures

During scheduled interviews at the patient's residence, caregivers completed a 57-item, investigator-generated, learning-needs checklist plus open-ended questions about the importance of information provided and frequency of use in providing care. The Caregiving Reaction Inventory was completed to measure factors that influence reactions to caring for family members in the home and reactions to caregiving.

Key Results

All 57 items on the Learning Needs Checklist were ranked "needed" or "very needed," but only 3 of 57 items had been taught to all caregivers. Fourteen items were taught to fewer than half the family caregivers. The Reaction Inventory revealed that as hours of ventilation per day increased, caregivers reported increased financial strain, schedule disruption, and negative reactions to caregiving. No significant correlation was noted between years of mechanical ventilation and caregiver reaction scores.

Study Strengths and Weaknesses

The small study sample is of concern and the possibility that subjects might check all content on a questionnaire as important without giving comments is a weakness; however, this study is another example of an attempt to learn from caregivers.

Clinical Implications

Items judged as needed or very needed were not taught to all caregivers, indicating that learning needs were not completely met. Perhaps a system of phase teaching would be more effective, with material prioritized to teach survival information first, delaying other topics until the patient and caregiver are comfortable with care at home. Subjects reported increased stress as ventilator hours per day increased, emphasizing the issues of respite and caregiver support.

12. Thomas VM, Ellison K, Howell EV, Winters K. Caring for the person receiving ventilatory support at home: caregivers' needs and involvement. *Heart Lung.* 1992;21:180–186.

Study Sample

Subjects were 44 caregivers 18 years and older who were responsible for the day-to-day care of 29 people receiving ventilatory support at home.

Purpose of Study

This study explored the needs of family members caring for people receiving ventilatory support.

Study Procedures

Trained nurse interviewers used a 77-item questionnaire to conduct in-home interviews with caregivers.

Key Results

Those interviewed ranked as highest the need for support services, education, attention to other family members, and handling of emergencies, finance, and respite. Caregiver needs varied depending on relationship to the person receiving ventilatory support, experience giving care, and the amount of time the person was involved in care.

Study Strengths and Weaknesses

It is unknown how well the sample represents all those receiving home ventilatory support and their caregivers, which limits generalizability; however, the authors offer insights into a variety of caregivers who were mostly the parents, spouse, or child living with the person receiving ventilatory support.

Clinical Implications

Learning what experienced caregivers need is important when decisions are made about home care and when preparation is made for discharge. Needs of caregivers and of the person receiving ventilatory support must be identified and met if home care is to succeed.

13. Thompson CL, Richmond M. Teaching home care for ventilator-dependent patients. The patients' perception. *Heart Lung.* 1990;19: 79–83.

Study Sample

The study population consisted of 13 ventilator-dependent patients (6 male, 7 female) living at home in the eastern United States and ranging in age from 17 to 70 (mean age 54.4 years) with diagnoses of kyphoscoliosis, neuromuscular diseases, and COPD. Subjects had been instructed and discharged from the medical intensive care unit of a large eastern US hospital within 5 years before the study.

Purpose of the Study

This study was conducted to identify perceptions of ventilator-dependent patients or family members providing care. Perceptions of the knowledge and skills required to prepare for home care and the ideal environment for learning that content were explored.

Study Procedures

A 61-item questionnaire was mailed to all subjects. Content variables were pulmonary hygiene, use and maintenance of equipment, and lung disease process. Environmental variables were media and methods of learning, length of a single session, location of the session, and who was present during the lesson.

Key Results

Content taught before discharge was rated "completely understood" by at least 85% of the subjects and basically understood by the remainder of subjects. Content taught was

considered essential or very important 79% of the time, with maintenance of nutrition, anatomy of the trachea and lungs, oxygen-carbon dioxide exchange in the lungs, and how other patients with the same disease manage at home listed by 2 subjects as only slightly important. The ideal setting for learning about home care was at the bedside with 1 or 2 family members present and only the team member teaching in 30-minute sessions using demonstration. No subjects thought pamphlets were appropriate for learning content.

Study Strengths and Weaknesses

Asking patients and caregivers what they needed to learn was vital in meeting their long-term needs; however, during the learning experience they may not know what is needed. This study provides insight into the perceptions of 1 group of patients. Because the sample size is small, replication is needed.

Clinical Implications

The patients' perception of the ideal environment and method for learning demonstrates the importance of asking patients and families their perception of what works best as the teaching progresses. Patients and their families in this study agreed with healthcare professionals on most of what is commonly taught before discharge. Information considered very important by patients and families may be retained better than content they consider less important.

14. Warren ML, Jarrett C, Senegal R, et al. An interdisciplinary approach to transitioning ventilator-dependent patients to home. *J Nurs Care Qual.* 2004;19:67–73.

The authors provide an overview, using the quality-improvement model, of how to prepare for and discharge a ventilator-dependent patient to the home. Algorithms for planning and a structured approach to teaching are described. A case study is presented to illustrate the process.

15. Wright SE, Van Dahm K. Long-term care of the tracheostomy patient. *Clin Chest Med.* 2003;24:473–487.

The authors provide an overview of the issues related to caring for the patient with a tracheostomy. The percutaneous tracheostomy is described and ongoing care of the patient is divided into an early period (up to 7 days after tracheostomy) and the established period (greater than 8 days after tracheostomy). Topics include airway management, stoma care, humidification, cuff care, communication, nutritional intake, management of complications, weaning and decannulation, and long-term care planning including teaching.

OTHER REFERENCES

1. Collard P, Rodenstein DO. Home mechanical ventilation and/or long-term oxygen therapy in chronic obstructive pulmonary disease. *Monaldi Arch Chest Dis.* 1994;49:441–444.

2. Curley, MAQ. Patient-nurse synergy: optimizing patients' outcomes. *Am J Crit Care.* 1998;7:64–72.

3. Donner CF, Howard P, Robert D. Patient selection and techniques for home mechanical ventilation. *Eur Respir J.* 1993;6:3–4.

4. Donner CF, Howard P, Robert D. Patient selection and techniques for home mechanical ventilation. *Monaldi Arch Chest Dis.* 1993;48:40–47.

5. Feldman J, Tueur PG. Mechanical ventilation: from hospital intensive care to home. *Heart Lung.* 1982;11: 162–165.

6. Ferns T. Home mechanical ventilation in a changing health service. *Nurs Times.* 1994;90:43–45.

7. Gajdos P. The French organization of mechanical ventilation at home for neuromuscular diseases. *Paraplegia.* 1993;31:147–149.

8. Glass CA. The impact of home-based ventilator dependence on family life. *Paraplegia.* 1993;31: 93–101.

9. Goldburg AI. Technology assessment and support of life-sustaining devices in home care. The home care physician perspective. *Chest.* 1994;105:1448–1452.

10. Mizumor NA, Nelson EJP, Prentice WS, Withey LW. Mechanical ventilation in the home. In: Turner J, McDonald GJ, Larter NL, eds. *Handbook of Adult and Pediatric Respiratory Home Care.* St Louis, Mo: Mosby; 1994:273–291.

11. Muir JF, Girault C, Cardinaud JP, et al. Survival and long-term follow-up of tracheotomized patients with COPD treated by home mechanical ventilation. A multicenter French study in 259 patients. *Chest.* 1994;106:201–209.

12. Pehrsson K, Olofson J, Larsson S, Sullivan M. Quality of life of patients treated by home mechanical ventilation due to restrictive ventilatory disorders. *Respir Med.* 1994;88:21–26.

13. Peters SG, Viggiano RW. Home mechanical ventilation. *Mayo Clin Proc.* 1988;63:1208–1213.

14. Sevick MA, Zucconi S, Sereika S, et al. Characteristics and health service utilization patterns of ventilator-dependent patients cared for within a vertically integrated health system. *Am J Crit Care.* 1992; 1:45–51.

15. Tablan OC, Anderson LJ, Besser RI, Bridges CA, Hajjeh RA. Guidelines for prevention of health-care associated pneumonia. *MMWR.* 2004;53:136.

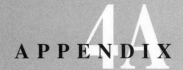
Algorithm for Home Mechanical Ventilation

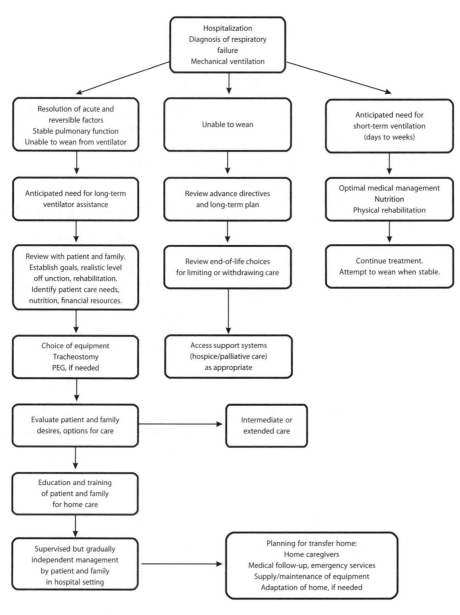

Adapted from Peters SC, Viggiano RW with permission (Other References: 12).

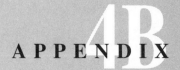
Responsibilities of Team Members: Education and Preparation for Home Mechanical Ventilation

Each hospital team matches the caregiver competency to patient/family need (See Other References: 1).

ADVANCED PRACTICE NURSE, CARE MANAGER, OR PRIMARY NURSE

- Plans and facilitates initial conference with family and attending physician (reviews need for home care and determines desire and ability of family to care for patient at home)
- Schedules, conducts, and documents initial conference with team members to identify problems and establish goals
- Completes and documents thorough nursing history and assessment
- Conducts necessary patient care conferences
- Establishes and documents teaching plan and patient education checklist
- Provides ongoing documentation of teaching activities in progress notes
- Provides ongoing communication:
  - Among members of team
  - With patient and family
  - In progress notes
  - With use of teaching checklist in bedside report
  - To orient physician and in-house staff to their responsibilities
- Coordinates services provided by other team members
- Maintains teaching checklist
- Organizes reference binder of information and teaching sheets for patient and family
- Reevaluates goals, problems, and teaching plan

- Coordinates home care resources for patient and family
- Projects and confirms discharge date
- Plans and conducts final conference with home care providers before discharge
- Writes discharge summary in medical record, sending copy home with patient

DESIGNATED STAFF NURSES

- Assists primary nurse in planning and caring for patient and family
- Attends initial conferences and other conferences as able
- Provides input into establishing teaching plan and documenting on patient education checklist
- Provides documentation of teaching activities in progress notes
- Documents teaching checklist
- Collaborates with primary nurse and other staff members on care of patient and family

CARE MANAGER/SOCIAL WORKER

- Consults with physician on appropriateness of candidate for program
- Assists patient and family in selection of home care company
- Contacts home care company
- Serves as liaison for equipment with home care company
- Attends conferences as needed
- Assists in communication with patient and family

- Collaborates with primary and associate nurses in establishing teaching plan, and consults with other health team members as needed
- Documents all teaching activities and other involvement in progress notes

ATTENDING PHYSICIAN

- Attends initial conference with patient and family (includes attending physician and fellow)
- Attends other conferences as needed
- Determines home care physician, makes referral, and provides necessary information for continuation of care at home
- Determines if flu and pneumococcal vaccines are needed and orders if appropriate
- Determines optimal ventilator settings 5 to 7 days before discharge
- Writes discharge orders 2 days before discharge

RESPIRATORY THERAPIST

- Receives referral from primary nurse when patient is identified as candidate for mechanical ventilation at home
- Provides input into establishing teaching plan and patient education checklist
- Provides documentation of teaching activities in progress notes
- Assists patient and family in selection of home care company
- Contacts home care company
- Serves as liaison for respiratory equipment with home care company

HOME CARE COMPANY AND PROVIDER OF DURABLE EQUIPMENT

- Evaluates home for use of ventilator and provides instruction to caregivers on use of ventilator
- Provides additional home care equipment (depending on company)
- Provides assistance in transportation home at time of discharge
- Provides service in home setting
- Conducts home safety evaluation for electrical supply and equipment

COMMUNITY HEALTH NURSE COORDINATOR

- Receives referral
- Conducts ongoing financial review
- Organizes home plan
- Develops discharge plan for community nursing resources and contacts
- Community health nurse assesses need and schedules speech therapy, occupational therapy, and physical therapy evaluation after discharge; secures nursing service coverage, or assistance with private duty coverage with family

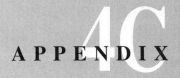

APPENDIX 4C

Checklists

Discharge skill list for: _____

Caregiver name: _____

Skill	Date Taught/initials	Date Observed/initials
Disease		
Name and list function of the parts of the respiratory system.		
Describe the air exchange in breathing.		
Describe the disease that has impacted breathing.		
Discuss underlying health issues contributing to the care of the patient.		
Airway Management		
Assess need for suctioning, including what to look for physically.		
Demonstrate listening for breath sounds.		
Demonstrate methods of preoxygenation.		
State the function of the tracheostomy tube.		
Describe the tracheostomy tube and size inserted.		
Demonstrate setup and operation of suctioning machine.		
Suction airway using sterile technique.		
Reevaluate effectiveness of suctioning, describing quality of sputum recovered.		
Demonstrate technique for checking cuff inflation and adding appropriate levels of air.		
Demonstrate troubleshooting cuff leak.		
Change tracheostomy tube holder.		
Demonstrate stoma care.		
Demonstrate correct plugging technique.		
Demonstrate ventilation with manual resuscitation bag.		
Oxygen Delivery		
Describe set up for nasal cannula or tracheostomy collar (if applicable).		
Describe schedule for changing tubing.		
Describe set up and checking of oxygen concentration.		

(Continues)

Skill	Date Taught/initials	Date Observed/initials
Describe function of ventilator.		
Describe operation of ventilator.		
Describe power sources for ventilator.		
Demonstrate set up of circuitry.		
Describe ventilator settings.		
Describe reason for humidification of inspired air.		
Demonstrate drainage of tubing condensate.		
Describe ventilator troubleshooting.		
Describe mechanism for oxygen supply.		
Demonstrate filling of oxygen strollers.		
Emergency Response		
Demonstrate troubleshooting techniques with tracheostomy and ventilator.		
Ventilate with manual resuscitation bag.		
Describe steps to take in case of accidental decannulation.		
Describe steps to troubleshoot tracheostomy tube failure.		
Identify support systems to use in case of emergency.		
Medication Management		
Demonstrate administration of nebulizers and MDIs via airway.		
Describe indications for giving as-needed medications.		
Evaluate response after administration of medication.		
Describe action, side effects, route, and dose of all discharge medications.		
Demonstrate appropriate technique in administering and documenting medication.		
Infection Control		
Describe importance of infection control practice.		
Demonstrate hand washing technique and indication for washing hands.		
Mix appropriate concentration of disinfectant solution (1 part chlorine bleach to 10 parts water).		
Demonstrate proper cleaning technique for:		
• Ventilator circuitry and airway equipment		
• Nebulizer equipment and suction apparatus		
• Commode		
Feeding		
State discharge diet and appropriate meal plans for diet.		
If altered liquid consistency recommended, demonstrate proper technique for mixing liquid with thickener.		
Discuss aspiration risk with an airway in place and prevention strategies.		
If patient is discharged with PEG and/or PEJ tube:		
• Explain anatomy of PEG and/or PEJ tube.		
• Name supplemental product for feeding.		
• Demonstrate residual check.		
• State reason to hold feeding if residual is > 100 mL.		
• Demonstrate process for feeding.		
• Demonstrate medication administration via PEG and/or PEJ.		
• Demonstrate site care for PEG and/or PEJ.		
• Demonstrate fluid flushes.		

(Continues)

Skill	Date Taught/initials	Date Observed/initials
PICC Care		
Demonstrate site check for any redness, swelling, or pain.		
Demonstrate dressing change.		
Demonstrate cap change.		
Advance Directives		
Discuss impact of advance decision making.		
Patient will complete a written advance directive.		
Physical Care		
Demonstrate safe physical care and transfer techniques.		
Caregiver Resources		
Identify roles of home care agency contacts:		
• Primary nurse		
• Agency nurses/coordinator		
• Durable equipment supplier contact		
Identify whom to call for assistance in different situations.		
List resource people for insurance/payment concerns.		
Identify contact at electric company for power outage emergency plan.		
Suggest strategies to provide caregiver respite from patient care.		

Abbreviations: MDI, metered dose inhaler; PEG, percutaneous endoscopic gastrostomy; PEJ, percutaneous endoscopic jejeunostomy; and PICC, peripherally inserted central catheter.

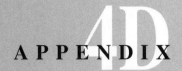
Sample Medication Administration Record

Medication and Dosage	Time	Sun	Mon	Tues	Wed	Thurs	Fri	Sat
Pantoprazole (Protonix) 40 mg	0800							
Ipratropium bromide and albuterol sulfate (Combivent) 6 puffs 4 times daily	0800							
	1200							
	1600							
	2000							
Aspirin 325 mg daily	0800							
Docusate sodium (Colace) 100 mg	0800							
	1600							
Albuterol nebulizer 2.5 mg every 4 hours as needed								
Acetaminophen (Tylenol) 650 mg as needed								

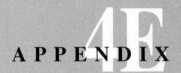
Decision Tree for Care

Situation	Possible Actions/Solutions	Contact for Assistance
Fever, change in secretion amount/volume	Increase fluid intake if necessary. Check for proper humidification of ventilator system.	Dr _____ NP _____
Ankle swelling	Check for decreased urine output or increased fluid intake. Check positioning of legs. Check for weight change.	Dr _____ NP _____
Less energy Less appetite Nausea/vomiting, diarrhea	Check temperature. Check food intake and record.	Dr _____ NP _____
Decreased responsiveness	Check oximetry and call if reaches agreed-upon lowest level. Write in: _____% Return patient to ventilator, and call appropriate contact.	Dr _____ NP _____
Filling tracheostomy cuff and it does not create a seal	Balloon rupture requires tracheostomy change. This is dependent on the individual. Plugging trach and using nasal prongs or return to ventilator are possible interventions. Call contact.	Dr _____ NP _____
Coughing beyond "normal"	Suction. Deflate and inflate cuff.	Dr _____ NP _____
Bloody secretions	Exercise caution with subsequent suctioning; try to go down gently and not as far. If bloody secretions continue and at large volume, may need to contact appropriate healthcare resource. May also need to use a different catheter.	Dr _____ NP _____
Low volume of supplies	Check amount weekly and order as needed.	Supply company
Ventilator malfunction	If patient is compromised, switch to backup ventilator and call healthcare resource. Selected patients may be able to use nasal prongs with a deflated cuff and plugged tracheostomy.	Supply company
Low-pressure alarm	Check all circuit connections and tighten. If cuff is not fully inflated, add more air. Try backup ventilator to see if same alarm situations repeat.	Supply company Dr _____ NP _____
High-pressure alarm	Check need for suctioning. Straighten any kinks in tubing. Drain water in tubing. Listen to lungs and give albuterol as needed.	Supply company Dr _____ NP _____

Abbreviation: NP, nurse practitioner

Nutritional Support for Mechanically Ventilated Patients

Carol Rees Parrish, MS, RD

Joe Krenitsky, MS, RD

Kate Willcutts, MS, RD, CNSD

Nutritional Support for Mechanically Ventilated Patients

CASE STUDY

Ms Tucker, a 62-year-old woman, was admitted to the medical ICU with a community-acquired pneumonia requiring mechanical ventilation. She was overweight, but had lost 9 kg (20 lbs) after a stroke 3 months ago. Her past medical history was significant for chronic obstructive pulmonary disease, atrial fibrillation, and hypertension. Laboratory results showed glucose, 8.9 mmol/L (160 mg/dL); potassium, 5.2 mmol/L (20.28 mg/dL); phosphate, 1.32 mmol/d (4.1 mg/dL); magnesium, 0.78 mmol/L (1.9 mg/dL); BUN, 7.14 mmol/d (20 mg/dL); creatinine, 97.24 μmol/L (1.1 mg/dL); sodium, 135 mmol/dL; carbon dioxide, 22 mmol/L; albumin, 23 g/L (2.3 g/dL).

An insulin drip was started on day 1 of hospitalization, per ICU protocol because of hyperglycemia. Potassium levels normalized with appropriate glucose control and hydration.

Enteral nutrition (EN) support was initiated by day 3 via orogastric tube. A 1.0 kcal/mL polymeric formula was infused via continuous drip to provide 20 total kcal/kg of adjusted body weight (see Table 5-1) and protein at 1.5 g/kg. A strict protocol for elevating the head of the bed at least 30° was maintained while EN was infused. Gastric residuals were checked every 6 hours, and EN was continued while gastric residuals remained < 250 mL.

Nursing flow sheets were evaluated after 3 days to determine if average nutrition provision was within the range of estimated needs. On day 3 of EN, Ms Tucker started to have frequent, liquid bowel movements. A review of her medication profile with the pharmacist revealed 3 liquid medications that contained sorbitol. The patient's diarrhea resolved within 24 hours after the medications were changed to crushed tablets.

Ms Tucker was very nervous, making weaning difficult. She had not been sleeping well so a propofol (Diprivan) infusion was initiated. The plan was to transition to oral anxiolytics via gastric tube after she slept and was more calm. Due to the lipid emulsion base in her propofol (1.1 kcal/mL), an average of 400 calories per 24 hours was provided. The EN rate was reduced to prevent resultant overfeeding. Ms Tucker ultimately required a tracheostomy. For her comfort (and by her choice) the orogastric tube was switched to a nasogastric tube. When it was appropriate, a speech evaluation was obtained to assess swallowing ability. Although she was cleared for the first stage of the dysphagia diet, EN continued at night until her diet was advanced and she was able to demonstrate she could meet nutritional needs orally.

GENERAL DESCRIPTION

The importance of proper nutritional support of mechanically ventilated patients has been well documented over the last 25 years. As early as 1950, it was shown that malnutrition could affect respiratory status.[1] Dockel and colleagues[2] demonstrated that a protein and calorie restricted diet could impair the ventilatory response to hypoxia. Several authors[3,4] have reported on the loss of diaphragm and intercostal muscle mass as a result of malnutrition and described the resulting effects on respiratory status. During the late 1970s and early 1980s, researchers demonstrated that providing nutrition support to mechanically ventilated patients improved ventilator weaning.[4,5] However, as the use of nutrition support in hospitalized patients became more common, the negative effects of excessive nutrition support began to be reported.[6] Clinicians began to realize that nutrition support could induce complications if not properly managed.

Table 5-1   Indications and Contraindications for Parenteral Nutrition

Parenteral nutrition (PN) is usually indicated in the following situations:

- Documented inability to absorb adequate nutrients via the gastrointestinal tract; this may be due to:

    Massive small-bowel resection or short bowel syndrome (at least initially)

    Radiation enteritis

    Severe diarrhea

    Steatorrhea

- Complete bowel obstruction or intestinal pseudo-obstruction

- Severe catabolism with or without malnutrition when gastrointestinal tract is not usable within 5–7 days

- Inability to obtain enteral access

- Inability to provide sufficient nutrients and fluids enterally

- Pancreatitis accompanied by abdominal pain with jejunal delivery of nutrients

- Persistent GI hemorrhage

- Acute abdomen/ileus

- Lengthy GI workup requiring nothing-by-mouth status for several days in malnourished patient

- High output enterocutaneous fistula and EN access cannot be obtained distal to the site

Parenteral nutrition may be indicated in the following situations:

- Enterocutaneous fistula

- Inflammatory bowel disease not responding to medical therapy

- Hyperemesis gravidarum when nausea and vomiting persist longer than 5–7 days and enteral nutrition (EN) is not possible

- Partial small bowel obstruction

- Intensive chemotherapy or severe mucositis

- Major surgery or stress when EN not expected to resume within 7–10 days

- Intractable vomiting when jejunal feeding is not possible

- Chylous ascites or chylothorax when EN does not decrease output adequately

Contraindications for parenteral nutrition:

- Functioning gastrointestinal tract

- Treatment anticipated for less than 5 days in patients without severe malnutrition

- Inability to obtain venous access

- A prognosis that does not warrant aggressive nutrition support

- When the risks of PN are judged to exceed the potential benefits

Used with permission from the University of Virginia Health System Nutrition Support Traineeship Syllabus; Other References: 196.

Within the last 5 to 10 years, accumulated evidence suggests the route of providing nutrition support, parenteral or enteral, could influence the incidence of complications related to providing nutrition. Increasingly, the gastrointestinal (GI) tract is emphasized for providing nutrition support, given the evidence of decreased infectious complications and improved outcomes with enteral support compared to total parenteral nutrition (PN).[7–9] Enteral nutrition (EN) has the additional advantage of being significantly less expensive than PN. New techniques, new devices, and improved clinical judgment allow the GI tract to be used earlier and more consistently than ever before.

COMPETENCIES

The nurse responsible for providing EN should demonstrate the ability to identify patients at nutrition risk, interpret clinical markers of malnutrition, identify patients at risk of refeeding syndrome, implement strategies for aspiration prevention, interpret indirect calorimetry measurements, and assess GI tract function.

ETHICAL CONSIDERATIONS

Nutritional support can be considered life sustaining in specific situations. In general, patients who choose to forego extraordinary life sustaining measures may refuse EN and PN support.

OCCUPATIONAL HAZARDS

There are no known occupational hazards associated with providing nutritional support.

FUTURE RESEARCH

Providing nutrition support to mechanically ventilated patients is considered standard practice. However, randomized controlled trials on a number of aspects of critical care (transfusions, tidal volumes, glucose control, etc) have yielded evidence that is contrary to conventional wisdom. These findings have prompted inquiry into the most basic questions of providing nutrition to the critically ill population. The best available evidence is that EN provides improved outcomes in the critically ill patient, compared to PN. Unfortunately, to date there are no large randomized trials to provide quality evidence on the best time to begin nutrition or what level of calories and protein are optimum in mechanically ventilated patients. Further, there are inadequate outcome data to provide *definitive* answers to questions about the best way to determine caloric needs, reduce aspiration pneumonia, and monitor nutritional status. Until there are prospective, blind randomized trials with adequate sample sizes to answer the outstanding questions, the selection of nutrition support will continue to be based on the best available evidence and clinical judgment.

The increased use of EN has prompted the introduction of a vast array of disease specific EN products. Controlled investigations have not supported the efficacy and the considerable cost of some of these specialized products.[10] Additional research is needed to determine if alterations in nutrient composition can affect outcome changes in mechanically ventilated patients.

It is imperative that clinicians continue to question practice to find ways to improve patient care, as the healthcare system can no longer afford to let folklore and tradition direct patient care. Consistent definitions and guidelines are needed for clinical dilemmas such as gastric residuals, aspiration pneumonia, diarrhea, etc. There also needs to be a clear distinction between theoretical, *statistically significant* standard of practice, and that which is *clinically significant.*

REFERENCES

1. Keys A, Brozek J, Henschel A, et al. *Biology of Human Starvation.* Minneapolis, Minn: University of Minnesota Press; 1950.

2. Dockel R, Zwillich CW, Scoggin C, et al. Clinical semi-starvation: depression of the hypoxic ventilatory response. *N Engl J Med.* 1976;295:356–361.

3. Arora NS, Rochester DF. Effect of general nutritional and muscular states on the human diaphragm [abstract]. *Am Rev Respir Dis.* 1977;115:84.

4. Askanazi J, Weissman C, Rosenbaum SH, et al. Nutrition and the respiratory system. *Crit Care Med.* 1982; 10:163–172.

5. Bassili HR, Deitel M. Effects of nutritional support on weaning patients off mechanical ventilators. *J Parenter Enteral Nutr.* 1981;5:161–163.

6. Askanazi J, Rosenbaum SH, Hyman AI, et al. Respiratory changes induced by the large glucose loads of total parenteral nutrition. *JAMA.* 1980;243: 1444–1447.

7. Braunschweig CL, Levy P, Sheean PM, et al. Enteral compared with parenteral nutrition: a meta analysis. *Am J Clin Nutr.* 2001;74:534–542.

8. Brennan MF, Pisters PW, Posner M, et al. A prospective randomized trial of total parenteral nutrition after major pancreatic resection for malignancy. *Ann Surg.* 1994;220:436–441.

9. Kudsk KA, Croce MA, Fabian TC, et al. Enteral versus parenteral feeding. Effects on septic morbidity after blunt and penetrating trauma. *Ann Surg.* 1992;215:503–515.

10. Veterans Affairs Total Parenteral Nutrition Cooperative Study. Perioperative total parenteral nutrition in surgical patients. The Veterans Affairs Total Parenteral Nutrition Cooperative Study Group. *N Engl J Med.* 1991;325:525–532.

CLINICAL RECOMMENDATIONS

The rating scales for the Level of Recommendation range from I to IV, with levels indicated as follows: I, manufactuer's recommendations only; II, theory based, no research data to support recommendations; recommendations from expert consensus group may exist; III, laboratory data only, no clinical data to support recommendations; IV, limited clinical studies to support recommendations; V, clinical studies in more than 1 or 2 different populations and situations to support recommendations; VI, clinical studies in a variety of patient populations and situations to support recommendations.

Period of Use	Recommendation	Rationale for Recommendation	Level of Recommendation	Supporting References	Comments
Selection of Patients	Enteral nutrition (EN) is the preferred route for nutritional support. Parenteral nutrition (PN) is not the recommended route for nutrition unless EN is not possible.	The reasons for using EN are specific and discussed in the methods section.	IV: Limited clinical studies to support recommendations	See Other References: 7, 10, 112	
	EN should be initiated for:				
	• Well-nourished adult patients who require mechanical ventilation (MV) for > 72 hours.	To maintain lean body mass (including diaphragmatic mass), provide adequate energy and protein for acute phase reactants, antimicrobial functions, and wound healing. There is evidence that mechanical ventilation required for 3 days is associated with prolonged ventilation (> 1 week). A malnourished state may make weaning more difficult.	V: Clinical studies in more than 1 or 2 different patient populations and situations to support recommendations	See Other References: 3, 5, 47, 102, 108, 110	
	Early EN (< 48 hours) may be beneficial as a means to reduce mucosal atrophy, increase intestinal permeability, and ultimately reduce the gut translocation and septic complications.	Early EN is associated with improved nitrogen balance, quicker normalization of C-reactive protein and cytokine levels, and a trend towards a decrease in infectious complications compared to PN.	V: Clinical studies in more than 1 or 2 different patient populations and situations to support recommendations	See Other References: 32, 52, 55, 104, 114, 217, 224	
		Methods of nutrition: parenteral vs enteral			
	PN should be avoided in well-nourished patients who are likely to tolerate EN in 7–10 days. See Table 5-1	PN use in well-nourished patients is associated with increased infections. Providing early PN to well-nourished patients does not improve hospital outcome or reduce surgical complications (compared to delayed EN).	IV: Limited clinical studies to support recommendations	See Other References: 8, 10, 112	There is a greater incidence of infectious episodes with PN than with EN. PN is significantly more expensive than EN.

Period of Use	Recommendation	Rationale for Recommendation	Level of Recommendation	Supporting References	Comments
		Methods of nutrition: parenteral vs enteral (cont.)			
Selection of Patients *(cont.)*	**PN should be used:**				
	1. For patients with a nonfunctional or inaccessible GI tract resulting from: • Massive intestinal hemorrhage • Acute abdomen • Short bowel syndrome with, 3 feet of small bowel remaining, or > 3 feet before adaptation takes place • Ileus/bowel obstruction 2. Patients with increased abdominal pain with pancreatitis following enteral feeding with a properly placed tube 3. Moderately or severely malnourished patients who cannot receive EN should receive PN.	PN prevents malnutrition in those patients who cannot receive or absorb enteral nutrients. PN use is associated with improved outcomes in significantly malnourished patients.	IV: Limited clinical studies to support recommendations	See Other References: 7, 10, 112, 184	Patients with pancreatitis who do not have ileus or small bowel obstruction should receive enteral feedings beyond the ligament of Treitz. Patients with new short gut should receive enteral feedings as soon as possible (in addition to PN) to support gut adaptation.
	Peripheral parenteral nutrition (PPN) Malnourished patients who cannot receive EN, and who temporarily are unable to have central access placed may benefit from short term (< 7 days) PPN.	PPN provides significant sparing of lean muscle mass compared to IV fluids alone. The duration of PPN is limited by peripheral access. Providing > 1200–1500 kcal/day requires large volumes (> 2.0 L) or a concentration (high osmolality) that increases the incidence of phlebitis.	IV: Limited clinical studies to support recommendations	See Other References: 17, 62 See Other References: 236	PPN use should generally be limited to < 7 days. Patients who require longer therapy may benefit from central PN. The addition of heparin or hydrocortisone to PPN may extend the life of peripheral lines
	Provide IV lipids with PPN continuously to reduce osmolality and as a calorie source.	Osmolality of IV lipid emulsions is ~ 290 mOsm.	II: Theory based, no research data to support recommendations; recommendations from expert consensus group may exist	See Other References: 17, 62	
	Central (total) parenteral nutrition (PN) PN may be provided via total nutrient admixtures (TNA) with all components in one bag, or IV lipids may be provided as a separate component.	There is no compelling data to support one method of PN preparation over another.	II: Theory based, no research data to support recommendations; recommendations from expert consensus group may exist	See Other References: 69, 76, 214,	

Period of Use	Recommendation	Rationale for Recommendation	Level of Recommendation	Supporting References	Comments
		Methods of nutrition: parenteral vs enteral (cont.)			
Selection of Patients *(cont.)*	PN provided as a TNA should be delivered through a 1.2–5-µ filter.	Calcium phosphate or other particulates cannot be visualized through opaque TNA solutions.	IV: Limited clinical studies to support recommendations	See Other References: 115, 219	Visible inspection of TNA solution for particulate matter is difficult with total nutrient admixtures.
	Lipid emulsions hang time should not be greater than 24 hours.	The Centers for Disease Control and Prevention (CDC) suggests a limit of a 12-hour hang time based on growth of microorganisms *introduced* into IV lipid emulsions. However, cultures from IV lipid emulsions in clinical settings do not support increased microbial growth in lipid emulsions infusing longer than 12 hours.	IV: Limited clinical studies to support recommendations	See Other References: 53, 79	There is inadequate data to provide outcome-based recommendations on the limit for intravenous lipid emulsion hang time.
	PN should be provided as a mixed fuel source from carbohydrates, amino acids, and lipids.	Providing excessive carbohydrate is associated with elevated hepatic enzymes, hyperglycemia, and CO_2 production. Current data are inadequate to determine if withholding IV lipid emulsion results in reduced complications from infection or improved outcomes.	IV: Limited clinical studies to support recommendations	See Annotated Bibliography: 22 See Other References: 30, 147, 238	
	Tapering PN rate when starting or stopping PN is not necessary for the vast majority of patients. Some patient conditions (eg, pregnancy, cirrhosis, long acting insulin therapy) may require tapering PN to prevent hypoglycemia.	Two studies have documented that sudden discontinuation of PN did not produce reactive hypoglycemia in patients free from hepatic or endocrine impairment.	IV: Limited clinical studies to support recommendations	See Other References: 80, 138, 188	Patients with cirrhosis, pregnancy, glycogen-storage disease, insulinoma, or those who have received long-acting insulin and do not have an enteral or parenteral carbohydrate source may require IV dextrose when TPN is discontinued to prevent transient hypoglycemia.
	Enteral Nutrition Institute EN within 72 hours of mechanical ventilation in patients with a functional GI (see Table 5-1). Exceptions are patients who will extubate within 3 days (unless malnourished on admission) or have a prognosis that does not warrant nutrition support.	Enteral Nutrition: • Maintains gut immunity • Provides a more complete nutrient profile than PN • Stimulates gallbladder contraction • Simplifies management of fluids and electrolytes • Less expensive than PN • Has fewer complications from infection than with PN	V: Clinical studies in more than 1 or 2 different patient populations and situations to support recommendations	See Other References: 7, 9, 16, 66, 67, 110, 119, 124, 151, 157, 175, 209, 247	A large, prospective, randomized controlled trial in critically ill patients comparing PN vs EN vs no nutrition in the setting of good glycemic control will be necessary to answer the question of whether early enteral nutrition improves outcome in critically ill patients.

Period of Use	Recommendation	Rationale for Recommendation	Level of Recommendation	Supporting References	Comments
		Methods of nutrition: parenteral vs enteral (cont.)			
Selection of Patients *(cont.)*		EN provides potential prophylaxis against stress ulcers; however, studies to date lack consistency between EN regimens, adequate power, and differ in definitions of bleeding. In addition they often have used other pharmacologic prophylaxis agents concurrently.			To date, evidence suggests early EN may be beneficial; however, the data are not rigorous. Lean body mass is lost daily when nutritional support is suboptimal or absent. PN is lacking in several nutrients including (but not limited to) fiber, glutamine, iron, nucleotides, mixed fat source, etc.
	Specific conditions In patients with pancreatitis without ileus, EN can be provided if enteral access is achieved past the ligament of Treitz. Note: It is necessary to ensure the feeding ports infuse beyond the ligament of Treitz to minimize stimulation of the pancreas (which occurs if EN is delivered in the second or third portion of the duodenum).	Jejunal feedings can be successfully administered in patients with acute and chronic pancreatitis. Both standard and elemental products have been used. See "Period of Use—Formula selection" in the "Elemental formulas" section.	V: Clinical studies in more than 1 or 2 different patient populations and situations to support recommendations	See Other References: 11, 35, 124, 171, 185, 190, 200, 202, 247, 251 See Other References: 272	The use of EN in the patient with pancreatitis has been discouraged in the past because it was thought to exacerbate enzyme release and further aggravate the condition. Therefore gut rest and the use of PN for nutrition has been the standard of practice until recently. Evidence challenging this practice suggests that EN, delivered past the ligament of Treitz in patients whose pain is severe enough to preclude oral feeding, is very successful and does not result in complications. Note: Often patients complain of abdominal pain with pancreatitis; hence, it is important to differentiate a change (an increase) in pain symptoms compared to baseline and to review adequacy of pain medications.
	Elevations in serum amylase and lipase levels do not necessarily correlate with severity of pancreatitis and therefore should not be the primary indicator used to withhold EN.	Serum lipase and amylase levels may be falsely elevated by other factors such as renal failure.	III: Laboratory data only, no clinical data to support recommendations	See Other References: 29, 142, 198	At this time, serial computed tomography scans are the gold standard for tracking resolution of pancreatitis.
	Patients with significant burns should receive feedings within 48 hours.	Burn patients have extremely high nutritional requirements. Early enteral nutrition blunts postburn hypermetabolic response. Delays in feeding are to be avoided.	IV: Limited clinical studies to support recommendations	See Other References: 72, 122	

Period of Use	Recommendation	Rationale for Recommendation	Level of Recommendation	Supporting References	Comments
		Methods of nutrition: parenteral vs enteral (cont.)			
Selection of Patients *(cont.)*	*Contraindications for EN* (See PN section above and Table 5-1).	GI tract nonfunctional by clinical criteria."	IV: Limited clinical studies to support recommendations	See Other References: 9, 99, 184	
	Unless there are clear medical/surgical reasons not to, a trial of EN is reasonable.	Unfortunately, current EN practices are entrenched in decades of traditional hearsay and not science. Many barriers in the hospital setting prevent adequate delivery of EN (see Table 5-2). Differing views on what constitutes GI function are one of the most common barriers.	II: Theory based, no research data to support recommendations; recommendations from expert consensus group may exist	See Other References: 13, 65, 172, 195	
	Absence of bowel sounds (BS) Lack of BS, flatus, or stool is not an absolute contraindication for EN. Objective assessment and clinical judgment (eg, abdominal exam and medical status) may be the best indicators of readiness to feed. (See Table 5-3). If abdominal exam is benign in a patient without BS, consider a trial of "trophic EN" (20 mL/h) and observe.	BS are a function of the air-fluid interface in the bowel and have not been demonstrated to consistently correlate with peristalsis. It is common for BS to return once EN is initiated. In the literature, the initiation of EN has been associated with the return of BS.	II: Theory based, no research data to support recommendations; recommendations from expert consensus group may exist	See Other References: 116, 148, 155, 195	Many institutions will start low dose EN (~ 20 mL/h) in patients without BS for a trial period if the abdominal exam is benign and no other contraindications exist. EN is increased as tolerated. If BS were a definitive indicator of peristalsis, then patients without BS would have a functional ileus/pseudo-obstruction and would require gastric decompression.

Table 5-2   Common Barriers to Optimizing Enteral Nutrition Delivery

- Diagnostic procedures (feedings are stopped)
- Diprivan (propofol) (calories from the lipid preparation must be calculated as part of the total kcal provided to prevent overfeeding)
- Enteral access issues (clogged or dislodged tubes or obtaining postpyloric access if needed)
- Feedings held due to drug-nutrient interactions
- Hypotensive episodes (patient is often flat in bed necessitating that feedings be turned off)
- Miscalculation of EN requirements (orders are hypocaloric etc)
- Patient has a nothing-by-mouth status from midnight on for tests, surgery, or procedures
- Conditioning regimes and or therapies that require the feedings to be turned off
- Transportation off the unit
- Hemodialysis (EN is often stopped during hemodialysis if the patient is deemed unstable by the nurse—often after the patient experiences hypotension.)
- Perceived or real GI intolerance or dysfunction (gastroparesis, ileus, diarrhea, lack of bowel sounds, residual volumes, aspiration risk, no gag reflex, etc)

Used with permission from the University of Virginia Health System Nutrition Support Traineeship Syllabus; Other References: 196.

Period of Use	Recommendation	Rationale for Recommendation	Level of Recommendation	Supporting References	Comments
		Methods of nutrition: parenteral vs enteral (cont.)			
Selection of Patients *(cont.)*	*Residual volumes (RV)* For lack of a better assessment tool, gastric aspirates, if used, should be used in conjunction with the patient's abdominal exam. As there has yet to be a volume identified that correlates with poor outcome, an RV > 300–500 mL may signal the need to avoid gastric feeding; however, small bowel feeding can usually proceed.	RVs represent not only EN infused, but medications, water to flush tube, and endogenous secretions (approx 1 L of saliva combined with 2–4 L of gastric secretions for a total of 3–5 L secreted daily above the pylorus). See Table 5-4. Although the checking of RV has been used for decades as an indicator of gastric EN tolerance, to date it has not been shown to correlate with physical exam, radiographic evidence, or aspiration events.	IV: Limited clinical studies to support recommendations	See Other References: 34, 103, 170	Little evidence exists to help identify a threshold for residual volumes. Practices that assign a specific volume (eg, as double the infusion rate) as a threshold for stopping feedings are illogical given the fact that saliva and gastric secretions account for 3 L (or 125 mL/hr). Also important is patient positioning. In the supine position, the contents of the stomach must reach a critical volume in order to "cascade" into the duodenum. It is reasonable to position the patient in a right lateral position to see if the residual diminishes before stopping the feeding.

Table 5-3   Suggested Guidelines in the Assessment of GI Function When Bowel Sounds Are Absent

- Assess need for, and volume of, gastric decompression (ie, compare volume aspirated to normal secretions above the pylorus expected over time frame between aspirations)
- Distinguish significance of volume by differentiating those patients requiring:
  - Low constant suction vs
  - Gravity drainage vs
  - An occasional gastric residual check every 4–6 hours
- Abdominal exam—firm, distended, tympanic
- Presence of nausea, bloating, feeling full, vomiting
- Assess whether patient is passing gas or stooling.
- Compare clinical exam with the differential diagnosis, specifically high suspicion for abdominal process.
- Finally, after determining low risk from above, consider a trial of total enteral nutrition (TEN) at low rate of 10–20 mL/h and clinically observe for any of the symptoms listed above.

Used with permission from the University of Virginia Health System Nutrition Support Traineeship Syllabus; Other References: 196.

Table 5-4   Absorption and Secretion of Fluid in the GI Tract

Gastrointestinal fluid movement

Additions	mL
Diet	2000
Saliva	1500
Stomach	2500
Pancreas/bile	2000
Intestine	1000
Subtractions	**mL**
Colointestinal	8900
Net stool loss	*100*

Reprinted with permission from Harig. See Other References: 103.

Period of Use	Recommendation	Rationale for Recommendation	Level of Recommendation	Supporting References	Comments
		Methods of nutrition: parenteral vs enteral (cont.)			
Selection of Patients *(cont.)*	In practice, RVs are typically checked every 4–12 hours.	See Table 5-5 for suggested guidelines to evaluate RV.	V: Clinical studies in more than 1 or 2 different patient populations and situations to support recommendations		Of interest, in one prospective, randomized study in noncritically ill patients, 34 patients were allowed oral intake postoperatively even when NG aspirates were > 1000 mL at the time of NG removal.
	Transpyloric feeding may be successful in patients with persistent nausea or high RV and should be attempted before switching to PN. If vomiting cannot be controlled, EN may be successful with an nasogastric-jejunal (NG J) tube (gastric port for suctioning, jejunal port for feeding).	Patients with increased aspirates can be fed via the small bowel with concurrent gastric decompression. Several studies have shown patients received a higher percentage of caloric requirements when fed jejunally.	IV: Limited clinical studies to support recommendations	See Other References: 126, 134, 154 See Annotated Bibliography: 15	Decompressing the stomach while continuing with small bowel feeding in patients who have significant RV is a reasonable approach.
	Hypotension/GI perfusion Patients with acute hypotension should receive adequate resuscitation before enteral feedings begin to reduce the risk of ischemia and small bowel necrosis. The use of vasopressors	Case studies of small bowel necrosis in hypotensive patients on enteral feedings have led some to withhold feedings in all patients on vasopressor medications. However, clinical studies suggest that EN improves splanchnic perfusion in patients on vasopressors.	IV: Limited clinical studies to support recommendations	See Annotated Bibliography: 19 See Other References: 77, 139, 169, 208, 254	

Table 5-5   Suggested Guidelines to Evaluate Residual Volume

1. Determine if it really is a residual (eg, assess if the volume aspirated is less than the flow rate of EN infusing).
2. Assess the appearance of the residual (formula, gastric secretions, bilious looking).
3. *Clinically* assess the patient for nausea, vomiting, abdominal distension, fullness, bloating, and discomfort.
4. Place the patient on his or her right side for 15–20 minutes before checking an RV to avoid the cascade effect.
5. Review *all* enterally given fluids including medications and water for flushes and medication delivery.
6. Try a prokinetic agent or antiemetic. Review orders for "as needed" vs standing vs elixir vs tablets. Typical doses for available prokinetics:
   – Metoclopramide: 5–20 mg 4 times a day (may need to give IV initially)
   – Erythromycin: 50–200 mg 4 times a day
   – Domperidone: 10–30 mg 4 times a day
7. Seek transpyloric access of feeding tube.
8. Switch to a more calorically dense product to decrease the total volume infused.
9. Tighten glucose control to less than 200 mg/dL to avoid gastroparesis from hyperglycemia.
10. Consider analgesic alternatives to opiates.
11. Consider a proton pump inhibitor (PPI) in order to decrease sheer volume of endogenous gastric secretions (eg, omeprazole, lansoprazole, esomeprazole, pantoprazole, rabeprazole). In patients whose increased gastric secretions are an issue, use of PPIs can decrease dependency/use of IV hydration. This option is typically used for those patients who will be going home on EN. It can decrease the sheer volume of gastric secretions and often allow discharge without IV hydration in addition to EN, or decrease it enough that reinfusion of gastric secretions through the j-port is manageable.
12. Consider increasing the threshold for what constitutes an RV for that particular patient.
13. Consider stopping the RV checks if the patient is *clinically stable*, has no abdominal issues, and the RV checks have been "acceptable" for 48 hours. Should the clinical status change, RV checks can be resumed.

Used with permission from the University of Virginia Health System Nutrition Support Traineeship Syllabus; Other References: 196.

Period of Use	Recommendation	Rationale for Recommendation	Level of Recommendation	Supporting References	Comments
		Methods of nutrition: parenteral vs enteral (cont.)			
Selection of Patients *(cont.)*	may not be a contraindication to enteral feeding. Tolerance of EN (abdominal distention) should be monitored closely.				
	Potential for aspiration Mechanically ventilated patients should receive intragastric (nasogastric, orogastric, gastrostomy) EN unless patient has a significant history of severe reflux, gastroparesis, refractory vomiting, or esophageal dysmotility. Patients who do not tolerate intragastric feedings may tolerate feedings into the small intestine. For steps to avoid aspiration, see "Prevention of complications" section and Table 5-6.	Over 10 studies have investigated aspiration risk in gastric versus small bowel feedings. There is no significant difference in aspiration rates between gastric and small bowel feeding. Interpretation of the studies is limited by varying definitions of aspiration, bias related to patient selection, differences of illness severity, location of feeding port in relation to pyloric sphincter, body positioning, poor differentiation of oropharyngeal vs gastric aspiration, and short follow-up intervals in some studies. Investigations with strict aspiration prevention protocols, including elevated head-of-bed, demonstrate very low rates of aspiration in patients that receive intragastric feeding. Jejunal feedings do not prevent aspiration of gastric or oropharyngeal secretions.	IV: Limited clinical studies to support recommendations	See Annotated Bibliography: 15, 16, 21 See Other References: 73, 81, 111, 126, 177, 186, 192	Aspiration can occur via either oropharyngeal secretions with or without food intake, or reflux of gastric contents. Placing a gastric vs a pyloric feeding tube is not helpful if aspiration pneumonia results from oropharyngeal secretions. Patients who are supine for hypotensive episodes, etc should have EN turned off. Note: Patients who have undergone a total laryngectomy cannot aspirate; therefore, gastric feedings are appropriate.
	Patients at risk for aspiration risk should not receive large and/or rapid bolus feedings. Consider continuous or cyclic feedings.	Patients who receive large or rapid intragastric feeding boluses have an increased likelihood of reflux.	IV: Limited clinical studies to support recommendations	See Annotated Bibliography: 22 See Other References: 57, 81, 218	

Table 5-6   Risk Reduction for Aspiration Pneumonia as a Result of GI Reflux

- Maintain a semirecumbent position with the head (shoulders) elevated > 30°–45° or placing patient in reverse Trendelenberg at 30°–45° if no contraindication to that position. Patients with femoral lines can be at 30°.
- Maintain good oral care.
- Minimize use of narcotics.
- Verify appropriate placement of feeding tube.
- Clinically assess GI tolerance:
  - Abdominal distention
  - Fullness/discomfort
  - Vomiting
  - Excessive residual volumes.
- Remove nasoenteric or oroenteric feeding tubes as soon as possible.

Used with permission from the University of Virginia Health System Nutrition Support Traineeship Syllabus; Other References: 196.

Period of Use	Recommendation	Rationale for Recommendation	Level of Recommendation	Supporting References	Comments
		Methods of nutrition: parenteral vs enteral (cont.)			
Selection of Patients *(cont.)*	Patients following a protocol for prone positioning may be at increased risk of emesis or increased gastric residuals. Consider jejunal feeding, or hold intragastric feedings while patient is in the prone position.	A nonrandomized study documented that patients fed while in the prone position had increased gastric residuals and an increased incidence of emesis compared to patients who were not placed in the prone position.	II: Theory based, no research data to support recommendations; recommendations from expert consensus group may exist	See Annotated Bibliography: 14 See Other References: 207, 240	It is unclear if the prone position itself increases the risk of emesis or if the study patients who met the criteria for prone position were at increased risk of feeding intolerance. One small, short-term trial found similar gastric residuals in the supine and prone position but did not investigate actual feeding intolerance or outcomes. (See Other References: 204)
		Determine nutrition needs			
Application and Initial Use	**Calories** Each patient's calorie needs should be individually calculated, based on nutrition status, clinical condition, and medical history.	Overfeeding can increase CO_2 production, exacerbate hyperglycemia, and cause fatty liver. Patients with a history of malnutrition may benefit from an initial period of *hypo*caloric feedings to minimize the effects of refeeding syndrome. Prolonged underfeeding may allow excessive catabolism of muscle and organ tissue (lean body mass).	IV: Limited clinical studies to support recommendations	See Annotated Bibliography: 12 See Other References: 4, 5, 27	Current data is inadequate to determine the "optimal" feeding regimen for ventilator patients.
	Total vs nonprotein calories When determining calorie needs, use protein as a component of total kcal provided.	If protein calories are not included, then critically ill patients may be overfed. In addition, formulas developed for estimation of calorie needs are based on total calories.	II: Theory based, no research data to support recommendations; recommendations from expert consensus group may exist	See Other References: 242	
	Calorie expenditure may be estimated via several methods.	There are no prospective studies on the use of different methods of calculating caloric expenditure in ventilated patients that demonstrate related outcomes (ie, ventilator time, lengths of stay).	II: Theory based, no research data to support recommendations; recommendations from expert consensus group may exist		
	Hypocaloric feeding in critical illness may improve outcomes in well-nourished patients.	Delivery of less than estimated calorie needs (9–18 kcals/kg) has been associated with higher likelihood of extubation when compared to lower or higher caloric delivery.	IV: Limited clinical studies to support recommendations	See Other References: 137	Hypocaloric feedings have never been studied in malnourished patients. Permissive underfeeding should be limited to well-nourished patients until further studies are available.

Period of Use	Recommendation	Rationale for Recommendation	Level of Recommendation	Supporting References	Comments
		Determine nutrition needs (cont.)			
Application and Initial Use *(cont.)*	Prolonged, or extremely low-calorie feeding (< 25% of estimated needs) may compromise outcome.	Very low-calorie provision for an extended period may result in increased loss of lean muscle mass, especially if inadequate protein is provided. A nonrandomized study reported an association between receiving < 25% of estimated calorie needs and increased nosocomial bloodstream infections.	IV: Limited clinical studies to support recommendations	See Annotated Bibliography: 20	Large randomized studies are necessary to determine if inadequate calorie provision in the critically ill patient population is a risk factor for increased infections and other outcomes.
	Predictive equations (see Table 5-7): Conservative estimates of calorie expenditure can be used to initiate nutrition support.	Studies with indirect calorimetry have allowed development of improved methods of estimating calorie expenditure. If enterally fed, the large variability in the amount of nutrition actually provided may negate the potential benefit of precisely estimating calorie expenditure (see Table 5-2). Indirect calorimetry cannot be used in all patients: Exclusions: • FIO_2 > 50%–80% (depending on the equipment used) • Air leaks (eg, chest tubes, bronchopleural fistulas, tracheal-esophageal fistulas) • Acid base abnormalities (including patients requiring hemodialysis with an acetate bath)	II: Theory based, no research data to support recommendations; recommendations from expert consensus group may exist	See Other References: 28, 82, 84, 92, 93, 128, 137, 231, 241	Most methods of predicting calorie expenditure are based on average energy expenditures and do not accurately predict 24-hour energy expenditure of individual patients.
	Indirect calorimetry can be used to measure energy expenditure.	Accurately predicts 24 hour energy expenditure Measures the effect of illness on resting energy expenditure Is not influenced by body alterations (eg, morbid obesity, amputations, and quadriplegia)	IV: Limited clinical studies to support recommendations	See Other References: 28, 231, 246	Not all facilities have access to indirect calorimetry. There are no prospective, cost effective data on the use of indirect calorimetry.
	Circulatory calorimetry: Calorie expenditure cannot be accurately estimated from oxygen consumption calculations as determined via pulmonary artery catheter thermodilution (Fick method).	Circulatory calorimetry measurements have not been shown to correlate with respiratory indirect calorimetry. Circulatory calorimetry assumes a standard, or average, respiratory quotient for all calculations.	IV: Limited clinical studies to support recommendations	See Other References: 8, 86, 91	Recent studies contradict the results of earlier studies that showed a correlation between the Fick equation and indirect calorimetry. Cannot determine CO_2 production or actual respiratory quotient with circulatory calorimetry.

Period of Use	Recommendation	Rationale for Recommendation	Level of Recommendation	Supporting References	Comments
		Determine nutrition needs (cont.)			
Application and Initial Use *(cont.)*	Without access to an indirect calorimeter, estimations of calorie needs include: • Harris-Benedict equation for basal energy expenditure × 1.25 • 20–35 kcals/kg	Many facilities do not have access to continuous indirect calorimetry. Energy needs are estimated based on data from studies using indirect calorimetry.	IV: Limited clinical studies to support recommendations		Estimating energy needs must include consideration of a patient's age, body mass, physiological stress, risk for refeeding syndrome, and overall nutrition goals.
	Use "adjusted body weight" in prediction equations when patients are > 130% above ideal weight. See Table 5-7.	Adipose tissue is significantly less metabolically active than lean mass. If actual body weight is used in standard equations then calorie needs will be overestimated. However, use of lean body weight for calculations will underestimate calorie and protein needs.	V: Limited clinical studies to support recommendations	See Other References: 25	

Table 5-7   Predictive Equations for Estimating Calorie Needs

Harris-Benedict equation

Predicts resting energy expenditure (REE) of nonstressed people:

Men: 66 + (weight in kg × 13.7) + (height in cm × 5) + (age × 6.8) = REE

Women: 655 + (weight in kg × 9.6) + (height in cm × 1.7) + (age × 4.7) = REE

Add metabolic activity factors ("stress factors") to the REE to estimate the calorie needs of hospitalized patients (Other References: 150):

Harris-Benedict metabolic activity factors

• Elective surgery: 1.0–1.1

• Multiple fractures: 1.1–1.3

• Severe infection: 1.2–1.6

• Burns: 1.5–2.1

Calories per kilogram

Most hospitalized patients will require between 25–35 kcal/kg.

• Mild stress or surgery: 25–30 kcal/kg

• Moderate to severe stress: 30–35 kcal/kg

• Sepsis, complicated surgery: 35–45 kcal/kg

Adjusted body weight (ABW)

(For patients > 130% IBW)

First estimate ideal body weight (IBW):

Males: 106 lbs for the first 5 feet of height
          plus 6 lbs for each additional inch (+/– 10% for frame size)

Females: 100 lbs for the first 5 feet of height
          plus 5 lbs for each additional inch (+/– 10% for frame size)

Use answer from above in calculation below (Other References: 19):
ABW = (Actual weight – IBW) × 0.5 + IBW

Hypocaloric feeding using adjusted weight (Other References: 196):

• 15–18 calories/kg of adjusted weight

• 1.3 g/kg of adjusted weight

Used with permission from the University of Virginia Health System Nutrition Support Traineeship Syllabus; Other References: 196.

Period of Use	Recommendation	Rationale for Recommendation	Level of Recommendation	Supporting References	Comments
		Determine nutrition needs (cont.)			
Application and Initial Use *(cont.)*	Patients > 130% of ideal weight may benefit from hypocaloric feedings with increased protein provision.	Obese patients fed hypocaloric, high-protein feeding had similar nitrogen balance and shorter ICU stay compared to similar patients who received full calories.	IV: Limited clinical studies to support recommendations	See Other References: 56, 68	Patients with severe hepatic or renal failure were excluded from hypocaloric feeding trials, and may not be appropriate for hypocaloric feeding.
	Use "estimated euvolemic weight" for calorie and protein calculations in patients with ascites. See Table 5-8.	Ascitic weight does not reflect metabolically active tissue.	II: Theory based, no research data to support recommendations; recommendations from expert consensus group may exist	See Other References: 196	
	Reassess calorie needs as clinical condition changes.	Patients can have significant day-to-day changes in energy expenditure.	II: Theory based, no research data to support recommendations; recommendations from expert consensus group may exist	See Annotated Bibliography: 8, 11	
	Protein needs vary according to the patient's condition: • Mild to moderate stress: 1.2–1.3 g/kg (of body weight) • Moderate to severe stress: 1.4–1.5 g/kg • Severe stress with wound healing: 1.6–2.0 g/kg	Protein turnover is increased in illness. Providing the body with increased protein can support synthetic functions and minimize catabolic losses.	II: Theory based, no research data to support recommendations; recommendations from expert consensus group may exist	See Other References: 15, 21, 150, 217 See Annotated Bibliography: 11	Protein intake of > 2 g/kg of body weight has been shown to increase respiratory drive compared to 1 g/kg of body weight; however, there is no outcome data to determine if this has any real clinical implication. (See Other References: 21)
	• Hemodialysis: 1.4–1.8 g/kg • Peritoneal dialysis: 1.4–1.8 g/kg Critically ill on continuous renal replacement therapy: 1.5–2.5 g/kg	Dialysis results in increased loss of nitrogen.	IV: Limited clinical studies to support recommendations		Protein restriction does not slow the progression of acute renal failure (ARF) but may be beneficial in chronic renal failure. Patients with ARF and critical illness need the highest levels of protein provision for hemodialysis.

Table 5-8   Weight Adjustment for Ascites (estimates)

To estimate euvolemic weight, determine degree of ascites and subtract the following amount from actual weight.

- Mild ascites   ~   3 kg
- Moderate ascites   ~   7–8 kg
- Severe/tense ascites ~   14–15 kg

Used with permission from the University of Virginia Health System Nutrition Support Traineeship Syllabus; Other References: 196.

Period of Use	Recommendation	Rationale for Recommendation	Level of Recommendation	Supporting References	Comments
		Determine nutrition needs (cont.)			
Application and Initial Use *(cont.)*	• End-stage liver disease • Hepatic coma/severe encephalopathy: 0.8–1.2 g/kg • Rehabilitative phase: 1.2–1.5 g/kg	Excessive protein in the GI tract may exacerbate encephalopathy. Use of lactulose or appropriate antibiotics can allow increased protein delivery. Increased protein provision supports the synthetic functions of the liver.	IV: Limited clinical studies to support recommendations	See Annotated Bibliography: 2 See Other References: 127, 135, 142	For information on branched-chain amino acids (BCAA) see "Formula Selection" section. BCAA formulations should be reserved for patients that do not have appropriate response to treatment with standard medications, adequate nutrition, and treatment of exacerbating conditions (GI bleed, infection).
	Carbohydrates (CHO) should not be provided in amounts that exceed the physiologic capacity for carbohydrate oxidation (7 g/kg of body weight). CHO should comprise 40%–60% of total calories.	Providing too much CHO can lead to fatty liver, hyperglycemia, increased CO_2 production, and further increase in calorie expenditure (futile cycling). Restricting CHO does not significantly affect CO_2 production if patients do not receive an excessive calorie load.	IV: Limited clinical studies to support recommendations	See Annotated Bibliography: 22 See Other References: 6, 181, 238	Changes in respiratory quotient cannot easily be translated into changes in ventilator weaning *Consider other factors that may hinder weaning process before restricting CHO:* • Infection (increases metabolic demand/minute ventilation) • Fluid overload (decreases compliance) • Atelectasis (ventilation-perfusion mismatch and decreased compliance) • Secretions • Bronchospasm • Pain/anxiety • Neuromuscular paralysis/weakness • Chest wall abnormalities • Increased CO_2 • Overfeeding
	Consider hidden sources of CHO: • 5% dextrose in IVs, medications • Dextrose in continuous venovenous hemo-dialysis (CVVHD) dialysate or replacement fluids.		IV: Limited clinical studies to support recommendations	See Other References: 94, 204	

Period of Use	Recommendation	Rationale for Recommendation	Level of Recommendation	Supporting References	Comments
		Determine nutrition needs (cont.)			
Application and Initial Use *(cont.)*	Fats (to be limited to ≤ 1.5 g/kg of body weight) should provide: • 20%–40% of total calories • At least 4% of total calories as omega 6 polyunsaturated fats to prevent essential fatty acid deficiency	Excessive polyunsaturated fats may compromise immune function. Increasing the percentage of lipid calories has not been shown to assist with glucose control or ventilator weaning in patients on nutrition support when total calories are not excessive.	IV: Limited clinical studies to support recommendations	See Other References: 90, 182, 238, 245, 253 See Annotated Bibliography: 22	IV lipid emulsions are primarily omega-6 polyunsaturated fats.
	Avoid rapid infusion of IV lipid emulsion in patients with ARDS.	Rapid administration of large volumes of IV lipid emulsion in patients with ARDS may lead to poorer oxygenation and pulmonary gas exchange.	IV: Limited clinical studies to support recommendations	See Other References: 230, 244	
	Consider fat sources in medications.	Propofol (Diprivan) is delivered in 10% lipid emulsion.	IV: Limited clinical studies to support recommendations	See Other References: 153, 212, 243	
	Monitor serum triglycerides levels in patients on IV lipids whether used alone or with propofol (Diprivan), if the patient has a history of dyslipidemia.	Inadequate lipid clearance can lead to dangerously high serum triglycerides levels (see Table 5-9).	II: Theory based, no research data to support recommendations; recommendations from expert consensus group may exist	See Other References: 64, 265	
	Gag vs cough reflex Do not include the presence (or absence) of an intact gag reflex when assessing a patient's ability to swallow or protect an airway.	The *cough reflex* protects the airway against aspiration by preventing entry of, or cleaning out, harmful material. The *gag reflex* is a protective response that prevents unwanted material (eg, noxious food bolus, foreign object) from entering the pharynx, larynx, and trachea. The gag reflex does not occur during swallowing.	IV: Limited clinical studies to support recommendations	See Other References: 63, 144, 145	The gag reflex is often routinely assessed as part of a bedside dysphagia evaluation despite the lack of evidence to support a relationship between swallowing ability and the gag reflex. It is often assumed that no gag reflex indicates the patient cannot protect their airway and hence is an aspiration risk.

Table 5-9   University of Virginia Health System Proposed Propofol Protocol

• Patients with a history of dyslipidemia will have triglyceride (TG) levels checked 24 hours after initiation of propofol if delivery exceeds 500 mL /day (= approx. 20 mL/h). If TG > 400 mg/dl, and high dose continues, levels to be rechecked again in 24 hours.

• Patients without a history of dyslipidemia will have TG levels checked 48 hours after initiation of propofol if delivery exceeds 500 mL/day, or if delivery exceeds 50% of estimated kcal needs for > 48 hours.

• If followed by one of the nutrition support teams and the TG level exceeds 400 mg/dl, the nutrition support team will discuss with the primary team. TG levels will continue to be monitored every 48 hours if infusion continues.

Period of Use	Recommendation	Rationale for Recommendation	Level of Recommendation	Supporting References	Comments
		Determine nutrition needs (cont.)			
Application and Initial Use *(cont.)*	Transpyloric feeding is not always necessary in patients who are at risk for aspiration as determined by modified barium swallow.	Patients can aspirate oropharyngeal secretions as well as gastric contents. Inability to swallow effectively does not mean that regurgitation and aspiration from the stomach will occur. In addition, transpyloric feeding has not been shown to decrease risk of aspiration. See "Potential for aspiration" under Recommendations.			
		Methods of feeding			
	Gastric feeding The preferred route for nutrient delivery	Takes advantage of normal gastric function and coordinates nutrient delivery to the small bowel for maximal assimilation with pancreatic enzymes and bile salts.	II: Theory based, no research data to support recommendations; recommendations from expert consensus group may exist	See Other References: 64	
	Orogastric (OG) tube vs nasogastric (NG) tube An OG tube is preferred over an NG tube in mechanically ventilated patients.	Decreased risk of sinusitis.	IV: Limited clinical studies to support recommendations	See Other References: 117, 213	When a patient has been extubated or has a tracheostomy, the OG tube may not be practical if the patient has begun to eat. Should the patient still require EN, consider switching patient to an NG tube (unless the patient prefers an OG tube).
	Percutaneous endoscopic gastrostomy (PEG) vs OG or NG • Patients who require extended EN may benefit from PEG placement. Consider PEG placement in patients expected to receive EN for > 4–6 weeks.	One study has shown (Annotated Bibliography: 17), that the early PEG feeding group at 6 weeks resulted in significantly lower mortality rates, improved nutritional status, and earlier discharge. Whether these results can be translated to all patients requiring enteral nutrition for 6 weeks or longer is unclear.	II: Theory based, no research data to support recommendations; recommendations from expert consensus group may exist	See Annotated Bibliography: 17 See Other References: 24	Norton's study (Annotated Bibliography: 17) was stopped early because the differences were so significant that it was deemed unethical to continue. Feeding tube size has not been shown to increase aspiration risk.
	Transpyloric feedings • May be indicated in patients with gastroparesis, high RV, scleroderma, reflux esophagitis, insufficient stomach from previous resection, or persistent emesis	Patients with gastric atony, postsurgical gastric ileus, gastric outlet obstruction, or severe reflux history can be successfully fed enterally when access past the pylorus has been achieved. Transpyloric placement commits patient to continuous or nocturnal feedings	IV: Limited clinical studies to support recommendations	See Other References: 50, 64, 126	CDC guidelines have reported that tube location and association with aspiration pneumonia is an unresolved issue.

Period of Use	Recommendation	Rationale for Recommendation	Level of Recommendation	Supporting References	Comments
		Methods of feeding (cont.)			
Application and Initial Use *(cont.)*		as the small intestine usually does not tolerate bolus feedings or sudden rate changes. See Table 5-10 for conditions that might warrant jejunal feedings.			
	PEG with jejunal extension (PEG-J) or a direct percutaneous endoscopic jejunostomy (PEJ) may be used for long-term jejunal feeding. Use of a PEG of at least 24F tube with a 12F jejunal tube may allow less clogging with PEG-J feedings.	PEG-J and PEJ generally do not require general anesthesia or the cost of a surgical suite. PEG-J allows simultaneous jejunal feeding and decompression of gastric secretions through a single site.	IV: Limited clinical studies to support recommendations	See Annotated Bibliography: 7 See Other References: 272, 273	Some groups have reported greater incidence of tube displacement and clogging in patients with PEG-J as compared to PEJ. Other groups have reported good long-term success with 12F jejunal extensions.
	• PEG-J may be a better option for those patients who are ultimately expected to transition to gastric feedings.	PEG J can be readily converted to a PEG as needed.	II: Theory based, no research data to support recommendations; recommendations from expert consensus group may exist		Conversion to a PEG for long-term feeding has the advantage of allowing bolus feedings for patients not at increased risk of reflux or aspiration.
	• PEG-J or PEJ should not be used as a preventive measure to decrease aspiration in patients with a normal anatomy and motility. Jejunal access should be reserved for patients who do not tolerate gastric feedings.	To date, no data clearly demonstrate that PEJ decreases aspiration risk. The J arm that is threaded through a PEG and placed down into the small bowel (preferably to the ligament of Treitz) can migrate back into the stomach.	IV: Limited clinical studies to support recommendations	See Annotated Bibliography: 7 See Other References: 108	
	Laparoscopic, surgical, or direct percutaneous endoscopic jejunostomy Jejunostomy is the preferred route for long term feeding of patients intolerant of gastric feedings or known to aspirate EN.	In particular, patients who will require EN postoperatively can be fed earlier through a jejunostomy if placed at the time of surgery. The small bowel recovers faster from the effects of anesthesia (< 12 hours) than the stomach or colon.	IV: Limited clinical studies to support recommendations	See Annotated Bibliography: 4, 25 See Other References: 143, 221	

Table 5-10   Potential Conditions That May Require Jejunal Feeding

• Neuromuscular disease involving aerodigestive tract

• Structural abnormalities of aerodigestive tract

• Gastroparesis or severely delayed gastric emptying

• Persistently high gastric residuals

• Patients who require supine positioning

Used with permission from the University of Virginia Health System Nutrition Support Traineeship Syllabus; Other References: 196.

Period of Use	Recommendation	Rationale for Recommendation	Level of Recommendation	Supporting References	Comments
		Initiation and advancement of enteral feedings			
Application and Initial Use *(cont.)*	***Initiation of enteral feedings*** *Osmolality and strength* All EN (isotonic or hypertonic) can be initiated at full strength.	There is no data to support the practice of diluting EN. Osmolality of formula has not been shown to be of clinical significance in enterally fed patients. Dilution of formula only acts to delay nutrient delivery. If hyperosmolar substances lead to clinical sequelae, then medications as well as hospital food and fluid would require dilution as many are significantly more hypertonic than enteral formulas. See Table 5-11.	IV: Limited clinical studies to support recommendations	See Annotated Bibliography: 8, 14, 26 See Other References: 105, 180, 206, 232	Dilution of EN may prove useful in patients who require significant amounts of additional water. EN can be diluted and run at a higher rate to provide nutrients and water simultaneously. Providing frequent water boluses is a time- and effort-intensive practice for nurses. Thus adding the water to the EN saves time and assures accurate water delivery. Several studies have initiated EN at full strength. (See Other References 206, 232; Annotated Bibliography: 14) Patients who experience dumping syndrome (gastric pull ups, partially gastrectomized patients, etc.) may be intolerant of hypertonic formula for the first 3 to 6 months postoperatively.
	Method of feeding **Continuous or cyclic:** Start most patients at 50 mL/h unless a 2.0 cal per mL is used; then start at a lower rate to avoid potential overfeeding in the malnourished patient.	There is very limited data on EN initiation; however, several studies have started EN at goal flow without apparent repercussions (see Table 5-12).	IV: Limited clinical studies to support recommendations	See Other References: 106, 205, 206, 232 See Other References: 57, 106, 132	Current starter regimens are based on traditional practice. Consider that 60 mL is the equivalent of 2 ounces infused over an hour; this volume is significantly less than a standard meal or even endogenous secretion production.
	Bolus or intermittent (gastric only): Initiate bolus or intermittent feedings at 125 mL every 3 hours × 2 feedings.		IV: Limited clinical studies to support recommendations		Although one study (see Other References: 57) showed that lower esophageal sphincter pressure was reduced with rapid bolus vs continuous infusion, it is not clear how this affects outcomes.
	Advancing to target volume • Continuous feeding: Progression of tube feeding may range from 10–30 mL every 4–24 hours until the desired volume is attained.	Rate advancement depends on severity of illness, length of time patient has been without enteral feeding, and condition of GI tract (resolving pancreatitis, ileus, etc.).	II: Theory based, no research data to support recommendations; recommendations from expert consensus group may exist	See Other References: 53, 99	Although discouraged by some clinicians, there are no data to support the contention that rate and strength should not be advanced concurrently.

Period of Use	Recommendation	Rationale for Recommendation	Level of Recommendation	Supporting References	Comments
		Initiaition and advancement of enteral feedings (cont.)			
Application and Initial Use *(cont.)*	• **Bolus or intermittent feeding (gastric only):** Advance by adding an additional 50–60 mL every 2 feedings given 3–4 hours apart, until the goal volume is attained.	There are no data that demonstrate the superiority of one infusion method over another in gastrically fed patients as related to GI complications or aspiration pneumonia. See "Potential for Aspiration" under Recommendations.	IV: Limited clinical studies to support recommendations	See Other References: 106, 107	In 2 different studies, (see Other References: 106, 117) Heitkemper infused 3 different volumes (200, 350, and 500 mL) of full strength, hypertonic EN at 30, 60 and 85 mL per minute into volunteers. GI intolerance occurred only at the 85 mL/minute rate.
	• Cyclic infusion: These are infusions that are provided for a set number of hours. Generally these are provided for less than 24 hours (typically 8–14 overnight). Occasionally daytime hours are more appropriate for some patients. Once the patient tolerates continuous feedings, consider switch-	Cyclic feedings allow for time off EN for procedures or "road trips" so common in critical care during the day. With the implementation of "tight glucose control" protocols that require continuous insulin infusions (261), cyclic infusions are now reserved for more stable patients who do not require insulin infusions.	II: Theory based, no research data to support recommendations; recommendations from expert consensus group may exist	See Other References: 121, 146, 227	A single trial (see Other Reference: 121) has suggested a decrease in nosocomial pneumonia incidence during cyclic feedings. Time off feedings may allow for a decrease in gastric pH to deter gastric colonization. Many patients are on proton pump inhibitors or an H_2 antagonist, which may negate this theoretical benefit.

Table 5-11   Osmolality of Selected Liquids and Medications

Typical Liquids	(mOsm/kg)	Drug	(mOsm/kg)
TEN formulas	250–710	Acetaminophen elixir	5400
Milk/eggnog	275/695	Diphenoxylate suspension	8800
Gelatin	535	KCl elixir (sugar free)	3000
Broth	445	Chloral hydrate syrup	4400
Sodas	695	Furosemide (oral)	3938
Popsicles	720	Metoclopramide	8350
Juices	~ 990	Multivitamin liquid	5700
Ice cream	1150	Sodium phosphate	7250
Sherbet	1225	Cimetidine liquid	4035

Used with permission from the University of Virginia Health System Nutrition Support Traineeship Syllabus; Other References: 196.

Table 5-12   Examples of Enteral Initiation

Continuous—standard textbook:
- Standard = 20–50 mL/h
  Note: 30 mL = 2 tablespoons
- Progression: by 10-25 mL/h every 6–24 h
- University of Virginia Health System:
  Initiation: Full strength (all products except 2 cal/mL) at 50 mL/h, and increase by 25 mL every 8 hours to goal rate. A 2.0 cal/mL product is started at 25 mL/h (as few patients need ≥ 50 mL/h to meet needs). The final goal rate is dependent on the patient's caloric requirements and GI comfort.

Intermittent/bolus—standard textbook:
- Typical: 120 mL every 4 hrs then,
- Progression: add 60 mL every 8–12 hours as tolerated
- University of Virginia Health System:
  Initiation: 125 mL, full strength (regardless of product) every 3 hours for 2 feedings; increase by 125 mL every 2 feedings to final goal volume per feeding during waking hours.

Used with permission from the University of Virginia Health System Nutrition Support Traineeship Syllabus; Other References: 196.

Period of Use	Recommendation	Rationale for Recommendation	Level of Recommendation	Supporting References	Comments
		Initiaition and advancement of enteral feedings (cont.)			
Application and Initial Use *(cont.)*	ing to a cyclic infusion (eg, 3 PM to 9 AM) to allow time off EN.				
	Formula selection				
	Standard polymeric formulas should be used for most patients. High-protein formulations may allow meeting protein goals without overfeeding calories. Formula selection is influenced by fluid status and renal function.	Disease-specific formulas generally cost more per calorie than standard formulas, and many disease specific formulas have yet to be shown to be superior to standard products by large, prospective clinical trials.	IV: Limited clinical studies to support recommendations	See Other References: 14, 19, 141, 237	
	In *syndrome of inappropriate antidiuretic hormone secretion or conditions where fluid overload is common*, a calorie dense product (1.5–2.0 calories per mL) may be useful.	A 1.5 or 2.0 calorie/mL formula will allow calorie requirements to be met with less free water delivery.			Patients who continue to receive calorie-dense products may be at risk of hypovolemia when the reason for the fluid-restriction is resolved.
	Renal failure A product with low phosphorus, potassium, and magnesium is advantageous if adjustments in dialysate do not sufficiently restore electrolyte balance. Standard enteral products may be used if patients do not experience elevated potassium, phosphorus, or magnesium levels (such as during continuous renal replacement therapy).	Chronic use of potassium or phosphate binding medication is less cost-effective than use of a reduced-electrolyte enteral formula. Patients who receive continuous dialysis (such as CVVHD) and those who experience refeeding syndrome may actually require increased electrolyte provision.	II: Theory based, no research data to support recommendations; recommendations from expert consensus group may exist	See Other References: 136	Identify and treat other underlying contributors to hyperkalemia, such as hyperglycemia or acidosis.
	Fiber supplement formulas These may be beneficial in patients with some types of constipation, diarrhea, or diverticular disease. A total of 15–30 g/d is generally well tolerated; > 35 g/d may decrease mineral absorption and increase stool volume.	Few data support clinical benefits of fiber containing formulas. However there is sufficient physiologic evidence to support empirical use of fiber containing formulas, such as normalization of colonic function by increasing fecal weight and bowel frequency. As a precursor to short chain fatty acids, fiber maintains small bowel and colonic mucosal structure and function as well as the colonic microflora. Studies in critically ill patients show reduced diarrhea using soluble fiber and no change in diarrhea using insoluble fiber.	II: Theory based, no research data to support recommendations; recommendations from expert consensus group may exist	See Other References: 71, 223, 226	

Period of Use	Recommendation	Rationale for Recommendation	Level of Recommendation	Supporting References	Comments
		Initiaition and advancement of enteral feedings (cont.)			
Application and Initial Use *(cont.)*	*Diabetes specific formulas* Insufficient data exists to support their use.	One small study in critically ill patients demonstrated that insulin needs were reduced; however, there was no improvement in clinical outcomes. Further trials that demonstrate outcome advantage and cost effectiveness will be required before these formulas can be recommended.	IV: Limited clinical studies to support recommendations	See Annotated Bibliography: 22 See Other References: 51, 176	Cost-benefit has yet to be shown.
	Hepatic formulas Standard tube feeding formulas should be routinely used for patients with cirrhosis and encephalopathy. Specialized, "hepatic" formulas high in branched-chain amino acids should be reserved for when encephalopathy remains a clinical problem after the usual measures for its prevention and treatment have failed—a very small minority of patients. Calorie dense, standard polymeric products may be helpful given the volume sensitivity seen in patients with ascites. Protein up to 1.5 g/kg can be used with adequate lactulose or other therapy to reduce encephalopathy.	Trials of formulas high in branched-chain amino acids have demonstrated marginal improvements in encephalopathy scores compared to standard formulas, and improvement may have resulted from providing increased nutrition.	IV: Limited clinical studies to support recommendations	See Other References: 127, 135, 152, 160, 189	There are no studies of the cost-effectiveness of specialized hepatic enteral formulas to justify routine use. Patients who have had a transjugular intrahepatic portosystemic shunt have increased risk of encephalopathy and may be more sensitive to dietary protein-induced encephalopathy. (See Other References: 215)
	Elemental formulas These products should be reserved for patients who have failed standard polymeric or semielemental formula trials (based on malabsorption studies and poor clinical response) prior to switching over to PN.	Elemental or semielemental tube feedings do not improve EN tolerance or hasten nutrition repletion compared to standard tube feedings. There is no evidence to suggest any clinical benefit associated with elemental formulas in patients without maldigestion/malabsorption.	IV: Limited clinical studies to support recommendations	See Other References: 36, 105, 203, 210, 228	Most of the studies done with elemental formulas have used PN (not standard EN feeds) as the control. Clinically, neither amino acid nor peptide-based EN formulas have been shown to be superior to standard polymeric formulas. Of note, the majority of immune-modulated formulas used in critical care studies are polymeric products, not elemental.

Period of Use	Recommendation	Rationale for Recommendation	Level of Recommendation	Supporting References	Comments
		Initiation and advancement of enteral feedings (cont.)			
Application and Initial Use *(cont.)*	Standard, polymeric EN can be used safely in patients with pancreatitis.	Elemental EN is often used in patients with pancreatic exocrine insufficiency, or presumed malabsorption (usually based on appearance of diarrhea). In patients with pancreatic insufficiency, standard polymeric products can be used with the addition of pancreatic enzymes (½ tsp to each can of tube feeding), or tube feedings can be interrupted and enzymes administered every 4–6 hours. An acid reducing agent may be necessary also to prevent denaturing of exogenous pancreatic enzymes from gastric acid. There is no data supporting the use of one product over the other; however, elemental products are significantly more expensive and labor intensive.	IV: Limited clinical studies to support recommendations	See Other References: 251	Although no data exist supporting the practice of adding pancreatic enzymes to enteral products, this practice is routine in some institutions. Patients who do not need an elemental diet, ie those with pancreatic insufficiency who are able to consume regular food with pancreatic replacement (eg, patients with cystic fibrosis).
	Immune modulating feedings "Immune-enhancing" enteral formulas should not be routinely used in all critically ill patients. Trauma patients (Acute Trauma Index [ATI] score ≥ 25) without existing sepsis may benefit from immune-enhancing enteral feedings.	Patients with sepsis who received arginine-supplemented enteral feedings had increased mortality in some studies and a trend towards increased mortality in other trials. Trauma patients (Acute Trauma Index [ATI] score ≥ 25) had significantly reduced infectious complications, antibiotic use, and hospital stay while receiving an immune modulating formula compared to patients receiving an isocaloric, isonitrogenous formula.	IV: Limited clinical studies to support recommendations	See Other References: 22, 33, 39, 97, 140	The addition of supplemental arginine, glutamine, omega 3 fatty acids, and nucleotides to enteral products decreases the incidence of infectious complications in critically ill patients. However, there are some groups of patients that appear to experience increased mortality with the use of these formulations. There is insufficient data to determine which of the "immunonutrients" are essential, or potentially harmful, in current immunonutrition formulas.
	Pulmonary formulas Standard enteral formulas can be used to feed patients with COPD.	Controlled trials have not demonstrated clinical benefits of specialized pulmonary formulas when patients do not receive an excessive calorie load.	IV: Limited clinical studies to support recommendations	See Annotated Bibliography: 22 See Other References: 238	
	ARDS-specific formulas There is inadequate data to recommend specialized formulas for acute respiratory distress syndrome (ARDS).	One study has demonstrated improvement in ARDS with a formula containing fish oils and borage oil when compared to a formula very high in polyun-	IV: Limited clinical studies to support recommendations	See Annotated Bibliography: 5	Further research is needed to determine if the combination of fish oil and oils containing gamma-linolenic acid offers outcome advan-

Period of Use	Recommendation	Rationale for Recommendation	Level of Recommendation	Supporting References	Comments
		Initiaition and advancement of enteral feedings (cont.)			
Application and Initial Use *(cont.)*		saturated fats (PUFA). It is unclear if the experimental formula was beneficial, or if providing 55% of calories as PUFA is detrimental to patients with ARDS.			tages compared to formulas without excessive PUFA.
		Routine assessment of gastrointestinal function			
Ongoing Monitoring	**Residual volumes** Routine checking of RV along with clinical assessment of abdominal symptoms may be of value in assessing gross intolerance of EN. Patients who continue to complain of gastric discomfort, bloating, fullness, or nausea may benefit from transpyloric passage of a feeding tube.	There are no data to suggest that aspiration risk is associated with a specific RV. However, current data suggest RV is not a reliable (or validated) tool to assess EN tolerance or aspiration risk. Common practice is to stop tube feedings when RVs exceed 100–250 mL or if the RV is twice the flow rate.	IV: Limited clinical studies to support recommendations	See Annotated Bibliography: 10, 13, 14 See Other References: 201	One small study (see Annotated Bibliography: 13) arbitrarily chose 200 mL as the RV that should raise concern about intolerance. The authors demonstrated that normal volunteers had RV as often as hospitalized patients. Of interest, one study (see Other Reference: 201) evaluated whether small bore gastric feeding tubes occlude more frequently when RV is checked. To prove their point, researchers *did not check* RV in one arm of the study. Perhaps the more important question is whether gastric RV correlates with aspiration events.
	If used as a gross marker, check every 6 hours for the first 48 hours and if < 200 mL, consider: • Decreasing frequency of RV checks or • Not checking if clinically stable (some institutions and clinicians may feel uncomfortable with this practice) For a stepwise approach to treat residuals see Table 5-5.	The RV must be greater than the flow rate of EN to be considered a RV. See Table 5-5. After EN is initiated it is common to see a rise in RV that usually tapers off and decreases over time.	IV: Limited clinical studies to support recommendations	See Annotated Bibliography: 13 See Other References: 13	
	Diarrhea assessment EN should not be stopped or slowed, nor should the patient be switched to PN. Instead a systematic workup should be accomplished. See Table 5-13 for suggested strategies to address diarrhea in the EN-fed patient.	EN rarely, if ever, is responsible for diarrhea. Although EN and diarrhea have been linked to the osmolality of EN, flow rate, formula composition, and serum hypoalbuminemia, current data supporting the relationships are not yet available. However, medications and C difficile infection have been associated with EN. The appearance of liquid stool requires a stepwise review of potential causes. When enteral feeding access is obtained, medications (previously given intravenously) are switched over to enteral delivery and	IV: Limited clinical studies to support recommendations	See Annotated Bibliography: 1, 3, 8 See Other References: 40, 49, 100, 125, 187, 255	Diarrhea rarely means malabsorption in the hospitalized patient. One small study (see Other References: 125) showed that normal adult men did not develop diarrhea until continuous duodenal infusion reached 198–340 mL/h.

Period of Use	Recommendation	Rationale for Recommendation	Level of Recommendation	Supporting References	Comments
		Routine assessment of gastrointestinal function (cont.)			
Ongoing Monitoring *(cont.)*		in doing so, are provided in a liquid form. Some medications, especially the sorbitol containing elixirs, induce osmotic diarrhea.			
		It is also important to rule out *C difficile* as a cause of diarrhea. Infection with *C difficile* is a medical emergency.			
	Avoid overfeeding Monitor for symptoms related to overfeeding (increased minute ventilation, significant hyperglycemia, etc).	Providing excess calories increases CO_2 production and may exacerbate hyperglycemia.	IV: Limited clinical studies to support recommendations	See Annotated Bibliography: 9, 22 See Other References: 6, 181	Measurement of calorie expenditure with indirect calorimetry can identify patients that are receiving excessive calories.
		Transitioning patients from tube to oral feeding			
	• Patients with a tracheostomy should have modified barium study prior to starting oral intake. Patients with a tracheostomy who have just started oral intake may benefit from nocturnal cycle tube feedings that provide 50%–75% of nutrition needs. Use calorie count to help direct TF taper.	Patients with a tracheostomy frequently have "silent" aspiration of oral intake that may be missed with bedside evaluations. A speech pathologist may recommend strategies and food consistencies that can reduce aspiration risk with oral intake. Patients with dysphagia who must consume a consistency-altered diet may have reduced oral intake. Both hydration and calories may be less than required.	II: Theory based, no research data to support recommendations; recommendations from expert consensus group may exist	See Other References: 81, 164, 191	There are no prospective, randomized controlled trials comparing the various dysphagia diets on clinical outcome. Thin liquids have been associated with an increased risk of aspiration. (See Other References: 81)

Table 5-13   Systematic Approach When Addressing Diarrhea in Enterally Fed Patients

1. Quantify stool volume—Determine if it is really diarrhea (> 200 mL/d).
2. Review medication list—Look for elixirs/suspensions with sorbitol (not always listed on the ingredient list; may need to contact manufacturer).
3. Try and correlate when diarrhea appeared in relation to start of new medication or switch of medications to enteral route once access obtained. Common offenders include:
   • Acetaminophen and theophylline elixir
   • Sodium phosphate and potassium phosphate
   • Lactulose
   • Standing orders for stool softeners/laxatives
4. Check for *C difficile* or other infectious cause (lactoferrin, leukocytes).
5. Try a fiber-containing formula or add a fiber powder.
   • Few clinical studies
   • Supports the health of colonocytes
6. When infectious causes are ruled out:
   • Try an antidiarrheal agent (may need standing order vs as needed).
7. Check for fecal impaction.
8. Check total hang time of EN (should not exceed 8 hours; open systems only).
9. Consider bolusing protein powders vs adding directly to formulas to decrease contamination risk.
10. Check qualitative fecal fat as last resort; if negative, it does not mean patient is not malabsorbing; however, if it is positive, investigate further.
11. Continue to feed.

Used with permission from the University of Virginia Health System Nutrition Support Traineeship Syllabus; Other References: 196.

Period of Use	Recommendation	Rationale for Recommendation	Level of Recommendation	Supporting References	Comments
		Transitioning patients from tube to oral feeding (cont.)			
Ongoing Monitoring *(cont.)*	• Carefully monitor hydration status of patients on dysphagia diets with thickened liquids, especially in patients with diabetes mellitus.				
		Serial weights			
	Patients should have serial weights monitored to assist with the assessment of fluid status and long-term nutrition trends.	Weight is one of the few accurate, noninvasive parameters available to help assess fluid status in ICU patients. Weight change does not reflect nutrition status in acutely ill patients, but in stable patients, weight change over time may indicate nutrition status (ie, too few or too many calories).	IV: Limited clinical studies to support recommendations	See Other References: 38, 199	Serial weights are not a sensitive indicator of nutritional status in the critical care setting. Involuntary weight loss is one of the few reliable tools in assessing a patient's long-term nutritional status.
	Subtract approximate ascitic weight to obtain an estimated euvolemic weight. See Table 5-8.	Including ascitic weight may overestimate true weight (and ultimately cause underappreciation of total weight loss and nutrition risk).	IV: Limited clinical studies to support recommendations	See Other References: 196	
	Hydration Hydration requirements of mechanically ventilated patients should be directed by the clinical goals of the medical team. Stable mechanically ventilated patients should be monitored for possible dehydration once IV fluids are decreased or discontinued. A combination of the following parameters may help identify dehydration in more stable ICU patients. • Increase in BUN: creatinine ratio from baseline • Rising serum sodium • Decrease in urine output or dark-colored urine • Input less than ouput (do not forget insensible losses!) • Weight loss with adequate nutrition support • Concurrent hyperglycemia	Dehydration may be underappreciated if insensible losses, diarrhea, or ostomy losses are not considered. Enteral feedings do not meet full hydration requirements. When mechanically ventilated patients have been stabilized and IVs are discontinued, patients need water in addition to tube feeding to meet hydration requirements. Defining optimal approaches to fluid management in mechanically ventilated patients is currently a clinical research priority. Traditional markers of intravascular volume such as BUN/creatine ratio, weight gain, or input/output do not necessarily determine hydration needs in critically ill patients.	IV: Limited clinical studies to support recommendations	See Other References: 38, 85, 179, 211	Enteral formulas are ~ 80% water. Additional water must therefore be given to meet fluid requirements, especially if the patient has a tracheostomy and is not on adequately humidified air. Frequently, patients are hydrated with IV fluids even though enteral water boluses would be just as successful. Insensible losses account for approximately 500–700 mL/day.

Period of Use	Recommendation	Rationale for Recommendation	Level of Recommendation	Supporting References	Comments
		Transitioning patients from tube to oral feeding (cont.)			
Ongoing Monitoring *(cont.)*	• Excess stool (especially in patients with decompensated liver disease on lactulose therapy) or those with high ostomy losses • Fever				
		Laboratory data			
Ongoing Monitoring	**Serum albumin** Albumin is a marker of the severity of illness and is not a valid indicator of nutrition status in acutely ill patients (see Table 5-14 for other factors that affect serum albumin).	Serum albumin level is a nonspecific marker of inflammatory disease. In the absence of disease, starvation may have little effect on albumin concentration.	IV: Limited clinical studies to support recommendations	See Other References: 74, 75, 95, 96, 151, 252	
	Serum prealbumin Prealbumin levels do not correlate with nutrition provision in critically ill patients and should not be used to determine adequacy of nutrition provision in this population. See Table 5-14 for other factors that affect serum albumin. In stable mechanically ventilated patients, prealbumin may be useful as part of nutrition assessment when limitations have been assessed.	Prealbumin is decreased in response to illness, injury, inflammation, and hyperglycemia, and therefore is rarely a good indicator of adequate nutrition in acutely ill patients. In stable patients, prealbumin may reflect nutritional repletion (48 hour half life); however, it is influenced by myriad factors including corticosteroid administration and ARF.	IV: Limited clinical studies to support recommendations	See Other References: 151	

Table 5-14 Factors Affecting Serum Albumin and Prealbumin Levels

Albumin		Prealbumin	
Increased in:	**Decreased in:**	**Increased in:**	**Decreased in:**
• Dehydration • Marasmus • Blood transfusion • Exogenous albumin	• Overhydration/ascites/ eclampsia • Hepatic failure • Inflammation/infection/metabolic stress • Nephrotic syndrome • Protein-losing states • Burns • Trauma/postoperative states • Kwashiorkor • Collagen diseases • Cancer • Corticosteroid use • Bed rest • Pregnancy • Zinc deficiency	• Severe renal failure • Corticosteroid use • Oral contraceptive use	• Acute catabolic states • Post-surgery • Liver disease/hepatitis • Infection/stress/inflammation • Dialysis • Hyperthyroidism • Sudden demand for protein synthesis • Nephrotic syndrome • Significant hyperglycemia (catabolic state) • Pregnancy

Period of Use	Recommendation	Rationale for Recommendation	Level of Recommendation	Supporting References	Comments
**Laboratory data (cont.)**					
Ongoing Monitoring *(cont.)*	**Hypophosphatemia** Maintain normal serum phosphorus levels.	Hypophosphatemia can worsen or precipitate acute respiratory failure. Low serum phosphorus also reduces diaphragmatic contractile strength.	IV: Limited clinical studies to support recommendations	See Other References: 23, 163	Also see "Prevention of complications—Refeeding syndrome" section
	Nitrogen balance Measurement of 24-hour total urine nitrogen (or urine urea nitrogen) allows the degree of catabolism to be estimated.	Protein is 16% nitrogen. Stool and sweat nitrogen losses can often be estimated using 4 g/24 hours.	IV: Limited clinical studies to support recommendations	See Other References: 149	It may not be possible to attain a positive nitrogen balance during critical illness, regardless of protein or calorie intake. Nitrogen balance cannot be estimated solely from urine nitrogen in patients with renal insufficiency or renal failure. (See Other Reference: 167)
	Hyperglycemia Maintain glucose level at or below 110 mg/dL. (See Table 5-15 for strategies to improve glucose control.)	Strict control of serum glucose with an insulin infusion protocol to maintain glucose under 110 mg/dL in the ICU setting has significantly decreased mortality, infectious complications, sepsis-related organ failure, transfusion requirements, and polyneuropathy. Hyperglycemia is associated with: • Decreased phagocytosis • Glycosylation of immune globulins • Poor wound healing • Altered collagen synthesis • Fluid and electrolyte abnormalities and increases in serum osmolality • Decreased lipoprotein lipase activity resulting in elevated triglycerides • Aggravated catabolic state • Aggravated gastroparesis— especially wide swings in glucose control • Attenuated effects of erythromycin in the treatment of gastroparesis	IV: Limited clinical studies to support recommendations	See Other References: 109, 123, 175, 197, 239	

Table 5-15   Suggested Strategies for Improving Glucose Control

• Do not overfeed the patient.

• Limit dextrose calories in total parenteral nutrition to 150 g/d initially.

• Increase units of insulin given at each step for sliding scale coverage.

• Increase frequency of glucose checks if necessary (every 4–6 hours).

• Add insulin drip if necessary.

• Once patient stabilizes, add longer acting insulin.

• Stop total parenteral nutrition for 24 hours, and get glucose under control.

Used with permission from the University of Virginia Health System Nutrition Support Traineeship Syllabus; Other References: 196.

Period of Use	Recommendation	Rationale for Recommendation	Level of Recommendation	Supporting References	Comments
		Laboratory data (cont.)			
Ongoing Monitoring *(cont.)*	**Hypercarbia** An increased arterial $PaCO_2$ may be a result of increased CO_2 production secondary to overfeeding. Rule out other potential causes first (dead space, inappropriate ventilator settings, etc). It is also important to note a patient's baseline $PaCO_2$ to assess true elevation (see "Carbohydrates" section above).	Excessive total calorie infusion may cause $PaCO_2$ to rise. Changing the percentage of substrate calories does not seem to affect CO_2 production adversely when patients are not overfed.	IV: Limited clinical studies to support recommendations	See Annotated Bibliography: 22 See Other References: 238	
Preventing Complications	**Nausea and vomiting** Consider postpyloric feedings or prokinetic medications for patients that experience persistent emesis during feeding. See Table 5-16 for strategies to address nausea and vomiting.	Ongoing nausea and vomiting will impede efforts to enterally feed patients. It is important that patients receive adequate treatment for these symptoms.	IV: Limited clinical studies to support recommendations	See Other References: 64, 98	Patients with significant gastric dysmotility or gastric outlet obstruction may require suction or drainage of gastric secretions to prevent emesis during jejunal feeding.
	Residual volume See "Ongoing Monitoring" section above.				Medication to enhance gastric emptying may need to be given by IV first to ensure delivery into the system if delayed emptying is severe, followed by oral or tube dosing.
	Diarrhea See "Ongoing Monitoring" section above.				
	Aspiration See Table 5-6 for strategies to avoid aspiration.	Avoiding a sustained supine position is one of the most effective interventions to decrease the incidence of aspiration in mechanically ventilated patients.		See Other References: 173	CDC guidelines list elevation of the head of the bed as an essential step in avoiding aspiration pneumonia.

Table 5-16   Suggested Management Strategies for Nausea and Vomiting in Enterally Fed Patients

1. Review medication profile; change suspicious agents to an alternative.
2. Try a prokinetic agent or antiemetic. Review orders for as needed" vs standing vs elixir vs tablets.
3. Switch to a more calorically dense product to decrease the total volume infused.
4. Seek transpyloric access of feeding tube.
5. Tighten glucose control to less than 200 mg/dL to avoid gastroparesis from hyperglycemia.
6. Consider analgesic alternatives to opiates.
7. Consider a proton pump inhibitor in order to decrease sheer volume of endogenous gastric secretions (eg, omeprazole, lansoprazole, esomeprazole, pantoprazole, or rabeprazole).
8. If bacterial overgrowth is a possibility, treat with enteral antibiotics.

Used with permission from the University of Virginia Health System Nutrition Support Traineeship Syllabus; Other References: 196.

Period of Use	Recommendation	Rationale for Recommendation	Level of Recommendation	Supporting References	Comments
		Laboratory data (cont.)			
Preventing Complications *(cont.)*	• Do not use blue food coloring or check tracheal aspirates for glucose to monitor for aspiration pneumonia.	Use of tracheal glucose and blue food coloring are not adequately specific and sensitive enough to reliably detect aspiration. Tracheal glucose can give false positive readings, resulting in unnecessary holding of enteral feeding. Depending on the carbohydrate source, many tube feedings may test negatively for glucose due to glucose polymer size. The Food and Drug Administration has released a Public Health Advisory regarding reports of toxicity associated with the use of FD&C Blue No. 1 in enteral feeding solutions.		See Annotated Bibliography: 10, 18 See Other References: 89, 129, 159	Glucose monitoring of tracheal aspirates and the use of food dyes in tube feedings, while often used clinically, are not valid indicators of aspiration pneumonia. Note: Methylene blue is used in some institutions instead of blue food coloring. It is vastly more expensive than blue food coloring and has the same sensitivity and specificity limitations.
	Clogged tubes To prevent clogged tubes: • Use elixir forms of medications rather than crushed pill forms (watch for diarrhea). If an elixir form is not available, crush and dissolve the pills before administration. (Note: Check contraindications for pill crushing and site of delivery before doing this.) • Flush feeding tube with water before and after administering medications.	Inadequate flushing of tubes after medication delivery is associated with clogging of feeding tubes. See Tables 5-17 and 5-18. Routine checking of RV from gastric small-bore feeding tubes has been associated with increased clogging of feeding tubes.	II: Theory based, no research data to support recommendations	See Other References: 161, 162, 201	

Table 5-17   Preventing Feeding Tube Occlusion and Declogging Techniques

Prevention of clogging

• Use liquid medications whenever possible.

• Adequately crush pills to powder form prior to administration.

• Irrigate feeding tube with water before and after administration of medications.

• Flush tube before and after aspirating for gastric residuals to eliminate acid precipitation of formula in the feeding tube.

• Avoid mixing tube feedings with liquid medications having a pH value of 5.0 or less.

Suggested technique for unclogging feeding tubes

• Attempt to unclog tube with lukewarm water.

• If unsuccessful, mix Viokase (pancrelipase) and sodium bicarbonate mixture (1 crushed Viokase tablet [or 1 teaspoon viokase powder], 1 non-enteric-coated 325 mg NaHCO₃ [or 1/8 teaspoon baking powder], dissolve in 5 mL lukewarm water).

• Gently aspirate the tube contents proximal to the clog to allow solution direct contact with clog.

• Inject the pancreatic enzyme solution into the feeding tube, clamp it and allow mixture to remain in tube for 30 minutes.

• Unclamp feeding tube and gently flush tube with warm tap water to restore patency.

Used with permission from the University of Virgina Health System Nutrition Support Traineeship Syllabus; Other References: 196.

Period of Use	Recommendation	Rationale for Recommendation	Level of Recommendation	Supporting References	Comments
		Laboratory data (cont.)			
Preventing Complications *(cont.)*	• Flush feeding tube with water after each check of gastric residuals.				
	Do not aspirate RV from transpyloric-placed tubes.	There is no benefit to checking RV from transpyloric feeding tubes as there is no reservoir in the small bowel to hold an RV.	II: Theory based, no research data to support recommendations; recommendations from expert consensus group may exist		Some facilities check RV from a jejunal-placed feeding tube in the event that a tube should migrate back into the stomach. One has to weigh the benefits (and "yield") to this approach as it increases nursing time and may clog feeding tubes (requiring a trip back to fluoroscopy, etc). This practice has no evidence to support its use.
	Feeding tube placement				
	To avoid complications, see Table 5-19.	Feeding tube placement is not a benign process. Many complications have been reported in the literature.	IV: Limited clinical studies to support recommendations	See Other References: 99	
	The use of a CO_2 monitoring device during placement of OG or NG tubes of any kind will decrease inadvertent pulmonary placement of enterally designated tubes.				
	To ensure placement of tubes into the duodenum or lower, X-ray or fluoroscopy is also necessary.		IV: Limited clinical studies to support recommendations	See Other References: 46, 194	

Table 5-18   Commercially Available Tube Decloggers

Product name	Description	Manufacturer contact details
DeCloggers	Soft, flexible screw-threaded device to be inserted down the tube to clear buildup or clog. Available in various lengths and sizes.	Bionix Development Corporation 5154 Enterprise Blvd Toledo, OH 43612 www.bionix.com 800-551-7096
Clog Zapper	Combines a "multienzyme cocktail," acids, buffers, and antibacterial agents in its formulation. Will break up formula clogs but may not work with clogs from medications. Kit contains chemical powder, syringe, and applicator. Unopened kit has a shelf life of 12 months. Reconstituted product should be used within 24 hours.	CORPAK Enteral Access Devices VIASYS Healthcare www.corpakmedsystems.com/products/enteral/zapper.htm 800-323-6305
PEG Cleaning Brush	Flexible catheter with feather cut brush at distal end # 000396	C. R. Bard, Inc. 730 Central Avenue Murray Hill, NJ 07974 www.crbard.com 800-367-2273

Used with permission from the University of Virgina Health System Nutrition Support Traineeship Syllabus; Other References: 26.

Period of Use	Recommendation	Rationale for Recommendation	Level of Recommendation	Supporting References	Comments
		Laboratory data (cont.)			
Preventing Complications (*cont.*)	**Refeeding syndrome** Be familiar with the syndrome. Identify patients at risk (see Table 5-20). Monitor electrolytes and replace as needed: • Phosphorus • Magnesium • Potassium Monitor glucose levels. Initiate nutrient delivery judiciously: 20 kcal/kg of actual (adjusted if obese) or estimated euvolemic weight in the presence of fluid overload. See Table 5-21 for more detailed guidelines on refeeding syndrome.	In semistarvation, energy is primarily derived from fat metabolism, which does not require phosphate-containing intermediates. A sudden infusion of glucose results in high demand for phosphate necessary for glycolysis, causing intracellular "trapping" of phosphate, severe hypophosphatemia can result. Magnesium is important in the transfer of high energy phosphate groups to generate adenosine triphosphate. In the setting of increased insulin secretion with refeeding, potassium is required for anabolism and hypokalemia can develop, much as in treatment of diabetic ketoacidosis.	IV: Limited clinical studies to support recommendations	See Annotated Bibliography: 24 See Other References: 43, 45, 61, 131, 163, 174, 225, 229	Note: Many factors can precipitate hypophosphatemia in addition to refeeding syndrome. (See Other References: 229) *Important:* Continue to increase calories to meet patient's nutrient goals once electrolytes are near normal or replaced. Although malnourished patients with renal failure may present with elevated serum potassium, phosphorus, and magnesium. With initiation of feeding, these patients may actually require electrolyte replacement (not restriction) during the first several days of increased nutrition. After 2–5 days of refeeding and electrolyte replacement they may again require a restriction in TPN or tube feeding electrolyte content.

Table 5-19   Avoiding Complications of Nasoenteric Feeding Tube Placement

Complications	Preventive Measures
Cranial	
Intracranial placement	Use caution with maxillofacial trauma or basilar skull fracture. Use oral route. Use endoscopic technique.
Nasal, laryngeal, pharyngeal	
Epistaxis, nasopharyngeal erosions, or pharyngitis	Use caution with placement. Discontinue procedure if resistance encountered.
Otitis media	Use smallest tube possible.
Sinusitis	Use polyurethane or silicone tube.
Vocal cord paralysis	Obtain permanent access if tube feeding is needed long term.
Esophageal	
Esophageal perforation	Use caution with placement.
Esophagitis	Discontinue placement if resistance encountered.
Esophageal varices rupture	Use caution with guidewire. Use smaller, softer tube.
Tracheal, pulmonary	
Intratracheal/bronchial placement	Use a CO_2 measurement device (capnograph or colormetric indicator) during placement.
Pneumothorax, bronchopleural fistula, or hemorrhage	Ensure radiographic confirmation before feedings. Discontinue procedure if resistance is met. Avoid replacing stylet once tube is in place.
Gastrointestinal	
Gastrointestinal perforation	Discontinue procedure if resistance is met. Avoid replacing stylet when tube is in place.

Reprinted with permission from WB Saunders. Other References: 99

Period of Use	Recommendation	Rationale for Recommendation	Level of Recommendation	Supporting References	Comments
		Laboratory data (cont.)			
Preventing Complications (*cont.*)		Hypophosphatemia causes a decrease in erythrocyte 2,3-diphosphoglycerate (2,3-DPG); a low level of 2,3-DPG may result in decreased peripheral oxygen delivery as hemoglobin will not release O_2 without phosphorus; ie, there is an increase in the hemoglobin-oxygen affinity that translates into ischemia at the cellular level.			

Table 5-20   Patients at Risk for Refeeding Syndrome

- Anorexia nervosa
- Chronic alcoholism
- Oncology patients
- Postoperative patients
- Residents admitted from skilled nursing facilities
- Geriatric patients with depression
- Uncontrolled diabetes mellitus (diabetic ketoacidosis)
- Chronic malnutrition:
  - Marasmus
  - Kwashiorkor
  - Prolonged hypocaloric feeding
  - Morbid obesity with profound weight loss
  - Prolonged fasting (including patients with nonnutritional IV fluids)
  - High stress patient not fed for more than 7 days
  - Hunger strikers
  - Victims of famine

(Other References: 57, 158, 165, 168)

Table 5-21   Summary Guidelines to Prevent Complications of the Refeeding Syndrome

1. Anticipate patients at risk for refeeding syndrome.
2. Check baseline electrolytes before initiating nutrition support, and replace any low levels promptly; however, do not withhold nutrition support until serum levels are corrected; rather, replete electrolytes concurrently with the nutrition support provided.
3. Slowly initiate nutrition support, including total calories and fluids (this does not mean that the enteral or parenteral nutrition has to progress slowly to meet the "refeeding level" that has been predetermined).

     For example, if a refeeding level of 20 kcal/kg is appropriate (which equates to a continuous tube feeding rate of 45 mL/h of a 1 kcal/mL product), there is no need to also start EN slower than this, as the amount of refeeding calories the patient is to receive in 24 hours has already been accounted for.
4. Consider additional sources of calories, such as dextrose in IV fluids, glucose or lipid calories from medications, etc, and include these in total calories.
5. Unless hemodynamically unstable, keep fluid and sodium to ~ 1 liter/d initially.
6. Monitor electrolytes daily for at least 3 days, and replace any low levels as needed. Be wary of the malnourished patient in renal failure with elevated serum electrolytes secondary to decreased clearance, as they may be a "late refeeder."
7. Be prepared for accelerated refeeding and the need for aggressive electrolyte replacement in the hyperglycemic patient while glucose control is pursued.
8. Routinely administer vitamins to malnourished patients, especially thiamin; consider a "loading dose" prior to initiation of nutrition support.
9. Increase calories cautiously in a stepwise manner. Continue to monitor electrolytes as calories are increased.
10. Outline a plan for nutrition advancement (especially if patient is to be discharged) to prevent the patient from remaining on refeeding levels longer than necessary, thereby delaying improvements in nutritional status over time.

Period of Use	Recommendation	Rationale for Recommendation	Level of Recommendation	Supporting References	Comments
		Laboratory data (cont.)			
Preventing Complications (*cont.*)		Patients presenting with diabetic ketoacidosis are at an accelerated risk of refeeding syndrome during and for some time after the catabolic process (hyperglycemia) and metabolic acidosis resolves.		See Other References: 168	
Quality Control	• Provide vitamins and minerals routinely, *especially* thiamine.	Infusion of carbohydrate in a thiamine deficient patient, especially if there is chronic alcohol use, may precipitate not only Wernicke's encephalopathy, but also lactic acidosis.		See Other References: 234	
	Enteral feeding delivery Ensure patients receive calorie needs that have been set. Monitor EN volume ordered vs received. It may be necessary to pad the hourly flow rate by basing flow rates on 20–22 hours vs 24 hours if a patient consistently receives < EN than ordered. See Table 5-22 to improve delivery of EN.	There are many impediments preventing patients from receiving EN volume ordered to meet their needs. See Table 5-2.	IV: Limited clinical studies to support recommendations	See Other References: 13, 65, 172, 220, 222	
	Consider using the "dose delivery mode" on enteral pumps if patients are on a < 24-hour (cyclic) feeding regimen.	Dose delivery presets the desired dose the patient is to receive per 24-hour period. When the full delivery has been infused, the pump shuts off, but not until then. This ensures better delivery compared to a set time frame such as, "run EN at 75 mL/hour from 1800–0600," so if the patient leaves the unit or	II: Theory based, no research data to support recommendations; recommendations from expert consensus group may exist		

Table 5-22 Suggested Orders to Improve Delivery of Enteral Nutrition

• ICU setting = 22 hours

• Floor beds = 16–20 hours (especially if protocol in place to hold for phenytoin suspension dosing)

• Stable medical ICU patients—The run time is changed to 3 PM – 9 AM to allow for planned trips off the unit for procedures unless on an insulin drip

• If TEN delivery still falls short of 100% of estimated needs, the following alternatives are tried (cyclic TEN defined as less than 24-hour infusion):

  – Run TEN at 75 mL/h from 7 PM – 7 AM for total of 900 mL.

  – Start TEN at 1900, and run at 75 mL/h until 5 cans infused.

  – Adjust pump setting to provide a "dose delivery" of TEN (eg, start TEN at 7 PM and run at 100 mL/hour until 1250 mL infused).

Used with permission from the University of Virginia Health System Nutrition Support Traineeship Syllabus; Other References: 196.

Period of Use	Recommendation	Rationale for Recommendation	Level of Recommendation	Supporting References	Comments
		Laboratory data (cont.)			
Quality Control (cont.)		requires a procedure, the EN can be turned off. The nurse can restart it regardless of the time frame. Patients may receive a greater percentage of EN throughout a 24-hour period with this method.			
	Set and monitor goals. Individualize nutritional goals and monitoring parameters for each patient.	Because tube feeding is often turned off, goal flow rates should be based on 20–22 hours depending on ICU versus ward setting. Tube feeding rates may need to be increased to ensure nutrient needs are met. For this reason, it is important to monitor the actual volume of EN delivered.	II: Theory based, no research data to support recommendations; recommendations from expert consensus group may exist		Nutritional needs and goals need to be continually reevaluated based on clinical status and metabolic monitoring.
		This problem is compounded by medications that require EN to be stopped before and after they are administered.			Many institutions stop tube feedings 1–2 hours before and 1–2 hours after enteral phenytoin dosing.
	Phenytoin (Dilantin) and EN Some institutions have protocols that require tube feedings to be held 1–2 hours before and after enteral administration of phenytoin. Other institutions do not hold tube feedings for phenytoin. Serum phenytoin levels should be monitored to ensure therapeutic levels.	The mechanism, if one exists, for the interaction between phenytoin and tube feedings is not known. Theories include reduced absorption of phenytoin during tube feeding or increased clearance.	II: Theory based, no research data to support recommendations; recommendations from expert consensus group may exist	See Other References: 31, 130	When tube feedings are discontinued, phenytoin levels should be monitored to avoid possible toxicity.
	Contamination of EN EN should be handled with the same aseptic technique as IV solutions.	Incidence of EN contamination may be underappreciated. There are several studies of microbial growth in enteral formula and a few case reports of pneumonias thought to be from the same source. See Table 5-23 for suggested guidelines.	IV: Limited clinical studies to support recommendations	See Other References: 18, 48, 113, 193, 235	

Table 5-23   Avoiding Contamination of Enteral Feeding

1. Wash hands before opening or preparing feeding solutions and after handling feeding systems for any reason.
2. Consider using disposable gloves during preparation.
3. Take care not to avoid touching parts of the container that contact the formula.
4. Minimize the number of times that the formula system is opened and handled.
5. Individual cans should be rinsed under tap water and dried before opening.
6. Prepared formulas should be refrigerated if not used immediately.
7. Consider blousing modular components instead of adding directly to formula to decrease handling.
8. Feeding sets should be changed as recommended or at least every 24 hours.
9. Prepared feedings that have been unopened on the ward can usually be hung safely at the bedside for 8–12 hours.
10. Flush tubing with water before adding more EN.
11. Powdered feedings can probably be hung safely for 6–8 hours.
12. Never add a new supply of formula to already-hung formula if it has been hanging for 8 hours.

(Other References: 48, 193)

ANNOTATED BIBLIOGRAPHY

1. **Benya R, Layden TJ, Mobarhan S. Diarrhea associated with tube feedings: the importance of using objective criteria.** *J Clin Gastroenterol.* **1991;13:167–172.**

Study sample

The study sample consisted of 9 malnourished patients (nothing-by-mouth [NPO] status longer than 5 days; albumin less than 30 g/L) who were started on an isosmolar enteral tube feeding.

Comparison Studied

The study compared subjective reports of diarrhea against actual stool weight and objective measures of diarrhea.

Study Procedures

Patients (or their nurses) were interviewed prior to tube feeding and daily for the 6 days of the study for subjective reports of diarrhea. Stool output was collected and weighed daily.

Key Results

Although patients who complained of diarrhea did, in fact, have more stool output than those who did not, none of the patients' stool output met the researchers' criteria for diarrhea (stool weight > 250 g/d).

Study Strengths and Weaknesses

This study made an interesting point concerning the difference in subjective and objective accounts of diarrhea and the need for a more consistent definition. The researchers were careful to exclude any patients with conditions predisposing them to diarrhea. However, the sample size is very small.

Clinical Implications

Subjective measures of diarrhea are difficult to interpret. If concern arises, diarrhea should be quantified and assessed for clinical significance. Tube feedings should not be held or discontinued before the facts are carefully evaluated.

2. **Cordoba J, Lopez-Hellin J, Planas M, et al. Normal protein diet for episodic hepatic encephalopathy: results of a randomized study.** *J Hepatol.* **2004;41:38–43.**

Study Sample

The study sample consisted of 20 cirrhotic patients with episodic hepatic encephalopathy who presented to the emergency department.

Comparison Studied

The study compared synthesis, protein degradation, and symptoms of hepatic encephalopathy while patients were on a low-protein tube feeding regimen with progressive increases in protein versus a normal protein tube feeding regimen.

Study Procedures

Patients were randomly assigned to 1 of the 2 enterally fed groups. The low-protein group received no protein for the first 3 days and then received protein in progressively higher amounts (12, 24, and 48 grams/d) up to 1.2 grams/kg/d. The normal protein group received 1.2 grams/kg/d from the beginning. Both groups received the same calories. Gastric retention was measured every 6 hours. Symptoms of hepatic encephalopathy were monitored daily, and protein synthesis and degradation were measured on days 2 and 14.

Key Results

There was no benefit found to limiting protein. The low-protein diet resulted in increased protein breakdown.

Study Strengths and Weaknesses

This is the first controlled study that randomized cirrhotic patients with encephalopathy to receive different amounts of protein. A weakness of the study is its small sample size.

Clinical Implications

Protein restriction for hepatic encephalopathy is still routine practice in many institutions. This study adds to the increasing body of literature that supports normal protein delivery to cirrhotic patients with hepatic encephalopathy.

3. **Edes TE, Walk BE, Austin JL. Diarrhea in tube-fed patients: feeding formula not necessarily the cause.** *Am J Med.* **1990;88:91–93.**

Study Sample

The study sample consisted of the 32 adult patients who experienced diarrhea (stool output > 500 mL for > 2 days) out of a total sample of 123 receiving nasoenteric tube feeding.

Comparison Studied

Researchers studied the causes of diarrhea in tube-fed patients.

Study Procedures

Stool samples were collected and analyzed for various factors including osmolality, which was analyzed by stool osmotic gap (> 100 mmol/L = osmotic diarrhea). If diarrhea was not judged to be osmotic, further diagnostic tests were done such as stool cultures, *C difficile* assay, and evaluation for ova or parasites. If diarrhea was thought to be osmotic, a change in enteral administration was made. If removal of a specific factor resulted in diarrhea subsiding and tube feedings continued without difficulty, this factor was determined to be the cause of the diarrhea. Diarrhea was associated with tube feedings after other causes were ruled out.

Key Results

Diarrhea was determined to be osmotic in 21 of 29 subjects, with the cause judged to be antacids in 3 patients (10%), enteral feedings in 6 patients (21%), and elixir medications in 14 patients (48%). Nonosmotic diarrhea was determined to be caused by *C difficile* (17%) or quinidine (3%).

Study Strengths and Weaknesses

This study evaluates the causes of diarrhea in an organized, stepwise method and shows that, in most cases, tube feedings can continue without difficulty when the factors to blame are removed. As is often the case, the sample size is small, and a larger study would be beneficial in confirming these results.

Clinical Implications

A variety of factors may contribute to diarrhea in hospitalized, tube-fed patients. Tube feedings themselves are rarely to blame. Nutrition should not be decreased or withheld automatically for reports of diarrhea; possible causes should be thoughtfully evaluated instead.

4. Fox KA, Mularski RA, Sarfati BS, et al. Aspiration pneumonia following surgically placed feeding tubes. *Am J Surg*. 1995;170: 564–566.

Study Sample

Study subjects were 155 adult patients who received a gastrostomy (n = 69) or jejunostomy (n = 86) tube placement. Patients who received a Roux-en-Y procedure were not included.

Comparison Studied

The study compared complication rates and incidence of aspiration pneumonia following gastrostomy versus jejunostomy placement.

Study Procedures

Data collected by retrospective chart review included preoperative state, procedure performed, and postprocedure complications including aspiration, which was defined as evidence of infiltrate on chest film, leukocytosis, and signs of respiratory problems.

Key Results

No significant differences in preoperative status were identified. There was no significant difference in the incidence of aspiration pneumonia between the gastrostomy and jejunostomy groups (6% vs 2%, respectively). No significant differences were observed in postoperative complication rates.

Study Strengths and Weaknesses

The study looked at a large sample population and showed that neither gastrostomy nor jejunostomy placements can completely prevent aspiration. The study was retrospective and relied on past documentation to obtain information and for a diagnosis of aspiration pneumonia. Patients were not randomized to gastrostomy versus jejunostomy tube placement, which may introduce bias.

Clinical Implications

Neither gastrostomy tubes (G-tubes) nor jejunostomy tubes can prevent aspiration pneumonia. This study indicates that both procedures carry similar complication rates and incidence of aspiration. Placement of a G-tube rather than a jejunostomy tube should be based on individual patient needs.

5. Gadek JE, DeMichele SJ, Karlstad MD, et al. Effect of enteral feeding with eicosapentaenoic acid, gamma-linolenic acid, and antioxidants in patients with acute respiratory distress syndrome. Enteral Nutrition in ARDS Study Group. *Crit Care Med*. 1999;27:1409–1420.

Study Sample

Subjects were 146 patients from intensive care units of 5 hospitals that had a condition known to be associated with ARDS and had bronchoalveolar lavage (BAL) evidence of severe acute lung injury.

Comparison Studied

The study compared an enteral formula enriched with fish oil, gamma-linolenic acid, and antioxidants (vitamin C, vitamin E, beta-carotene, and taurine) to an isocaloric, isonitrogenous enteral formula.

Study Procedures

The subjects were randomized to a tube feeding formula, and the study was double-blind. Patients received the enteral feedings within 24 hours of randomization and continued for at least 4 days. The primary outcomes were time on the ventilator, time in the intensive care unit (ICU), and time on supplemental oxygen.

Key Results

Data was presented on the 98 patients who completed the study; 47 received the control formula, and 51 received the study formula. The subjects who received the enteral formula enriched with fish oil, gamma-linolenic acid, and antioxidants had significantly decreased total cells and neutrophils on BAL, days on the ventilator, days on oxygen, days in the ICU, and significantly less new organ failure.

Study Strengths and Weaknesses

The study strengths are that it is a double-blind, randomized trial and that the subjects received similar amounts of calories and macronutrients. One weakness of this study is that the enriched formula contained a number of different ingredients from the control formula; there is no way to know if all nutrients are required, or if just 1 of these components is responsible for the improved outcomes. Another weakness is that the control formula provided 55% of the calories as polyunsaturated fats, and high intakes of polyunsaturated fats have the potential to increase production of prostaglandins, thromboxanes, and leukotrienes that may exacerbate ARDS.

Clinical Implications

This study demonstrates that either fish oil, gamma-linolenic acid, or antioxidants, or some combination of these nutrients, may have the potential to improve clinical outcome in ARDS. However, the enriched formula needs to be compared to a formula with moderate fat content from mixed lipid sources in order to know if the experimental formula was beneficial or if the control formula was detrimental.

6. Ibrahim EH, Mehringer L, Prentice D, et al. Early vs. late enteral feeding of mechanically ventilated patients: results of a clinical trial. *J Parenteral Enteral Nutr.* 2002;26:174–181.

Study Sample

189 medical ICU patients admitted to a university-affiliated urban teaching hospital requiring mechanical ventilation (MV). Exclusion criteria included: prior nutrition support (enteral nutrition [EN] or parenteral nutrition [PN]), diagnosis of pancreatitis, or malnourished as determined by ICU nutrition support criteria at time of admission.

Comparison Studied

This was a prospective, controlled clinical trial to determine whether provision of early EN to mechanically ventilated medical patients was associated with beneficial or detrimental outcomes compared with delayed feeding; and, to study the occurrence of hospital-acquired infections including ventilator-associated pneumonia (VAP) among patients receiving EN.

Study Procedures

All patients had an orogastric tube placed on day 1 of MV. The heads of the patients' beds were kept at 30° except during procedures or hypotensive episodes. Patients were assigned to receive either early EN, (scheduled to meet their total estimated nutrient requirements on day 1 of MV) or delayed EN, (scheduled to meet 20% of their estimated nutritional requirements for the first 4 days of MV, then increase to goal on day 5). All patients were fed a 1.0 cal/mL

polymeric formula (Osmolite HN) based on 25 kcal/kg of ideal body weight. Early EN protocol: EN bolused by gravity every 4 hrs starting with 60 mL every 3 feedings, then 120 mL every 3 feedings, then increased by 60 mL every 3 feedings until established needs were met. Gastric residuals were checked every 4 hours before the next feeding and held if the residual volumes exceeded 150 mL. After 3 consecutive feedings were held, a small bowel feeding tube was placed and continuous EN provided. The study period encompassed the first 5 days of MV.

Key Results

The early EN group had more VAP (P < .02), antibiotic days (P = .001) and *Clostridium difficile* infections (P < .042). Of note, the study groups differed in that the EN group had a statistically lower total lymphocyte count (P < .01) at study entry. Hospital and ICU length of stay was greater in the early EN group (P < .023) and (P < .043) respectively. More patients in the early group required small bowel tube placement, but it did not reach statistical significance; however, use of Reglan was significantly greater in the early EN group (P < .005). Early EN patients *averaged* 474 versus 126 calories (P < .001) and 20 versus 5.0 g/kg of protein daily (P < .001).

Study Strengths and Weaknesses

All definitions were prospectively selected (malnutrition, diarrhea, VAP, leukocytosis, residual volume, etc) as were the patients in the study population. Although the authors spent a good deal of time on detail, the quasi-randomized design may have introduced bias. The fact that the early group appeared more immunosuppressed at the outset based on a lower total lymphocyte count, begs the question whether sicker patients are more prone to pneumonia, hence more antibiotics, hence more *C difficile* infections and longer ICU and hospital stays. Furthermore, *C difficile* was diagnosed by rectal swab cultures, not sending stool samples for toxin A and B, which may have resulted in a much higher incidence of *C difficile* infections compared with the normally expected incidence because 2% to 8% of elderly persons in nursing homes and up to 20% of hospitalized patients. As both groups were fed early, they were the same with regard to orogastric and nasogastric (NG) tubes and the clinical implications of same—it is hard to imagine that a mere 348 kcal average difference was responsible for the difference in outcomes. Most clinicians would argue that *both* groups were fed inadequately. VAP was based on a clinical diagnosis, which may explain the high rate of 49%. Of note, the early EN group was to receive full kcal needs day 1 (estimated average goal = 1700 kcal/d); however, the study design would not allow that:

60 mL bolus each of 3 feedings every 4 hours (180 kcal first 12 hours), then 120 mL at each of 3 feedings (360 kcal the next 12 hours), and so on.

Hence, in the first 24 hours the *most* a patient could receive per protocol would be 540 kcal or 31% of the average total kcal estimated needs. The *late* EN group was to receive 20% of estimated needs (or 340 kcal) for the first 4 days of MV-hence for day 1 the goals were essentially identical.

Clinical Implications

It is also possible that feeding well-nourished patients in the first 5 days of MV may lead to deleterious consequences. What is most surprising is how little EN 150 patients in a university-affiliated urban teaching hospital actually received.

It is also possible that bolusing EN in mechanically ventilated medical patients may be detrimental. This study has sufficient limitations such that changing practice on the results would be premature.

7. Kadakia SC, Sullivan HO, Starnes E. Percutaneous endoscopic gastrostomy or jejunostomy and the incidence of aspiration in 79 patients. *Am J Surg*. 1992;164:114–118.

Study Sample

Of the total sample of 79 adult patients, 72 underwent percutaneous endoscopic gastrostomy (PEG) placement, and 7 underwent percutaneous endoscopic jejunostomy (PEJ) placement.

Comparison Studied

Researchers reviewed the incidence of aspiration after PEG or PEJ placement.

Study Procedures

Data were collected by retrospective chart review. All patients had a PEG tube placed by the gastroenterology staff on an inpatient basis. Patients with a history of aspiration had a jejunostomy tube placed through the PEG tube into the small bowel. Full-strength tube feedings were initiated 24 hours after the procedure and advanced to goal within 24 hours.

Key Results

The rate of aspiration (defined as presence of tube feeding in the bronchial tree or by infiltrate on chest film with symptoms) after the procedure was 11.4%. All 6 patients who were known to aspirate before PEJ tube placement continued to aspirate; 3 other patients without history of aspiration were judged to aspirate after the PEG procedure.

Study Strengths and Weaknesses

The format of the study—retrospective chart review—is not ideal as researchers were forced to rely on old charts to determine aspiration and complication rates. Study subjects were not randomized; in fact, all patients who had PEJ placed had a history of aspiration of unknown origin. As with other studies evaluating aspiration, the definition used

is subjective and not consistent in the literature. It is possible that patients aspirated oropharyngeal secretions rather than gastric or small bowel contents.

Clinical Implications

This study indicates that neither PEG or PEJ tube can completely prevent aspiration.

8. Keohane PP, Attrill H, Love M, et al. Relation between osmolality of diet and gastrointestinal side effects in enteral nutrition. *Br Med J*. 1984;288:678–680.

Study Sample

The study population consisted of 118 patients who required EN. Patients with fluid restrictions, diabetes, nitrogen losses greater than 17 g, or known GI disorders were excluded.

Comparison Studied

Researchers studied diet osmolality and GI side effects.

Study Procedures

In this double-blind study, patients were randomized to receive 1 of 3 feeding regimens: group 1 (n = 40) received a hypertonic diet (430 mmol/kg); group 2 (n = 39) initially received a diluted diet, which was advanced over 4 days to the same hypertonic diet as group 1 (145 mmol/kg advancing to 420 mmol/kg over 4 days); group 3 (n = 39) received an isotonic diet (296 mmol/kg). Diets were administered via NG tube by gravity drip continuously over 24 hours. Patients were monitored daily for tolerance; nitrogen balance studies were also performed daily.

Key Results

Nitrogen losses were comparable in all groups, even though group 1 received significantly more protein than the other 2 groups (given actual volume received). There were no significant differences in incidence of bloating, cramping, or nausea. Of the patients fed a hypertonic diet, 5% reported diarrhea (defined simply as changes in bowel habits, loose frequent stool); 21% of group 2 developed diarrhea, as did 18% of patients receiving an isotonic diet (group 3). All patients who developed diarrhea were concurrently receiving antibiotic therapy.

Study Strengths and Weaknesses

This randomized, double-blind study looked at a large sample population. Antibiotic therapy seems to have interfered with the diagnosis of GI side effects. The definition of diarrhea used is rather vague. Study groups 2 and 3 received considerable less tube feeding than group 1, which may have altered results. Enteral feedings greater than 500 mOsm are not considered hypertonic by some clinicians.

Clinical Implications

This study indicates that hypertonic formula can be administered continuously with few side effects. It does not appear necessary to dilute formulas during initiation of tube feedings even with hyperosmolar formula.

9. Kreyman G, Grosser S, Buggish P, et al. Oxygen consumption and resting metabolic rate in sepsis, sepsis syndrome, and septic shock. Crit Care Med. 1993;21:1012–1019.

Study Sample

The sample population consisted of 30 surgical patients treated for presumed bacterial infection in an ICU.

Comparison Studied

The study compared estimated resting energy expenditure (Harris-Benedict equation, see Table 5-1) with measured resting energy expenditure during transition from sepsis, sepsis syndrome (current term is *SIRS*), and septic shock.

Study Procedures

The study population was selected from patients admitted to an ICU (mean stay 5.2 days; range 1–22 days) for presumed bacterial infection. Metabolic measurements to determine resting energy expenditure were conducted on a total of 118 treatment days. Patients were classified into either sepsis, sepsis syndrome, or septic shock on each day of metabolic measurements.

Key Results

The mean resting metabolic rate was +55% ± 14% in sepsis, +24% ± 12% in sepsis syndrome, and +2% ± 24% in septic shock. Daily variation in measured energy expenditure was significant; some patients had a change in degree of metabolic rate as high as 90%.

Study Strengths and Weaknesses

The results of this study are influenced by the criteria for sepsis, sepsis syndrome, and septic shock. Study results may also be influenced by the use of actual body weight to calculate estimated energy expenditure; the use of actual weight in obese patients falsely increases calculations of estimated energy expenditure.

Clinical Implications

The results of this study have important implications. The large daily variability in energy expenditure demonstrates the difficulty in predicting caloric needs of critically ill patients. The results demonstrate how a single (or several) metabolic measurements can lead to the provision of an inappropriate caloric load. Providing nutrition that meets the average calorie expenditure (25–35 kcal/kg) may be appropriate for this patient population.

10. Lukan J, McClave S, Lowen C, et al. Poor validity of residual volume as a marker for risk of aspiration. Am J Clin Nutr. 2002;75: 417S–418S.

Study Sample

Twenty-eight critically ill patients with a mean age of 51 years (37% male) requiring MV were fed with Probalance at 25 kcal/kg intragastrically via NG tube or PEG.

Comparison Studied

This was a prospective study to validate the use of residual volumes (RV) as a marker for risk of aspiration in critically ill patients.

Study Procedures

Yellow microspheres and blue food color were added to enteral feeding. APACHE III, bowel function score, and aspiration risk score were evaluated by measuring RV, detecting blue food color, and collecting oropharynx and tracheal specimens every 4 hours for 3 days. Aspiration and regurgitation events were defined by detection of yellow color on fluorometry.

Key Results

RV, aspiration risk score, and blue food coloring did not correlate with incidence of aspiration or regurgitation events. Blue food coloring was detected on only 0.2% of samples. A low RV did not ensure lack of events.

Study Strengths and Weaknesses

Only the abstract is available, hence it is difficult to truly assess the significance of the results. A small sample size of 28 patients over a short span of 3 days was included. The study was not designed to detect pneumonias (aspiration and regurgitation (aspiration pneumonia); therefore, it is unclear how many patients subsequently developed clinically important pneumonia. Finally, can NG tube and PEG aspirates be viewed as the same?

Clinical Implications

Blue food dye is of limited clinical value. RV may be an insensitive marker for aspiration risk for values less than 400 mL. It may be better to direct efforts at clinical prevention instead of measuring frequent RV.

11. Macias WL, Alaka KJ, Murphy HM, et al. Impact of the nutritional regimen on protein catabolism and nitrogen balance in patients with acute renal failure. J Parenter Enteral Nutr. 1996;20:56–62.

Study Sample

The sample population consisted of 40 patients with acute renal failure (ARF).

Comparison Studied

The study compared the protein catabolic rate (PCR) and net nitrogen balance with the nutritional regimen of the patients.

Study Procedures

Patients were monitored during 357 treatment days (average treatment duration 8.9 ± 6 days) of continuous venovenous hemofiltration. Patients with ARF who required continuous venovenous hemofiltration had their PCR and net nitrogen balance calculated daily. The daily intake of calories and protein (via total parenteral nutrition [TPN], tube feedings, oral intake, or a combination) were calculated daily.

Key Results

Patients with a low protein intake (< 1 g/kg/d) remained in negative nitrogen balance. Providing increased levels of protein (1.5 g/kg/d) did not significantly increase the PCR but did allow nitrogen balance. Other potential catabolic variables such as APACHE II score, presence of infection, and administration of corticosteroids were not associated with the PCR. A predictive equation based on regression analysis of the data was developed to determine the nutrition regimen that would provide the most positive nitrogen balance with the least influence on the PCR. The authors propose that 1.5 to 1.8 g of protein and 25 to 35 kcal/kg would be the optimal nutritional regimen for patients with ARF.

Study Strengths and Weaknesses

The patients in study were all critically ill (APACHE II 28.0 $\pm$ 6.7) and 75% had infectious episodes during the study. The potential catabolic factors (other than nutrition) were investigated over a very narrow range; therefore, the study had limited power to detect the influence of nondietary factors on PCR. The homogeneous nature of the nondietary catabolic factors did allow examination of the nutritional influence on catabolism and nitrogen balance.

This study was noninterventional; decisions regarding nutritional support were determined by the primary physicians, possibility introducing selection bias. Additional studies that randomize patients to a nutrition regimen are needed to confirm the accuracy of the regression equation.

Clinical Implications

This study demonstrates that many critically ill patients with ARF have a significantly negative nitrogen balance, and that it is possible to decrease net nitrogen losses by improved nutritional support (providing increased protein). Many specialized renal nutritional products will contain inadequate protein to provide the nutritional needs recommended by the authors.

12. Makk LJ, McClave SA, Creech PW, et al. Clinical application of the metabolic cart to the delivery of total parenteral nutrition. *Crit Care Med.* 1990:18:1320–1327.

Study Sample

The sample population consisted of 26 patients (18 surgical, 8 medical) admitted to an acute care facility who were monitored by indirect calorimetry.

Comparisons Studied

This study compared the results of measured energy expenditure with a common method of estimating energy expenditure (Harris-Benedict equation, see Table 5-7) in critically ill patients.

Study Procedures

Patients who were monitored by indirect calorimetry had the Harris-Benedict equation calculated using both ideal and actual weight. The results of the metabolic cart study were adjusted for the metabolic effects of feeding (10% subtracted in patients who received nutrition during the study), activity (10% added for bed rest), and fever (7% subtracted for each degree > 100°F) to determine the true resting energy expenditure (TREE). The TREE was compared to the Harris-Benedict equation results, with and without the addition of stress factors.

Key Results

The Harris-Benedict equation without the addition of stress-factors underestimated the TREE, while the adjusted Harris-Benedict equation overestimated the TREE. However, the Harris-Benedict equation was significantly correlated with the measured resting expenditure.

Study Strengths and Weaknesses

This study is significantly weakened by the use of only one indirect calorimetry measurement per patient. The day-to-day variability of energy expenditure in critically ill patients can be significant (Annotated Bibliography: 12), and a single measurement may be misleading about the average needs of patients. In addition, the measured metabolic rate was adjusted for activity while the prediction equation was not. The authors did not elaborate on the specific stress factor chosen for each patient; the use of more conservative stress factors may have allowed greater correlation with metabolic measurements.

Clinical Implications

The results of this study need to be interpreted with caution. The use of indirect calorimetry can be useful in measuring hypermetabolism and substrate use in critically ill patients. However, the results of a single study can be misleading. Repeated measurements should be considered when clinical condition of the patient changes, but this can increase the costs of providing care. No investigation to date has adequately examined the cost-effectiveness, or potential to affect outcome (such as time to vent weaning), of indirect calorimetry to individualize nutrition provision for critically ill patients.

13. McClave SA, Snider HL, Lowen CC, et al. Use of residual volume as a marker for enteral feeding intolerance: retrospective blinded comparison with physical examination and radiographic findings. *J Parenter Enteral Nutr.* 1992;16:99–105.

Study Sample

The study sample was composed of 18 adult men receiving EN, either stable ward patients (n = 8, mean age 67.4 years) with G-tubes or ICU patients (n = 10, mean age 69.6 years) with NG feeding tubes.. Patients with a history of feeding intolerance were excluded. Twenty healthy adult volunteers (10 men, 10 women; mean age 28.7 years) served as controls. Of the ICU patients 3 had diabetes, compared with none in the gastrostomy or control groups.

Comparison Studied

The study evaluated RV as a marker for gastric tolerance of EN versus physical exam and radiography.

Study Procedures

Subjects were not fed for 12 hours prior to initiation of the study period. Patients received a 10F NG tube with placement confirmed by abdominal film. A full-strength, elemental formula designed to provide 25 kcal/kg was administered. Patients with G-tubes and the ICU patients were fed for 8 hours; healthy volunteers were kept NPO for 2 hours and then fed for 6 hours. Residual volumes were checked at the beginning of the study and then every 2 hours during the 8-hour period. RVs were checked in the supine and right lat-

eral decubitus positions. Physical exams were carried out during the last 2 hours of the study while tube feedings continued; the examiners were blind to gastric residuals or abdominal film results. Supine and cross-table lateral abdominal films were taken at the beginning of the study and at 6 hours.

Key Results

None of the subjects showed significant signs of intolerance. Increasing EN flow rate correlated with increasing gastric RV. Most subjects showed a peak in RV near the initiation of the study that decreased throughout the remaining residual volume checks. The range of volumes reported was 2 to 375 mL without obvious intolerance. The group with gastrostomy placement had lower residual volumes than the other 2 groups. No significant difference in RV in the 2 different positions were noted. Physical examinations did not correlate with residual levels nor did radiographic readings. There was a correlation between physical exam and radiographic findings.

Study Strengths and Weaknesses

This is the first study to try to correlate RV with subjective or objective data. The short study duration (8 hours) is not sufficient for it to be clinically significant. The groups were not matched and had differing enteral access (NG tube vs. G-tube). Healthy volunteers were fed for only 6 hours, patients for 8 hours. Some patients were not consistently assessed in both positions. It is unclear what effect hyperglycemia had on gastric emptying in the ICU patients with diabetes mellitus. There is no mention of H_2 blockers, proton pump inhibitors, or prokinetic agents that may influence RV. It would be interesting to see if results would have differed with a standard polymeric formula.

Clinical Implications

Abnormalities on radiography can occur in normal volunteers with scattered air fluid levels and dilated loops of small bowel with no clinical significance. Residual volumes of up to 400 mL may be seen in critically ill patients at times, with no obvious clinical significance. Higher residual volumes may be seen with higher infusion rates. The authors arbitrarily conclude that the appropriate level of RV that should raise concern about inadequate gastric emptying is 200 mL in patients with NG tubes and 100 mL in patients with G-tubes. The most important outcome of this limited study is a question: are residual volumes a useful marker in the clinical setting?

14. Mentec H, Dupont H, Bocchetti M, et al. Upper digestive intolerance during enteral nutrition in critically ill patients: frequency, risk factors, and complications. *Crit Care Med.* **2001;29:1955–1961.**

Study Sample

This was a prospective, descriptive survey of 153 critically ill patients (93% medical).

Comparison Studied

The frequency of and risk factors associated with increased gastric aspirate volume (GAV) and upper digestive intolerance (UDI) and their complications during enteral nutrition in critically ill patients were studied.

Study Procedures

Patients were fed 25 kcal/kg via 14F NG tube infused by pump or gravity over 20–24 hours (24 if on insulin drip). Ninety-eight percent of the patients received a polymeric formula. No starter regimen was used for EN (ie, all feedings were started at goal flow rate). Primary outcomes monitored were vomiting and nosocomial pneumonia up until ICU discharge. UDI was defined as the following:

- GAV between (150–500 mL) on 2 occasions at 2 consecutive measurements (which justified the use of prokinetics),
- GAV greater than 500 mL (which led to EN discontinuation) or,
- Vomiting

GAV was measured before starting EN and every 4 hours the first 5 days, then every 12 hours, days 6 to 20. Aspirate was returned unless it was greater than 500 mL.

Key Results

49 (32%) of patients experienced GAV
- 20 greater than 500 mL
- 29 with 150 to 500 mL on 2 consecutive occasions

40 (26%) of patients vomited
- 19 (12%) had an elevated GAV
  - 6 before increased GAV
  - 13 at the time of increased GAV
- 21 (14%) patients with normal GAV (< 150 mL)
  - 10 patients during EN
  - 11 patients after EN stopped

Increased GAV was significantly associated with male gender ($P < .003$), catecholamine and sedation use ($P < .01$ and .0006) and percentage of days in the prone position ($P < .0009$). Nosocomial pneumonias were significantly associated with vomiting ($P < .02$), a greater number of days with sedation ($P < .03$), and a greater ICU length of stay ($P < .007$). Those patients without UDI received more EN ($P < .01$)

Study Strengths and Weaknesses

This study was well designed with great attention to detail. The maximum GAV reported in the study was 328 mL in the patients who vomited; it is unclear what happened to the 20 patients with GAV *greater than* 500 mL. Of the 49 patients with GAV, 33 continued EN, 7 went on to PN—it is unclear what happened to these patients in the results. It is unclear what the GAV was of the patients who went on to develop pneumonia. GAV on 2 occasions justified the use of prokinetics agents; it was not reported how many patients in each group actually received them.

Clinical Implications

This study sets out to answer an important question and is the most liberal RV study to date. RV was allowed to range between 150 to 500 mL, yet vomiting, and hence worse outcomes did not necessarily correlate with GAV. What is apparent is that sicker patients (those requiring catecholamines, sedation, and being kept in a prone position) warrant extra care with regards to potential vomiting. Perhaps one of the findings of this study may be not to start very sick ICU patients at goal flow of EN as these patients were more likely to be sedated and receiving catecholamines at the beginning of EN (when the majority of patients had adverse events). Of note, it has been demonstrated that RV will initially increase with the start of EN, then level off and ultimately decrease over time.

15. Montecalvo MA, Steger DA, Farber HW, et al. Nutritional outcome and pneumonia in critical care patients randomized to gastric versus jejunal tube feedings. *Crit Care Med.* **1992;20:1377–1387.**

Study Sample

The study population was 38 ICU patients receiving either gastric (n = 19) or jejunal (n = 19) feedings. Patients had to receive tube feedings for more than 3 days, have no evidence of GI bleeding, and have no contraindications to gastric or jejunal feeding.

Comparison Studied

Nutritional status, bacterial colonization of the stomach, and incidence of aspiration in patients fed gastrically versus patients fed into the jejunum.

Study Procedures

Patients were randomly assigned to either the gastric or jejunal feeding group. Both groups had 12F feeding tubes placed. Jejunal placement was achieved by endoscopic placement over a guide wire and confirmed by abdominal roentgenogram. Patients were fed estimated nutritional needs with a 1.2 kcal/mL formula unless clinical situation required otherwise. Stress ulcer prophylaxis (carafate, antacids, H_2 antagonist, or a combination regimen) was administered to both groups. Following an initial assessment each patient was followed daily by researchers. The study also included a survey of ICU nurses evaluating tube-feeding practices in the ICU setting.

Key Results

There were no significant differences in age, sex, race, number of postoperative patients, days of intubation, number of tracheostomy tubes, Glasgow Coma Scale, severity of illness, or type of ICU between the 2 groups. There were no significant differences found in gastric pH or number of GI bleeds between the 2 groups. Patients in the jejunal feeding group received significantly more tube feeding and had an increase in prealbumin level. There were no significant differences in incidence of diarrhea, vomiting, gastric colonization, average number of ICU days, days of ventilation, or mortality rates. No significant difference in number of tube occlusions was seen, although several patients in the jejunally fed group did not have tubes replaced after occlusion and crossed over to the gastric group. There were 2 confirmed cases of aspiration in the gastric group, none in the jejunal tube feeding group, and 4 cases of "possible" aspiration in each group. The nurses' survey revealed that nurses stop gastric tube feedings more frequently than jejunal feedings for vomiting, absent bowel sounds, 8 hours prior to surgery, and for flat or Trendelenburg position (although many nurses reported treating gastric and jejunal tubes similarly).

Study Strengths and Weaknesses

The sample size was not large enough to evaluate significance of aspiration pneumonia in this study, which was one of the original objectives. Many of the patients had infiltrates on chest radiograph at time of randomization (gastric group 73.7%; jejunal group 63.2%), which may have affected diagnosis of aspiration pneumonia. Several patients from the jejunal group had to cross over to gastric feeds after tubes occluded and were not replaced. There was no mention of whether corticosteriods could have affected the change in prealbumin levels. It is also unclear whether the increase in prealbumin has clinical significance.

Clinical Implications

Jejunally fed patients received significantly more tube feeding than the gastric group. The nursing survey indicates that this may be due to different practices for gastric versus jejunal feedings.

16. Mullan H, Roubenoff RA, Roubenoff R. Risk of pulmonary aspiration among patients receiving enteral nutrition support. *J Parenter Enteral Nutr*. 1992;16:160–164.

Study Sample

The sample population consisted of 276 hospital patients receiving EN (various routes).

Comparison Studied

Aspiration and pneumonia events were studied in patients receiving EN via nasoenteric, gastrostomy, or jejunostomy feedings.

Study Procedures

In this prospective study, all patients who were assessed by the nutrition support team and received EN were entered into the study. Tube feedings were administered continuously using a feeding pump. Rate, formulas, and feeding routes were chosen based on clinical situation. Patients were monitored daily for complications, including aspiration— witnessed event, radiographic infiltrate, blue dye in tube feeding suctioned, or symptoms such as fever, dyspnea, etc without other cause.

Key Results

Of the 12 patients (4.4%) thought to aspirate during the study, 6 were confirmed by chest radiogram or blue dye in enteral feeding suctioned (2.2%). This translates to 2.4 aspiration events per 1000 days of tube feeding. There was no significant difference in mortality between those who aspirated and those who did not. Older patients had more aspiration events, and floor patients had significantly more episodes than ICU patients. The number of patients with gastrostomy and jejunostomy tubes was not large enough to determine any significant difference in risk in patients fed with or without an NG tube in place. No significant difference was noted based on size of feeding tube.

Study Strengths and Weaknesses

It would have been interesting to know more about where feeding tubes were placed (gastric vs. small bowel) and the aspiration and complication rate of various tube placements. However, the study goal was to look at enteral feeding in general in a variety of patients and clinical situations.

Clinical Implications

This study indicates a low rate of aspiration among enterally fed patients. Significant risk factors include age and location in the hospital. It may be helpful to investigate further the conditions in the ICU such as positioning and tube care that put this high-risk population at lower risk for aspiration (or in acute care where there is increased risk).

17. Norton B, Homer-Ward M, Donnelly MT, et al. A randomized prospective comparison of percutaneous endoscopic gastrostomy and nasogastric tube feeding after acute dysphagic stroke. *Br Med J.* 1996;312:13–16.

Study Sample

Thirty adult patients, mean age 77 years, who had experienced a severe stroke and resultant persistent dysphagia received NG feedings (n = 14) or underwent PEG placement (n = 16).

Comparison Studied

Researchers studied NG feeding versus PEG placement after stroke.

Study Procedures

Following random assignment to receive either a PEG tube or NG feedings for nutritional support, patients were fed while semirecumbent using a standard formula administered by feeding pump (average 100 mL/h). Mortality, length of stay, nutritional state, and incidence of complications were monitored.

Key Results

There was a significant difference in mortality at 6 weeks between the groups: 2 patients (12.5%) in the gastrostomy-fed group died, while 8 (57%) of the NG-fed group died, with bronchopneumonia being the cause of death for 50%. PEG-fed patients received significantly more feeding than did the NG-fed group. Gastrostomy-fed patients required only 1 tube placement, whereas NG-fed patients had tubes replaced an average of 6 times (range 1–10). Patients with PEG tube gained significantly more weight than did patients fed via NG tubes. Albumin levels were also significantly improved in PEG-fed patients. No significant differences in complication rates between routes of feeding were observed. Of the PEG-fed group, 6 patients were discharged within 6 weeks; another 6 were discharged by 3 months. None of the NG-fed group was discharged by 3 months, a significant difference.

Study Strengths and Weaknesses

The study was well-designed—prospective and randomized, although it could not be a blind study. A larger group is needed to confirm these results.

Clinical Implications

PEG tubes may be a safe and efficacious route for administering tube feedings after an acute stroke. This preliminary study suggests PEG tubes carry less risk for mortality while improving nutritional status compared to NG feeding. Implications for other patient populations are unknown.

18. Potts RG, Zaroukian MH, Guerrero PA, Baker CD. Comparison of blue dye visualization and glucose oxidase test strip methods for detecting pulmonary aspiration of enteral feedings in intubated patients. *Chest.* 1993;103:117–121.

Study Sample

The study sample comprised adult, tracheally intubated patients in an ICU. Patients in the experimental group (n = 15) received EN; patients in the control group (n = 14) did not receive EN. Five patients from the control group crossed over when nutrition was started.

Comparison Studied

The study tested whether it was possible to detect pulmonary aspiration of enteral feedings by using either blue dye or glucose oxidase test strips.

Study Procedures

Patients admitted to the ICU were studied prospectively. The decision to begin enteral feedings or to hold feedings was made by the patient's primary doctor (patients were not randomized). All patients were NPO. Sufficient blue food dye was added to enteral tube feedings to color the feedings visibly. Patients were tracheally suctioned every 8 hours. Specimens were examined for visible blue dye and were tested for glucose concentration using a glucose oxidase test strip. A glucose reading greater than 1.1 mmol/L was considered positive based on tests performed on the enteral formulas. Patients were also monitored for positioning, gastric residual volume, and clinical signs of pulmonary aspiration.

Key Results

In the control group 18% of samples were positive for glucose, and of these 90% were also positive for visible blood, which the researchers felt explained the positive glucose readings. Monitoring for blue dye in the control group was not applicable as none received enteral feeding. In the experimental group, 16% of samples were positive for glucose, of which 47% were positive for *visible* blood. Therefore, 8% of the specimens from the experimental group were positive for glucose, which was not explained by *visible* blood. Blue dye was seen in only 2.6% of the specimens. Eight patients in the experimental group were labeled with *presumptive aspiration* (positive glucose reading *and* other clinical symptoms of aspiration). It is not stated whether any of the control group developed symptoms of aspiration. In the experimental group, aspiration appeared to occur significantly more often in the supine position.

Study Strengths and Weaknesses

The study population was relatively small and was not randomized. It is unclear what impact oropharyngeal secretions may have had on the results: is the incidence of detecting blue dye lower than positive glucose reading due to oropharyngeal aspiration? It is not stated whether any control-group patients developed symptoms of aspiration. It would be interesting to know whether systemic blood glucose levels could affect glucose readings in pulmonary secretions. The specimens were monitored only for visible blood in secretions, meaning no method to test for blood such as test strips was used.

Clinical Implications

To date there is no sensitive, reliable method for detecting aspiration of enteral formula. If a positive glucose reading of tracheal secretions is used to determine the need to withhold feedings or use postpyloric feeding, more research is needed to determine the effectiveness of these variations (ie, are there fewer positive glucose readings and a lower incidence of aspiration pneumonia in patients fed with postpyloric tubes?). Body positioning (head of bed > 30°) is again shown to protect against aspiration.

19. Rokyta R Jr, Matejovic M, Krouzecky A, et al. Post-pyloric enteral nutrition in septic patients: effects on hepato-splanchnic hemodynamics and energy status. *Intensive Care Med.* 2004;30:714–717.

Study Sample

The study sample was 10 mechanically ventilated patients with sepsis in a medical ICU on day 2 to day 5 of ICU admission.

Comparison Studied

The effects of starting and then stopping low-dose postpyloric EN on splanchnic blood flow, metabolic response, and gastric mucosal P_{CO_2} in septic patients.

Study Procedures

To gauge intestinal perfusion all subjects had a catheter placed into the hepatic vein via the internal jugular, and hepatosplanchnic blood flow was estimated with primed continuous indocyanine green. In addition, gastric mucosal P_{CO_2} was measured with gastric tonometry. Arterial and hepatic blood lactate and pyruvate, blood gasses, blood glucose, heart rate, cardiac index, and indirect calorimetry were measured before, during, and after the feedings. The subjects received a semielemental, 1 calorie/mL formula (Survimed OPD) via a postpyloric feeding tube. The feeding was provided as a 40 mL bolus, then 40 mL/hr for 2 hours; then the feedings were held for 2 hours for further data collection.

Key Results

The authors reported that hepato-splanchnic blood flow significantly increased during enteral feeding and returned to baseline after feedings were stopped. The splanchnic lactate, pyruvate, and mucosal P_{CO_2} did not change during the feedings. The authors concluded that enteral nutrition may not be harmful during sepsis, even in patients requiring norepinephrine.

Study Strengths and Weaknesses

One strength of this study is that each patient served as their own control as feedings were started and then held again. In a diverse group of ICU patients, with different degrees of stress and comorbidities, it is difficult to compare results between patients. The use of each patient as their own control allows an examination of the effects of changing only one variable (feeding).

There are, however, a number of limitations to this study. One major limitation is the small number of patients studied. Another factor that limits application of the results is that patients who were deemed to be hemodynamically unstable, or who had a cardiac index less than 2.5 L/min, were excluded from the study. Those patients who were included were able to have their blood pressure controlled with a *modest* dose of a single vasopressor drug (2 required no vasopressors during the study). In addition, patients only received enteral feedings for *2 hours*, and all feedings were designed to be hypocaloric (40 mL bolus, followed by 40 mL per hour for 2 hours, which totals 120 kcal).

Clinical Implications

This study has a limited clinical applicability because of the short duration and limited amount of the feedings and because of the *stable* nature of the patients. The results would not necessarily apply to a much more unstable patient, or a patient with significant prior cardiovascular disease with severe hypotension. However, this study is valuable to let us know that it is *not* necessarily correct to make statements "that patients on vasopressors should not receive enteral feedings." The results of this study suggest that it would be safe to provide enteral feedings to relatively stable patients who have their blood pressure controlled with modest doses of vasopressor medications.

20. Rubinson L, Diette GB, Song X, et al. Low caloric intake is associated with nosocomial bloodstream infections in patients in the medical intensive care unit. *Crit Care Med.* **2004 Feb;32:350–357.**

Study Sample

This was a prospective cohort study that enrolled all patients admitted to a medical ICU who were NPO greater than 96 hours.

Comparison Studied

The primary outcome was the development of bloodstream infections during the study and the patient's percentage of calorie goals that were provided via enteral nutrition (EN).

Study Procedures

Calorie goals were based on the American College of Chest Physicians (ACCP) guidelines of 25 calories/kg (27.5 calories/kg for SIRS) based on ideal body weight. The actual amount of nutrition that was provided to each patient was monitored.

Key Results

The authors reported that the overall mean calories provided by EN were approximately 50% of the ACCP guidelines (49.4 +/– 29.3%). They also reported that those patients who received less than 25% of the ACCP goals had a significantly increased frequency of bloodstream infections. There was no significant difference in bloodstream infections between the groups that received 25%–49%, 50%–74%, or greater than 75% of calorie goals. There was no significant difference in mean serum glucose between groups. There was no difference in the number of PN days between groups; however, the groups who received less EN calories had a greater percentage of calories provided via the parenteral route.

Study Strengths and Weaknesses

This was not an intervention study; the investigators only observed what happened to patients. Therefore, it has a similar potential for selection bias as a retrospective study; ie, patients who are sicker are likely to receive less calories. In addition, the authors state that they did not prospectively decide the calorie groups until *after* the data was collected (post hoc)—essentially they looked to see what cut-off point in calorie goals would be different in terms of infections, and then divided the groups. The authors state that they did not monitor ventilator-associated pneumonia, antibiotic use, or intravascular catheters.

Clinical Implications

This is an observational study that reports an *association* between reduced calorie provision and bloodstream infections; however, it would be inappropriate to state that the study demonstrates that the decreased calorie provision *caused* the infections. In nonrandomized studies, it is possible that some factor other than enteral calorie provision was responsible for the increased infections. It is worth noting that those patients who received more than 75% of calorie provision did not have fewer infections than those patients who received 25%–50% of calorie requirements. It is possible that the short-term benefits of EN may be achieved without meeting full calorie requirements. Randomized trials are required to determine the amount of calories that results in the best outcomes for critically ill patients.

21. Strong RM, Condon SC, Solinger MR, et al. Equal aspiration rates from postpyloric and intragastric-placed small-bore nasoenteric feeding tubes: a randomized , prospective study. *J Parenteral Enteral Nutr.* **1992;16:59–63.**

Study Sample

In this sample of 33 malnourished adults receiving either gastric feeds (n = 17) or jejunal feeds (n = 16), patients were to be fed for at least 3 days and needed to have chest and abdominal radiographs every 3 days.

Comparison Studied

Researchers compared the incidence of aspiration in patients receiving gastric versus postpyloric enteral feedings.

Study Procedures

Patients were randomized to receive either gastric or postpyloric (duodenal) enteral feedings through a 10F feeding tube. Patients were fed estimated nutritional needs with a polymeric formula administered by feeding pump. The head of the bed was elevated at least 30°. Patients were observed daily for signs of aspiration or other complications. Aspiration was evaluated using a point score and radiographic assessment. Chest and abdominal radiographs were reviewed every 3 days. Weight was monitored weekly.

Key Results

Indications for tube feeding, mean age, Glasgow Coma Scale, and albumin levels were comparable in both groups. There were no significant differences in duration of feeding, time to goal rate, number of bowel movements, or number of tube displacements between the groups. There was no significant difference in the rate of aspiration, as defined by radiographic changes; overall, 11 patients (33%) aspirated (5 in the gastrically fed group and 6 in the postpyloric group). Clinical aspiration assessment scores were significantly higher in the group that had radiographic changes.

Study Strengths and Weaknesses

The study was prospective and randomized; however, the sample group was small. Radiographic evaluation is a sensitive marker of aspiration and, when correlated with daily aspiration scores, may provide a more accurate assessment of aspiration. This may lead to a higher rate of aspiration reported compared with studies that use a less sensitive parameter.

Clinical Implications

This study indicates that transpyloric feeding tube placement does not prevent aspiration. Achieving postpyloric feeding is often labor intensive and time consuming and may lead to increased cost (procedures, nursing time, etc) and to delayed nutrition while awaiting correct placement. The study also concludes that many of the aspiration events were silent and were not evident to researchers on a daily basis. It is unclear what effect these aspirations have on outcome and whether they are clinically significant.

22. Talpers SS, Romberger DJ, Bunce SB, et al. Nutritionally associated increased carbon dioxide production. *Chest.* 1992:102:551–555.

Study Sample

The sample population consisted of 20 stable patients (average APACHE II score 9) requiring MV.

Comparison Studied

This study compared the carbon dioxide production (Vco_2) from isocaloric parenteral feedings with low, moderate, and high percentages of calories from carbohydrates. The study also examined the effects of increasing calorie load on carbon dioxide (CO_2) production when a standard level of carbohydrate (60% of calories) was used.

Study Procedures

The 20 patients in this study were divided into 2 equal groups. Group 1 (n = 10) received isocaloric parenteral feedings that differed in only carbohydrate and fat percentage. Each nutritional regimen was based on the resting energy expenditure (REE) as determined by the Harris-Benedict equation times 1.3, and it provided 20% of the total calories as protein. The 3 nutritional regimens were 40% carbohydrate (CHO), 40% fat; 60% CHO, 20% fat; and 75% CHO, 5% fat. Each regimen was given for 48 hours before CO_2 production was measured. Group 2 (*n* = 10) received a *standard* mix of fuels (60% CHO, 20% fat, 20% protein), but total calories were increased every 48 hours. The patients received PN equal to the REE (as estimated by the Harris-Benedict equation), at 1.5 times the REE, and at 2.0 times the REE.

Key Results

In group 1 patients, who received isocaloric nutrition at varied percentages of CHO and fat, there was no significant difference in Vco_2 between the 3 regimens. In group 2, Vco_2 was significantly influenced by calorie level. Vco_2 was significantly increased above fasting during each of the feeding levels. The highest calorie level, 2.0 times the REE, resulted in a significant increase in Vco_2 level compared to the other 2 feeding groups.

Study Strengths and Weaknesses

The results of this study are somewhat weakened by the low number of patients. In addition, only 30% of the patients involved in the study had a history of restrictive chronic lung disease, where CO_2 retention would be expected to be a limiting factor. However, the use of PN as a nutrition source did allow the various regimens to be administered in a controlled fashion without being influenced by tolerance factors. Patients who received the isocaloric nutrition were fed at a level appropriate for the degree of metabolic stress.

Clinical Implications

The results of this study demonstrate that changes in the carbohydrate-fat ratio have minimal influence in CO_2 production in mechanically ventilated patients who are fed at an appropriate level. In addition, this study demonstrates the significant increase in CO_2 production that results when excessive calories are provided. Other clinical trials (Other References: 111) have demonstrated similar results; changing the carbohydrate-fat ratio does not affect ventilator weaning when patients are not grossly overfed.

23. Torres A, Serra-Batlles J, Ros E, et al. Pulmonary aspiration of gastric contents in patients receiving mechanical ventilation: the effect of body position. Ann Int Med. 1992;116: 540–543.

Study Sample

The sample comprised 19 patients with acute respiratory failure, mean age 60 years, requiring MV who were admitted to the respiratory ICU.

Comparison Studied

The study compared the risk of aspiration of gastric contents while in the supine position versus the semirecumbent position.

Study Procedures

Patients recovering from abdominal surgery or with ileus were excluded from the study. All patients had NG tubes; gastric contents were labeled and radioactive counts in endobronchial secretions measured. Samples of endobronchial secretions, gastric juice, and pharyngeal contents were obtained for bacterial cultures. The 2 positions, supine and semirecumbent, were studied 48 hours apart. Patients were monitored for pneumonia until discharge from the ICU.

Key Results

Mean radioactive counts in endobronchial secretions were higher in the supine position. In addition, the aspiration pattern was time dependent, more so for the supine position— that is, the likelihood of aspiration increased with the length of time the head was lowered.

Study Strengths and Weaknesses

The study sample was small. Enteral feeding was stopped 12 hours prior to the study. All patients received stress ulcer prophylaxis. It would have been interesting to have a group that did not receive an H_2 blocker. Lastly, waiting 7 days rather than 48 hours before crossing over might have shown that all pneumonia developed in the supine position.

Clinical Implications

Placing patients in the semirecumbent position is a simple and potentially effective measure to minimize aspiration of gastric contents.

24. Weinsier RL, Krumdieck PH, Krumdieck CL. Death resulting from overzealous total parenteral nutrition: the refeeding syndrome revisited. *Am J Clin Nutr.* 1980;34:393–399.

Description

This article reviews 2 case studies of severely malnourished, cachectic patients who were treated with aggressive PN support.

Case 1: A 28-year-old woman with a long history of malnutrition, diarrhea, abdominal pain, nausea, and vomiting presented at 23 kg, which is about 40% of ideal weight for her height of 162 cm. The patient, who was stable at time of admission, was treated with TPN providing 500 g glucose, 80 g amino acids, and 2 L fluid. The patient began to complain of chest pain approximately 20 hours after initiation of TPN; an electrocardiogram reading was consistent with acute myocardial infarction. The patient was transferred to the ICU with metabolic acidosis and acute respiratory distress syndrome (ARDS) requiring intubation. Chemistries revealed a phosphorus level of 0.129 mmol/L. The patient's status continued to decline and she died 3 weeks after admission.

Case 2: A 66-year-old woman admitted with abdominal pain, anorexia, and an unknown amount of weight loss weighed 36 kg, about 70% of ideal weight for her height of 155 cm. Central TPN was initiated to provide 750 g glucose, 120 g amino acids, and 3 L fluid. After 48 hours of TPN infusion, she became lethargic; a blood chemistry revealed a phosphorus level of 0.7 mg/dL. She soon became apneic, requiring intubation. The patient developed ARDS, hypotension, and peritonitis; she died on hospital day 6.

Clinical Implications

Severe malnutrition and cachexia are not uncommon in the hospital. It is therefore important to recognize patients who are at risk for refeeding syndrome. These patients should be refed cautiously and monitored frequently for electrolyte abnormalities, especially decreases in serum potassium, magnesium, and phosphorus, as well as other clinical symptoms. In most cases, these abnormalities can be corrected, but in rare instances, increased morbidity or even death may occur.

25. Weltz CR, Morris JB, Mullen JL. Surgical jejunostomy in aspiration risk patients. *Ann Surg* 1992;215:140–145.

Study Sample

In this study, 100 adult patients, mean age 66 years, required long-term, postpyloric feeding. All patients had jejunostomy tubes placed as the primary procedure.

Comparison Studied

Researchers measured the incidence of aspiration pneumonia after surgically placed jejunostomy tubes.

Study Procedures

Jejunostomy tubes were placed in the operating room according to standard procedure. Tubes were put to drainage for 12 hours; dextrose 5% in water was administered for the next 24 hours, followed by tube feedings, which were advanced to individual goals (determined by indirect calorimetry). Patients were monitored for complications until discharge or death.

Key Results

It was determined that 94% of patients who had a jejunostomy tube placed needed postpyloric feeding due to aspiration risk. After tube placement, 10 patients were diagnosed with aspiration, of which 2 had a history of aspiration. Four patients were thought to aspirate prior to initiation of jejunostomy feedings. Complications other than aspiration (n = 12) after tube placement included: inadvertent removal, drainage around the tube, small bowel obstruction, wound infection or dehiscence, and clogging of the tube. The 30-day mortality rate was 21%, with 1 death directly related to jejunostomy (witnessed aspiration).

Study Strengths and Weaknesses

The study eliminated patients who aspirated prior to tube feeding infusion, suggesting that if patients are fed via a jejunostomy, aspiration must have something to do with enteral feedings. The researchers compared their results to studies involving G-tubes, which may not have defined aspiration in the same way. It would have been interesting to see patients with G-tubes involved in the study as comparison.

Clinical Implications

All patients can aspirate; a jejunostomy does not ensure freedom from aspiration. The only way to prevent all aspiration is to create a spit fistula, which would be clinically inappropriate.

26. Zarling EJ, Parmar JR, Mobarhan S, et al. Effect of enteral formula infusion rate, osmolality, and chemical composition upon clinical tolerance and carbohydrate absorption in normal subjects. *J Parenteral Enteral Nutr.* 1986;10:588–590.

Study Sample

The study sample consisted of 20 healthy adult males.

Comparison Studied

The researchers studied the effect of rate, osmolality, and composition on tube feeding tolerance.

Study Procedures

Subjects were randomized to receive either an elemental (1.0 kcal/mL) formula or a complex (2.0 kcal/mL) tube feeding product via a nasoduodenal tube (placement confirmed by fluoroscopy). Tube feedings were run for 8 h/d for 4 days and were run at full strength for the first 3 days. During this time, half the group had the tube-feeding rate increased incrementally from 50 to 100 and then to 150 mL/h, while the other half received decreasing amounts of tube feeding starting from 150 and decreasing to 100 then 50 mL/h. On the fourth day, tube feedings were diluted with water to half strength and run at 100 mL/h. Subjects were allowed one small meal at the end of each feeding, but were otherwise kept NPO. Subjective complaints of abdominal pain, bloating, gas, and diarrhea were evaluated every 30 minutes during the tube feedings.

Key Results

Both formulas appeared to be tolerated well. There were no significant differences in GI complaints between the low and high infusion rates with either formula. Diluted tube feeding was not associated with a decrease in symptoms.

Study Strengths and Weaknesses

This study looked at young, healthy volunteers; it is unclear how this would carry over into the hospitalized patient. The study looked at a small sample size over a short period of time. In many facilities, 8-hour feedings are not standard practice.

Clinical Implications

In healthy patients it does not appear necessary to begin feedings using a diluted formula or at a very low rate. Healthy patients typically tolerate both elemental and complex formulas equally well. It is unclear how this translates into patient care.

OTHER REFERENCES

1. Keys A, Brozek J, Henschel A, et al. *Biology of Human Starvation.* Minneapolis, Minn: University of Minnesota Press; 1950.

2. Dockel R, Zwillich CW, Scoggin C, et al. Clinical semi-starvation: depression of the hypoxic ventilatory response. *N Engl J Med.* 1976;295:356–361.

3. Arora NS, Rochester DF. Effect of general nutritional and muscular states on the human diaphragm [abstract]. *Am Rev Respir Dis.* 1977;115:84.

4. Askanazi J, Weissman C, Rosenbaum SH, et al. Nutrition and the respiratory system. *Crit Care Med.* 1982;10:163–172.

5. Bassili HR, Deitel M. Effects of nutritional support on weaning patients off mechanical ventilators. *J Parenter Enteral Nutr.* 1981;5:161–163.

6. Askanazi J, Rosenbaum SH, Hyman AI, et al. Respiratory changes induced by the large glucose loads of total parenteral nutrition. *JAMA.* 1980;243:1444–1447.

7. Braunschweig CL, Levy P, Sheean PM, et al. Enteral compared with parenteral nutrition: a meta analysis. *Am J Clin Nutr.* 2001;74:534–542.

8. Brennan MF, Pisters PW, Posner M, et al. A prospective randomized trial of total parenteral nutrition after major pancreatic resection for malignancy. *Ann Surg.* 1994;220:436–441.

9. Kudsk KA, Croce MA, Fabian TC, et al. Enteral versus parenteral feeding. Effects on septic morbidity after blunt and penetrating trauma. *Ann Surg.* 1992;215:503–515.

10. Veterans Affairs Total Parenteral Nutrition Cooperative Study. Perioperative total parenteral nutrition in surgical patients. The Veterans Affairs Total Parenteral Nutrition Cooperative Study Group. *N Engl J Med.* 1991;325:525–532.

11. Abou-Assi S, Craid K, O'Keefe SJ. Hypocaloric jejunal feeding is better than total parenteral nutrition in acute pancreatitis: results of a randomized comparative study. *Am J Gastroenterol.* 2002;97:2255–2262.

12. Abou-Assi S, O'Keefe SJ. Nutrition in acute pancreatitis. *J Clin Gastroenterol.* 2001;32:203–209.

13. Adam S, Batson S. A study of problems associated with the delivery of enteral feed in critically ill patients in five ICUs in the UK. *Intensive Care Med.* 1997;23:261.

14. Adrogue HJ, Madias NE. Hyponatremia. *N Engl J Med.* 2000;342:1581–1589.

15. Alexander JW, MacMillan BG, Sinnett JD, et al. Beneficial effects of aggressive protein feeding in severely burned children. *Ann Surg.* 1980;192:505–517.

16. Alverdy J, Chi HS, Shedon GF. The effect of parenteral nutrition on gastrointestinal immunity: the importance of enteral stimulation. *Ann Surg.* 1985;202:681–684.

17. Anderson AD, Palmer D, MacFie J. Peripheral parenteral nutrition. *Br J Surg.* 2003;90:1048–1054.

18. Anderton A. Bacterial contamination of enteral feeds and feeding systems. *Clin Nutr.* 1993;12 (Suppl 1): S16–S32.

19. Andris DA, Krzywda EA. Nutrition support in specific diseases—back to basics. *Nutr Clin Pract.* 1994; 9:28–32.

20. Askanazi J, Weisman C, La Sala PA, Charlesworth PM. Nutrients and ventilation. *Adv Shock Res.* 1983;9:69–79.

21. Askanazi J, Weissman C, LaSala PA, et al. Effect of protein intake on ventilatory drive. *Anesthesiology.* 1984;60:106–110.

22. Atkinson S, Sieffert E, Bihari D. A prospective, randomized, double-blind, controlled clinical trial of enteral immunonutrition in the critically ill. Guy's Hospital Intensive Care Group. *Crit Care Med.* 1998;26:1164–1172.

23. Aubier M, Muciano D, Lecoguic Y, et al. Effect of hypophosphatemia on diaphragmatic contractility in patients with acute respiratory failure. *N Engl J Med.* 1985;313:420–424.

24. Baeten C, Hoefnagels J. Feeding via nasogastric tube or percutaneous endoscopic gastrostomy. A comparison. *Scand J Gastroenterol Suppl.* 1992;194:95–98.

25. Barak N, Wall-Alonso E, Sitrin MD. Evaluation of stress factors and body weight adjustments currently used to estimate energy expenditure in hospitalized patients. *J Parenter Enteral Nutr.* 2002;26:231–238.

26. Barnadas G. Navigating home care: enteral nutrition—part one. *Pract Gastroenterol.* 2003;27:13. Available at: http://www.healthsystem.virginia.edu/ internet/digestive-health/nutrition/resources.cfm. Accessed June 22, 2005.

27. Barr J, Hecht M, Flavin KE, et al. Outcomes in critically ill patients before and after the implementation of an evidence-based nutritional management protocol. *Chest.* 2004;125:1446–1457.

28. Bartlett RH, Dechert RE, Mault JR, Ferguson SK, Kaiser AM, Erlandson EE. Measurement of metabolism in multiple organ failure. *Surgery.* 1982;92: 771–779.

29. Bastani B, Mifflin TE, Lovell MA, et al. Serum amylases in chronic renal and end-stage renal failure. Effects of mode of therapy, race, diabetes and peritonitis. *Am J Nephrol.* 1987;7:292–299.

30. Battistella FD, Widergren JT, Anderson JT, et al. A prospective, randomized trial of intravenous fat emulsion administration in trauma victims requiring total parenteral nutrition. *J Trauma.* 1997;43:52–58.

31. Bauer LA. Interference of oral phenytoin absorption by continuous nasogastric feedings. *Neurology.* 1982; 32:570–572.

32. Beier-Holgersen R, Boesby S. Influence of postop enteral nutrition on postsurgical infections. *Gut.* 1996; 39:833–835.

33. Bertolini G, Iapichino G, Radrizzani D, et al. Early enteral immunonutrition in patients with severe sepsis: results of an interim analysis of a randomized multicentre clinical trial. *Intensive Care Med.* 2003;29:834–840.

34. Bickel A, Shtamler B, Mizrahi S. Early oral feeding following removal of nasogastric tube in gastrointestinal operations: a randomized, prospective study. *Arch Surg.* 1992;127:287–289.

35. Bodocky G, Harsanyi L, Pap A, et al. Effect of enteral nutrition on exocrine pancreatic function. *Am J Surg.* 1991;161:144–148.

36. Borgstrom B, Dahlquist G, Lundh G, et al. Studies of intestinal digestion and absorption in the human. *J Clin Invest.* 1957;36:1521–1536.

37. Bourgault AM, Heyland DK, Drover JW, et al. Prophylactic pancreatic enzymes to reduce feeding tube occlusions. *Nutr Clin Pract.* 2003;18:398–401.

38. Boussat S, Jacques T, Levy B, et al. Intravascular volume monitoring and extravascular lung water in septic patients with pulmonary edema. *Intensive Care Med.* 2002;28:712–718.

39. Bower RH, Cerra FB, Bershadsky B, et al. Early enteral administration of a formula (Impact) supplemented with arginine, nucleotides, and fish oil in intensive care unit patients: results of a multicenter, prospective, randomized, clinical trial. *Crit Care Med.* 1995;23:436–449.

40. Bowling TE, Silk DBA. Diarrhea and enteral nutrition. In: Rombeau JL, Rolandelli RH, eds. *Enteral and Tube Feeding.* Philadelphia. Pa: WB Saunders Co; 1997:540–553.

41. Bozzetti F, Gavazzi C, Miceli R, et al. Perioperative total parenteral nutrition in malnourished, gastrointestinal cancer patients: a randomized, clinical trial. *J Parenter Enteral Nutr.* 2000;24:7–14.

42. Brandi LS, Bertolini R, Santini L. Calculated and measured oxygen consumption in mechanically ventilated surgical patients in the early post-operative period. *Eur J Anaesthesiol.* 1999;16:53–61.

43. Brooks MJ, Melnik G. The refeeding syndrome: am approach to understanding its complications and preventing its occurrence. *Pharmacother.* 1995;15: 713–726.

44. Brown GR, Greenwood JK. Drug-induced nutrition-induced hypophosphatemia: mechanisms and relevance in the critically ill. *Ann Pharmacother.* 1994;28:626–632.

45. Brozek J, Chapman CB, Keys A. Drastic food nutrition: effects on cardiovascular dynamics in normotensive and hypertensive conditions. *JAMA.* 1948;137: 1569–1574.

46. Burns SM, Carpenter R, Truwit J. Report on the development of a procedure to prevent placement of feeding tubes into the lungs using end-tidal CO_2 measurements. *Crit Care Med.* 2001;29:936–939.

47. Burns SM, Clochesy JM, Hanneman SK, et al. Weaning from long-term mechanical ventilation. *Am J Crit Care.* 1995;4:4–22.

48. Campbell SM. *Preventing microbial contamination of enteral formulas and delivery systems.* Columbus, Ohio: Ross Products Division, Abbott Laboratories; 1995:1–28.

49. Cataldi-Betcher EL, Seltzer MH, Slocum BA, et al. Complications occurring during enteral nutrition support: a prospective study. *J Parenter Enteral Nutr.* 1983;7:546–552.

50. CDC guidelines for prevention of nosocomial pneumonia. *Resp Care.* 1994;39:1191–1236.

51. Malone AM. Enteral formula selection: a review of selected product categories. Practical Gastroenterology 2005;29(6):44. Available at: http://www.healthsystem.virginia.edu/internet/digestive-health/nutrition/resources.cfm. Accessed November 30, 2005.

52. Charash WE, Kearney PA, Annis KA, et al. Early enteral feeding is associated with an attenuation of the acute phase/cytokine response and improved outcome following multiple trauma. *J Trauma.* 1994;37:1015.

53. Charney P. Enteral nutrition: indications, options, and formulations. In: Gottslchlich MM, ed. *The Science and Practice of Nutrition Support.* Dubuque, Iowa: American Society for Parenteral and Enteral Nutrition, Kendall/Hunt Publishing Co; 2001:146.

54. Chendrasekhar A. Jejunal feeding in the absence of reflux increases nasogastric output in critically ill trauma patients. *Am Surg.* 1996;62:887–888.

55. Chiarelli A, Enzi G, Casadei A, et al. Very early nutrition supplementation in burned patients. *Am J Clin Nutr.* 1990;51:1035–1039.

56. Choban PS, Burge JC, Scales D, et al. Hypoenergetic nutrition support in hospitalized obese patients: a simplified method for clinical application. *Am J Clin Nutr.* 1997;66:546–550.

57. Coben RM, Weintraub A, Dimarino AJ, et al. Gastroesophageal reflux during gastrostomy feeding. *Gastroenterology.* 1994; 106:13–18.

58. Cordoba J, Lopez-Hellin J, Planas M, et al. Normal protein diet for episodic hepatic encephalopathy: results of a randomized study. *J Hepatol.* 2004; 41:38–43.

59. Crocker KS, Noga R, Filibeck DJ, et al. Microbial growth comparisons of five commercial parenteral lipid emulsions. *J Parenter Enteral Nutr.* 1984;8:391–395.

60. Crook M. Lipid clearance and total parenteral nutrition: the importance of monitoring plasma lipids. *Nutrition.* 2000;16:774–775.

61. Crook MA, Hally V, Panteli JV. The importance of the refeeding syndrome. *Nutrition.* 2001;17:632–637.

62. Culebras JM, Martin-Pena G, Garcia-de-Lorenzo A, et al. Practical aspects of peripheral parenteral nutrition. *Curr Opin Clin Nutr Metab Care.* 2004;7:303–307.

63. Davies AE, Kidd D, Stone SP. Pharyngeal sensation and gag reflex in healthy subjects. *Lancet.* 1995;345:487–488.

64. Davies AR, Bellomo R. Establishment of enteral nutrition: prokinetic agents and small bowel feeding tubes. *Curr Opin Crit Care.* 2004;10:156–161.

65. De Jonghe B, Appere-De-Vechi C, Fournier M, et al. A prospective survey of nutritional support practices in intensive care unit patients: what is prescribed? what is delivered? *Crit Care Med.* 2001;29:8–12.

66. de Ledinghen V, Beau P, Mannant PR, et al. Early feeding or enteral nutrition in patients with cirrhosis after bleeding from esophageal varices? A randomized controlled study. *Dig Dis Sci.* 1997;42:536–541.

67. de Ledinghen V, Beau P, Mannant PR, When should patients with bleeding peptic ulcer resume oral intake? A randomized controlled study. *Gastroenterol Clin Biol.* 1998;22:282–285.

68. Dickerson RN, Boschert KJ, Kudsk KA, Brown RO. Hypocaloric enteral tube feeding in critically ill obese patients. *Nutrition.* 2002;18:241–246.

69. Didier ME, Fischer S, Maki DG. Total nutrient admixtures appear safer than lipid emulsion alone as regards microbial contamination: growth properties of microbial pathogens at room temperature. *J Parenter Enteral Nutr.* 1998;22:291–296.

70. DiSario JA, Foutch PG, Sanowski RA. Poor results with percutaneous endoscopic jejunostomy. *Gastrointest Endosc.* 1990;36:257–260.

71. Dobb GJ, Towler SC. Diarrhoea during enteral feeding in the critically ill: a comparison of feeds with and without fibre. *Intensive Care Med.* 1990;16:252–255.

72. Dominioni L, Trocki J, Mochizuki H, et al. Prevention of severe postburn hypermetabolism and catabolism by intermediate intragastric feeding. *J Burn Care Rehab.* 1984;5:106–112.

73. Dotson RG, Robinson RG, Pingleton SK. Gastroesophageal reflux with nasogastric tubes. *Am J Respir Crit Care Med.* 1994;149:1659–1662.

74. Doweiko JP, Nompleggi DJ. Role of albumin in human physiology and pathophysiology. *J Parenter Enteral Nutr.* 1991;15:207–211.

75. Doweiko JP, Nompleggi DJ. The role of albumin in human physiology and pathophysiology: albumin and disease states. *J Parenter Enteral Nutr.* 1991;15:476–483.

76. Driscoll DF, Bacon MN, Bistrian BR. Effects of in-line filtration on lipid particle size distribution in total nutrient admixtures. *J Parenter Enteral Nutr.* 1996;20:296–301.

77. Duranteau, J Sitbon P, Teboul JL, et al. Effects of epinephrine, norephinephrine, or the combination of norephinephrine and dopamine on gastric mucosa in septic shock. *Crit Care Med.* 1999;27:893–900.

78. Dvorak MF, Noonan VK, Belanger L, et al. Early vs late enteral feeding in patients with acute cervical spinal cord injury. *Spine.* 2004;29:E175–E180.

79. Ebbert ML, Farraj M, Hwang LT. The incidence and clinical significance of intravenous fat emulsion contamination during infusion. *J Parenter Enteral Nutr.* 1987;11:42–45.

80. Eisenberg PG, Gianino S, Clutter WE, Fleshman JW. Abrupt discontinuation of cycled parenteral nutrition is safe. *Dis Colon Rectum.* 1995;38:933–939.

81. Elpern EH, Scott MG, Petro L, et al. Pulmonary aspiration in mechanically ventilated patients with tracheostomies. *Chest.* 1994;105:563–566.

82. Elpern EH, Stutz L, Peterson S, et al. Outcomes associated with enteral tube feedings in a medical intensive care unit. *Am J Crit Care.* 2004;13:221–227.

83. Elpern EH. Pulmonary aspiration in hospitalized adults. *Nutr Clin Pract.* 1997;12:5–13.

84. Elwyn DH, Kinney JM, Askanazi J, et al. Energy expenditure in surgery patients. *Surg Clin North Amer.* 1981;61:545–556.

85. Ely EW, Haponik EF. Using the chest radiograph to determine intravascular volume status: the role of vascular pedicle width. *Chest.* 2002;121:942–950.

86. Epstein CD, Peerless JR, Martin JE, et al. Comparison of methods of measurement of oxygen consumption in mechanically ventilated patients with multiple trauma: the Fick method versus indirect calorimetry. *Crit Care Med.* 2000;28:1363–1369.

87. Eyer SD, Micon LT, Konstantinides FN, et al. Early enteral feeding does not attenuate metabolic response after blunt trauma. *J Trauma.* 1993;34:639–644.

88. Fang JC, DiSario JA. Strategies in managing chronic pancreatitis—placement of direct percutaneous endoscopic jejunostomy feeding tubes. *Nutr Clin Pract.* 2004;19:50–55.

89. US Food and Drug Administration (FDA). Reports of blue discoloration and death in patients receiving enteral feedings tinted with the dye, FD&C Blue No. 1. FDA Public Health Advisory, FDA/Center for Food Safety & Applied Nutrition. September 29, 2003. Available at: http://www.cfsan.fda.gov/~dms/col-ltr2.html. Accessed November 1, 2004.

90. Fischer GW, Wilson SR, Hunter KW, et al. Diminished bacterial defenses with intralipid. *Lancet.* 1980;2:819–820.

91. Flancbaum L, Choban PS, Sambucco S, et al. Comparison of indirect calorimetry, the Fick method, and prediction equations in estimating the energy requirements of critically ill patients. *Am J Clin Nutr.* 1999;69:461–466.

92. Frankenfield D, Smith JS, Cooney RN. Validation of 2 approaches to predicting resting metabolic rate in critically ill patients. *J Parenter Enteral Nutr.* 2004;28:259–264.

93. Frankenfield DC, Muth ER, Rowe WA. The Harris-Benedict studies of human basal metabolism: history and limitations. *J Am Diet Assoc.* 1998;98:439–445.

94. Frankenfield DC, Reynolds HN. Nutritional effect of continuous hemofiltration. *Nutrition.* 1995;11:388–393.

95. Friedman RB, Young DS. *Effects of Disease on Clinical Laboratory Tests.* Washington, DC: American Association of Clinical Chemistry Press; 1989.

96. Fuhrman MP, Charney P, Mueller CM. Hepatic proteins and nutrition assessment. *J Am Diet Assoc.* 2004;104:1258–1264.

97. Galban C, Montejo JC, Mesejo A, et al. An immune-enhancing enteral diet reduces mortality rate and episodes of bacteremia in septic intensive care unit patients. *Crit Care Med.* 2000;28:643–648.

98. Garrett K, Tsurata K, Walker S, et al. Managing nausea and vomiting. *Crit Care Nurse.* 2003;23:31–55.

99. Guenter P, Jones S, Sweed MR, et al. Delivery systems and administration of enteral nutrition. In: Rombeau JL, Rolandelli RH, eds. *Enteral and Tube Feeding.* 3rd ed. Philadelphia, Pa: WB Saunders; 1997:240–267.

100. Guenter PA, Settle RG, Perlmutter S, et al. Tube-feeding-related diarrhea in acutely ill patients. *J Parenter Enteral Nutr.* 1991;15:277–280.

101. Gurr MI. The role of lipids in the regulation of the immune system. *Prog Lipid Res.* 1983;22:257–287.

102. Hanneman SK, Ingersoll GL, Knebel AR, et. al. Weaning from short-term mechanical ventilation: a review. *Am J Crit Care.* 1994;3:421–441.

103. Harig JM. Pathophysiology of small bowel diarrhea. In: Kahrilas PJ, Vanagunas A, eds. *American Gastroenterological Association Postgraduate Course.* Boston, Mass: American Gastroenterological Association; 1993:199–203.

104. Hasse JM, Blue LS, Liepa GU, et al. Early enteral nutrition in patients undergoing liver transplantation. *J Parenter Enteral Nutr.* 1995;19:437–443.

105. Hecketsweiler P, Vidon N, Emonts P, Bernier JJ. Absorption of elemental and complex nutritional solutions during a continuous jejunal perfusion in man. *Digestion.* 1979;19:213–217.

106. Heitkemper M, Hanson R, Hansen B. Effects of rate and volume of tube feeding in normal subjects. *Commun Nurs Res.* 1977;10:71–89.

107. Heitkemper ME, Martin DL, Hansen BC, et al. Rate and volume of intermittent enteral feeding. *J Parenter Enteral Nutr.* 1981;5:125–129.

108. Henderson JM, Strodel WE, Gilinsky NH. Limitations of percutaneous endoscopic jejunostomy. *J Parenter Enteral Nutr.* 1993;17:546–550.

109. Hennessey PJ, Black CT, Andrassy RJ. Nonenzymatic glycosylation of immunoglobulin G impairs complement fixation. *J Parenter Enteral Nutr.* 1991;15:60–64.

110. Heyland DK, Dhaliwal R, Drover JW, et al. Canadian clinical practice guidelines for nutrition support in mechanically ventilated, critically ill adult patients. *J Parenter Enteral Nutr.* 2003;27:355–373.

111. Heyland DK, Drover JW, MacDonald S, Novak F, Lam M. Effect of postpyloric feeding on gastroesophageal regurgitation and pulmonary microaspiration: results of a randomized controlled trial. *Crit Care Med.* 2001;29:1495–1501.

112. Heyland DK, Montalvo M, MacDonald S, et al. Total parenteral nutrition in the surgical patient: a meta-analysis. *Can J Surg.* 2001;44:102–111.

113. Heyland DK, Wood G. Effect of acid feeds on feeding system contamination. *Nutr Clin Pract.* 1998;13: S33–S37.

114. Hill D, Kearney P, Magnuson, et al. Effects of route and timing of nutrition in critically ill patients. *Gastroenterology.* 2002;122:A-38.

115. Hill SE, Heldman LS, Goo ED, et al. Fatal microvascular pulmonary emboli from precipitation of a total nutrient admixture solution. *J Parenter Enteral Nutr.* 1996;20:81–87.

116. Holte K, Kehlet H. Postoperative ileus: a preventable event. *Brit J Surg.* 2000;87:1480–1493.

117. Holzapfel L, Chevret S, Madinier G, et al. Influence of long-term oro- or nasotracheal intubation on nosocomial maxillary sinusitis and pneumonia: results of a prospective, randomized, clinical trial. *Crit Care Med.* 1993;21:1132–1138.

118. Ibañez J, Penafiel A, Raurich JM, et al. Gastroesophageal reflux in intubated patient receiving enteral nutrition: effects of supine and semirecumbent positions. *J Parenter Enteral Nutr.* 1992;16:419–422.

119. Jackson WD, Grand RJ. The human intestinal response to enteral nutrients: a review. *J Am Coll Nutr.* 1991;10:500–509.

120. Jacobs DG, Jacobs DO, Kudsk A, et al. Practice Management Guidelines for Nutritional Support of the Trauma Patient. *J Trauma.* 2004;57:660–679.

121. Jacobs SJ, Chang RWS, Lee B, Bartlett FW. Continuous enteral feeding: a major cause of pneumonia among ventilated intensive care unit patients. *J Parenter Enteral Nutr.* 1990;14:353–356.

122. Jenkins M, Gottschlich M, Alexander JW, et al. Effect of immediate enteral feeding on the hypermetabolic response following severe burn injury [abstract]. *J Parenter Enteral Nutr.* 1989;13(Suppl):12S.

123. Jones KL, Berry M, Kong MF, Kwiatek MA, Samsom M, Horowitz M. Hyperglycemia attenuates the gastrokinetic effect of erythromycin and affects the perception of postprandial hunger in normal subjects. *Diabetes Care.* 1999;22:339–344.

124. Kalfarentzos F, Kehagias J, Mead N, et al. Enteral nutrition is superior to parenteral nutrition in severe acute pancreatitis: results of a randomized prospective trial. *Br J Surg.* 1997;84:1665–1669.

125. Kandil HE, Opper FH, Switzer BR, et al. Marked resistance of normal subjects to tube feeding-induced diarrhea: the role of magnesium. *Am J Clinical Nutr.* 1993;57:73–80.

126. Kearns PJ, Chin D, Mueller L, et al. The incidence of ventilator-associated pneumonia and success in nutrient delivery with gastric versus small intestinal feeding: a randomized clinical trial. *Crit Care Med.* 2000;28:1742–1746.

127. Kearns PJ, Young H, Garcia G, et al. Accelerated improvement of alcoholic liver disease with enteral nutrition. *Gastroenterology.* 1992;102:200–205.

128. Kemper M, Weissman C, Hyman AI. Caloric requirements and supply in critically ill surgical patients. *Crit Care Med.* 1992;20:344–348.

129. Kinsey GC, Murray MJ, Swensen SJ, et al. Glucose content of tracheal aspirates: implications for the detection of tube feeding aspiration. *Crit Care Med.* 1994;22:1557–1562.

130. Kitchen K, Smith D. Problems with phenytoin administration in neurology/neurosurgery ITU patients receiving enteral feeding. *Seizure.* 2001;10:265–268.

131. Knochel JP. The pathophysiology and clinical characteristics of severe hypophosphatemia. *Arch Intern Med.* 1977;137:203–220.

132. Kocan M, Hickisch SM. A comparison of continuous and intermittent enteral nutrition in NICU patients. *J Neurosci Nurs.* 1986;18:333–337.

133. Kondrup J, Müller MJ. Energy and protein requirements of patients with chronic liver disease. *J Hepatol.* 1997;27:239–247.

134. Kortbeek JB, Haigh PI, Doig C. Duodenal versus gastric feeding in ventilated blunt trauma patients: a randomized controlled trial. *J Trauma.* 1999;46:992–996.

135. Krenitsky J. Nutritional guidelines for patients with hepatic failure. Pract Gastroenterol. 2003;27:23. Available at: http://www.healthsystem.virginia.edu/internet/digestive-health/nutrition/resources.cfm. Accessed June 22, 2005.

136. Krenitsky J. Nutrition in renal failure: myths and management. *Pract Gastroenterol.* 2004;28:40. Available at: http://www.healthsystem.virginia.edu/internet/digestive-health/nutrition/resources.cfm. Accessed January 4, 2005.

137. Krishnan JA, Parce PB, Martinez A, et al. Caloric intake in medical ICU patients. *Chest.* 2003;124:297–305.

138. Krzywda EA, Andris DA, Whipple JK, et al. Glucose response to abrupt initiation and discontinuation of total parenteral nutrition. *J Parenter Enteral Nutr.* 1993;17:64–67.

139. Kudsk K. Enteral feeding in bowel necrosis: an uncommon but perplexing problem. *Nutr Clin Pract.* 2003;18:277–278.

140. Kudsk KA, Minard G, Croce MA, et al. A randomized trial of isonitrogenous enteral diets after severe trauma. An immune-enhancing diet reduces septic complications. *Ann Surg.* 1996;224:531–540.

141. Kumar S, Berl T. Electrolyte quintet: sodium. *Lancet.* 1998;352:220–228.

142. Lankisch PG, Haseloff M, Becher R. No parallel between the biochemical course of acute pancreatitis and morphologic findings. *Pancreas.* 1994;9:240–243.

143. Lazarus BA, Murphy JB, Culpepper L. Aspiration associated with long-term gastric versus jejunal feeding: a critical analysis of the literature. *Arch Phys Med Rehabil.* 1990;71:46–53.

144. Leder SB. Videofluoroscopic evaluation of aspiration with visual examination of the gag reflex and velar movement. *Dysphagia.* 1997;12:21–23.

145. Leder SB. Gag reflex and dysphagia. *Head Neck.* 1996;18:138–141.

146. Lee B, Chang WS, Jacobs S. Intermittent nasogastric feeding: a simple and effective method to reduce pneumonia among ventilated ICU patients. *Clin Int Care.* 1990;1:100–102.

147. Lenssen P, Bruemmer BA, Bowden RA, et al. Intravenous lipid dose and incidence of bacteremia and fungemia in patients undergoing bone marrow transplantation. *Am J Clin Nutr.* 1998;67:927–933.

148. Livingston EH, Passaro EP. Postoperative ileus. *Dig Dis Sci.* 1990;35:121–132.

149. Loder PB. Validity of urinary urea nitrogen as a measure of total urinary nitrogen in adult patients requiring parenteral nutrition. *Crit Care Med.* 1989;17:309–312.

150. Long C, Schaffel N, Geiger JW, et al. Metabolic response to injury and illness: estimation of energy and protein needs from indirect calorimetry and nitrogen balance. *J Parenter Enteral Nutr.* 1979;3:452.

151. Lopez-Hellin J, Baena-Fustegueras JA, Schwartz-Riera S, Garcia-Arumi E. Usefulness of short-lived proteins as nutritional indicators surgical patients. *Clin Nutr.* 2002;21:119–125.

152. Lowell JA. Nutritional assessment and therapy in patients requiring liver transplantation. *Liver Transplantation Surg.* 1996;2:79–88.

153. Lowrey TS, Dunlap AW, Brown RO, et al. Pharmacologic influence on nutrition support therapy: use of propofol in a patient receiving combined enteral and parenteral nutrition support. *Nutr Clin Prac.* 1996;11:147–149.

154. Lucey BC, Gervais DA, Titton RL, et al. Enteric feeding with gastric decompression: management with separate gastric accesses. *Am J Roentgenol.* 2004;183:387–390.

155. Luckey A, Livingston E, Tache Y. Mechanisms and treatment of postoperative ileus. *Arch Surg.* 2003;138:206.

156. MacLaren R. Intolerance to intragastric enteral nutrition in critically ill patients: complications and management. *Pharmacotherapy.* 2000;20:1486–1498.

157. MacLaren R, Jarvis CL, Fish DN. Use of enteral nutrition for stress ulcer prophylaxis. *Ann Pharmacother.* 2001;35:1614–1623.

158. Mallet M. Refeeding syndrome. *Age Aging.* 2002;31:65–66.

159. Maloney JP, Halbower AC, Fouty BF, et al. Systemic absorption of food dye in patients with sepsis. *N Engl J Med.* 2000;343:1047–1048.

160. Marchesini G, Bianchi G, Merli M, et al, Italian BCAA Study Group. Nutritional supplementation with branched-chain amino acids in advanced cirrhosis: a double-blind, randomized trial. *Gastroenterology.* 2003;124:1792–1801.

161. Marcuard SP, Stegall KL, Trogdon S. Clearing obstructed feeding tubes. *J Parenter Enteral Nutr.* 1989;13:81.

162. Marcuard SP, Stegall KS. Unclogging feeding tubes with pancreatic enzyme. *J Parenter Enteral Nutr.* 1990;14:198–200.

163. Marik PE, Bedigian MK. Refeeding hypophosphatemia in critically ill patients in an intensive care unit. *Arch Surg.* 1996;131:1043–1047.

164. Marik PE, Kaplan D. Aspiration pneumonia and dysphagia in the elderly. *Chest.* 2003;124:328–336.

165. Marinella MA. The refeeding syndrome and hypophosphatemia. *Nutr Rev.* 2003;61:320–323.

166. Masclans JR, Iglesia R, Bermejo B, et al. Gas exchange and pulmonary haemodynamic responses to fat emulsions in acute respiratory distress syndrome. *Intensive Care Med.* 1998;24:918–923.

167. Masud T, Manatunga A, Cotsonis G, et al. The precision of estimating protein intake of patients with chronic renal failure. *Kidney Int.* 2002;62:1750–1756.

168. Matz R. Parallels between treated uncontrolled diabetes and the refeeding syndrome with emphasis on fluid and electrolyte abnormalities. *Diabetes Care.* 1994;17:1209–1213.

169. McClave SA, Chang W. Feeding the hypotensive patient: does enteral feeding precipitate or protect against ischemic bowel? *Nutr Clin Pract.* 2003;18:279–284.

170. McClave SA, Snider HL. Clinical use of gastric residual volume as a monitor for patients on enteral tube feedings. *J Parenter Enteral Nutr.* 2002;26 (Suppl 6):S43–S57.

171. McClave SA, Greene LM, Snider HL, et al. Comparison of the safety of early enteral vs. parenteral nutrition in mild acute pancreatitis. *J Parenter Enteral Nutr.* 1997;21:14–20.

172. McClave SA, Sexton LK, Spain DA, et al. Enteral tube feeding in the intensive care unit: factors impeding adequate delivery. *Crit Care Med.* 1999;27:1252–1256.

173. McClave SA, DeMeo MT, DeLegge MH, et al. North American Summit on Aspiration in the Critically Ill Patient: consensus statement. *J Parenter Enteral Nutr.* 2002;26:S1–S85.

174. McCray S, Walker S, Parrish CR. Much ado about refeeding. *Pract Gastroenterol.* 2004;28:26. Available at: http://www.healthsystem.virginia.edu /internet/digestive-health/nutrition/resources.cfm. Accessed June 22, 2005.

175. McMahon MM, Farnell MB, Murray MJ. Nutritional support of the critically ill patient. *Mayo Clin Proc.* 1993;68:911–920.

176. Mesejo A, Acosta JA, Ortega C, et al. Comparison of a high-protein disease-specific enteral formula with a high-protein enteral formula in hyperglycemic critically ill patients. *Clin Nutr.* 2003;22:295–305.

177. Metheny N. Minimizing respiratory complications of nasoenteric tube feedings: state of the science. *Heart Lung.* 1993;22:213–223.

178. Metheny NA, Eisenberg P, Spies M. Aspiration pneumonia in patients fed through nasoenteral tubes. *Heart Lung.* 1986;15:256–261.

179. Metheny NM. *Fluid and electrolyte balance; nursing considerations.* 4th ed. Philadelphia, Pa: Lippincott; 2000.

180. Miller LJ, Malagelada JR, Go VLW. Postprandial duodenal function in man. *Gut.* 1978;19:699–706.

181. Mizock BA. Alterations in carbohydrate metabolism during stress: a review of the literature. *Am J Med.* 1995;98:75–84.

182. Mochizuki H, Trocki O, Dominioni L, et al. Optimal lipid content for enteral diets following thermal injury. *J Parenter Enteral Nutr.* 1984;8:638–646.

183. Montejo JC, Grau T, Acosta J, et al. Multicenter, prospective, randomized, single-blind study comparing the efficacy and gastrointestinal complications of early jejunal feeding with early gastric feeding in critically ill patients. *Crit Care Med.* 2002;30:796–800.

184. Moore FA, Moore EE, Jones TN, et al. TEN versus TPN following major abdominal trauma-reduced septic morbidity. *J Trauma.* 1989:29:916–922.

185. Nakad A, Piessevaux H, Marot J, et al. Is early enteral nutrition in acute pancreatitis dangerous? About 20 patients fed by an endoscopically placed nasogastrojejunal tube. *Pancreas.* 1998;17:187–193.

186. Neumann DA, DeLegge MH. Gastric versus small-bowel tube feeding in the intensive care unit: a prospective comparison of efficacy. *Crit Care Med.* 2002;30:1436–1438.

187. Niemiec PW, Vandervenn TW, Morrison JI, et al. Gastrointestinal disorders caused by medication and electrolyte solution osmolality during enteral nutrition. *J Parenter Enteral Nutr.* 1983;7:387–389.

188. Nirula R, Yamada K, Waxman K. The effect of abrupt cessation of total parenteral nutrition on serum glucose: a randomized trial. *Am Surg.* 2000;66:866–869.

189. Nompleggi DJ, Bonkovsky HL. Nutritional supplementation in chronic liver disease: an analytical review. *Hepatology.* 1994;19:518–533.

190. Olah A, Pardavi G, Belagyi T, et al. Early nasojejunal feeding in acute pancreatitis is associated with a lower complication rate. *Nutrition.* 2002;18:259–262.

191. O'Neil-Pirozzi TM, Lisiecki DJ, Jack Momose K, et al. Simultaneous modified barium swallow and blue dye tests: a determination of the accuracy of blue dye test aspiration findings. *Dysphagia.* 2003;18:32–38.

192. Orozco-Levi M, Torres A, Ferrer M, et al. Semirecumbent position protects from pulmonary aspiration but not completely from gastroesophageal reflux in mechanically ventilated patients. *Am J Respir Crit Care Med.* 1995;152:1387–1390.

193. Padula CA, Kenny A, Planchon C, et al. Enteral Feedings: what the evidence says. *Am J Nurs.* 2004;104:62–69.

194. Parrish CR, Burns SM, Carpenter R, et al. Keeping patients safe: assuring that feeding tubes stay out of the lung [abstract]. *Nutr Clin Pract* 2005;20:139–N048.

195. Parrish CR, Enteral Feeding: The art and the science. *Nutr Clin Pract.* 2003;18:76.

196. Parrish CR, Krenitsky J, McCray S. University of Virginia Health System Nutrition Support Traineeship Syllabus, January 2003. Available at: http://www.healthsystem.virginia.edu/internet/dietitian/dh/syllabus.cfm. Accessed January 17, 2006.

197. Petrakis IE, Chalkiadakis G, Vrachassotakis N, Sciacca V, Vassilakis SJ, Xynos E. Induced-hyperglycemia attenuates erythromycin-induced acceleration of hypertonic liquid-phase gastric emptying in type I diabetic patients. *Dig Dis Sci.* 1999;17:241–247.

198. Pezzilli R, Billi P, Miglioli M, et al. Serum amylase and lipase concentrations and lipase/amylase ratio in assessment of etiology and severity of acute pancreatitis. *Dig Dis Sci.* 1993;7:1265–1269.

199. Phang PT, Aeberhardt LE. Effect of nutritional support on routine nutrition assessment parameters and body composition in intensive care unit patients. *Can J Surg.* 1996;39:212–219.

200. Powell JJ, Murchison JT, Fearon KCH, et al. Randomized controlled trial of the effect of early enteral nutrition on markers of the inflammatory response in predicted severe acute pancreatitis. *Br J Surg.* 2000;87:1375–1381.

201. Powell KS, Marcuard SP, Farrior ES, et al. Aspirating gastric residuals causes occlusion of small-bore feeding tubes. *J Parenter Enteral Nutr.* 1993;17:243–246.

202. Pupelis G, Selga G, Austrums E, et al. Jejunal feeding, even when instituted late, improves outcomes in patients with severe pancreatitis and peritonitis. *Nutrition.* 2001;17:91–94.

203. Raimundo AH, Rogers J, Filden P, et al. Influence of intraduodenal infusion of polymeric enteral diets on human pancreatic enzyme function [abstract]. *Gastroenterology.* 1990;98:427.

204. Ravasco P, Camilo ME. The impact of fluid therapy on nutrient delivery: a prospective evaluation of practice in respiratory intensive care. *Clin Nutr.* 2003;22:87–92.

205. Rees RPG, Hare WR, Grimble GK, et al. Do patients with moderately impaired gastrointestinal function requiring enteral nutrition need a predigested nitrogen source? A prospective crossover controlled trial. *Gut.* 1992;33:877–881.

206. Rees RPG, Keohane PP, Grimble GK, et al. Tolerance of elemental diet administered without starter regimen. *Br Med J.* 1985;290:1869–1870.

207. Reignier J, Thenoz-Jost N, Fiancette M, et al. Early enteral nutrition in mechanically ventilated patients in the prone position. *Crit Care Med.* 2004;32:94–99.

208. Revelly JP, Tappy L, Berger MM, et al. Early metabolic and splanchnic responses to enteral nutrition in postoperative cardiac surgery patients with circulatory compromise. *Intensive Care Med.* 2001;27:540–547.

209. Rochester DF. Nutrition repletion. *Semin Respir Med.* 1992;13:44–52.

210. Romano, TJ, Dobbins JW. Evaluation of the patient with suspected malabsorption. *Gastroenterol Clin North Am.* 1989;18 467–483.

211. Rosenberg AL. Fluid management in patients with acute respiratory distress syndrome. *Respir Care Clin North Am.* 2003;9:481–493.

212. Roth MS, Martin AB, Katz JA. Nutritional implications of prolonged propofol use. *Am J Health Syst Pharm.* 1997;54:694–695.

213. Rouby JJ, Laurent P, Gosnach M, et al. Risk factors and clinical relevance of nosocomial maxillary sinusitis in the critically ill. *Am J Respir Crit Care Med.* 1994;150:776–783.

214. Rubin M, Bilik R, Mor R, et al. Alteration of pulmonary function by filtration of intravenous nutrient mixture. *Nutrition.* 1993;9:153–155.

215. Russo MW, Sood A, Jacobson IM, et. al. Transjugular intrahepatic portosystemic shunt for refractory ascites: an analysis of the literature on efficacy, morbidity, and mortality. *Am J Gastroenterol.* 2003;98:2521–2527.

216. Sagar S, Harland P, Shields R. Early postoperative feeding with elemental diet. *Br Med J.* 1979;1:293–295.

217. Scheinkestel CD, Kar L, Marshall K, et al. Prospective randomized trial to assess calorie and protein needs of critically ill, anuric, ventilated patients requiring continuous renal replacement therapy. *Nutrition.* 2003;19:909–916.

218. Shang E, Geiger N, Sturm JW, Post S. Pump-assisted enteral nutrition can prevent aspiration in bedridden percutaneous endoscopic gastrostomy patients. *J Parenter Enteral Nutr.* 2004;28:180–183.

219. Shay DK, Fann LM, Jarvis WR. Respiratory distress and sudden death associated with receipt of a peripheral parenteral nutrition admixture. *Infect Control Hosp Epidemiol.* 1997;18:814–817.

220. Sherman BW, Hamilton C, Panacek EA. Adequacy of early nutrition support by the enteral route in patients with acute respiratory failure. *Chest.* 1990;98:104S.

221. Shike M, Latkany L, Gerdes H, Bloch A. Direct percutaneous endoscopic jejunostomies for enteral feeding. *Gastrointest Endosc.* 1996;44:536–540.

222. Shuster M. Do patients receive ordered enteral feeding? [abstract]. *Am J Crit Care.* 1997;6:254.

223. Silk DB, Walters ER, Duncan HD, et al. The effect of a polymeric enteral formula supplemented with a mixture of six fibres on normal human bowel function and colonic motility. *Clin Nutr.* 2001;20:49–58.

224. Singh G, Ram P, Khanna SK. Early postoperative enteral feeding in patients with nontraumatic intestinal perforation and peritonitis. *J Am Coll Surg.* 1998;187:142–146.

225. Soloman SM, Kirby DF. The refeeding syndrome: a review. *J Parenter Enteral Nutr.* 1990;14:90–97.

226. Spapen H, Diltoer M, Van Malderen C, et al. Soluble fiber reduces the incidence of diarrhea in septic patients receiving total enteral nutrition: a prospective, double-blind, randomized, and controlled trial. *Clin Nutr.* 2001;20:301–305.

227. Spilker CA, Hinthorn DR, Pingleton SK. Intermittent enteral feeding in mechanically ventilated patients. *Chest.* 1996;110:243–248.

228. Steinhardt JH, Wolf A, Jakober B, et al. Nitrogen absorption in pancreatectomized patients: protein vs. protein hydrolysate as substrate. *J Lab Clin Med.* 1989;113:162–167.

229. Subramanian R, Khardori R. Severe hypophosphatemia. *Medicine.* 2000;79:1–8.

230. Suchner U, Katz DP, Furst P, et al. Effects of intravenous fat emulsions on lung function in patients with acute respiratory distress syndrome or sepsis. *Crit Care Med.* 2001;29:1569–1574.

231. Swinamer DL, Phang PT, Jones RL, et al. Twenty-four hour energy expenditure in critically ill patients. *Crit Care Med.* 1987;15:637–643.

232. Taylor SJ, Fettes SB, Jewkes C, et al. Prospective, randomized controlled trial to determine the effect of early enhanced enteral nutrition on clinical outcome in mechanically ventilated patients suffering head injury. *Crit Care Med.* 1999;27:2525–2531.

233. Thompson B, Robinson LA. Infection control of parenteral nutrition solutions. *Nutr Clin Pract.* 1991;6:49–54.

234. Thomson AD, Cook CC, Touquet R, et al. Guidelines for managing Wernicke's encephalopathy in the accident and emergency department. *Alcohol Alcoholism.* 2002;37:513–521.

235. Thurn J, Crossley K, Gerdts, et al. Enteral hyperalimentation as a source of nosocomial infection. *J Hosp Infect.* 1990;15:203–217.

236. Tighe MJ, Wong C, Martin IG, McMahon MJ. Do heparin, hydrocortisone, and glyceryl trinitrate influence thrombophlebitis during full intravenous nutrition via a peripheral vein? *J Parenter Enteral Nutr.* 1995;19:507–509.

237. Vachharajani TJ, Zaman F, Abreo KD. Hyponatremia in critically ill patients. *J Intensive Care Med.* 2003;18:3–8.

238. Van den Berg B, Bogaard JM, Hop WC. High fat, low carbohydrate, enteral feeding in patients weaning from the ventilator. *Intensive Care Med.* 1994;20:470–475.

239. Van den Berghe G, Wouters P, Weekers F, et al. Intensive insulin therapy in critically ill patients. *N Engl J Med.* 2001;345:1359–1367.

240. van der Voort PH, Zandstra DF. Enteral feeding in the critically ill: comparison between the supine and prone positions: a prospective crossover study in mechanically ventilated patients. *Crit Care.* 2001;5:216–220.

241. van Lanschot JJ, Feenstra BW, Looijen R, et al. Total parenteral nutrition in critically ill surgical patients: fixed vs. tailored caloric replacement. *Intensive Care Med.* 1987;13:46–51.

242. Van Way C. Total calories vs. nonprotein calories [editorial]. *Nutr Clin Pract.* 2001;16:271–272.

243. Vasile B, Rasulo F, Candiani A, et al. The pathophysiology of propofol infusion syndrome: a simple name for a complex syndrome. *Intensive Care Med.* 2003;29:1417–1425.

244. Venus B, Smith RA, Patel C, et al. Hemodynamic and gas exchange alterations during intralipid infusion in patients with adult respiratory distress syndrome. *Chest.* 1989;95:1278–1281.

245. Waitzberg DL, Lotierzo PH, Logullo AF, et al. Parenteral lipid emulsions and phagocytic systems. *Br J Nutr.* 2002;87(Suppl 1):S49-S57.

246. Weissman C, Kemper M, Askanazi J, et al. Resting metabolic rate of the critically ill patient: measured versus predicted. *J Anesthesiol.* 1986;64:673–679.

247. Windsor ACJ, Kanwar S, Li AGK, et al. Compared with parenteral nutrition, enteral feeding attenuates the acute phase response and improves disease severity in acute pancreatitis. *Gut.* 1998;42:431–435.

248. Windus DW. Fluid and electrolyte management. In: Orland MJ, Saltman RJ, eds. *Manual of Medical Therapeutics.* Boston, Mass: Little, Brown; 1986:40–56.

249. Wolfe RR. Carbohydrate metabolism in the critically ill patient: implications for nutrition support. *Crit Care Clin.* 1987;3:11–24.

250. Yoder A. Nutrition support in pancreatitis: beyond parenteral nutrition. *Pract Gastroenterol.* 2003;27:19. Available at: http://www.healthsystem.virginia.edu/internet/digestive-health/nutrition/resources.cfm. Accessed January 4, 2005.

251. Yoder AJ, Parrish CR, Yeaton P. A retrospective review of the course of patients with pancreatitis discharged on jejunal feedings. Nutr Clin Pract 2002;17:314–320.

252. Young DS. *Effects of Drugs on Clinical Laboratory Tests.* 3rd ed. Washington, DC: American Association Clinical Chemistry Press; 1990.

253. Zaloga GP, Marik P. Lipid modulation and systemic inflammation. *Crit Care Clin.* 2001;17:201–217.

254. Zaloga GP, Roberts PR, Marik P. Feeding the hypotensive unstable patient: a critical evaluation of the evidence. *Nutr Clin Pract.* 2003;18:285–293.

255. Zimmaro D, Guenter PA, Settle RG. Defining and reporting diarrhea in tube-fed patients—what a mess! *Am J Clin Nutr.* 1992;55:753–759.

Sedation and Neuromuscular Blockade in Mechanically Ventilated Patients

Jill Luer, PharmD

CHAPTER SIX

Sedation and Neuromuscular Blockade in Mechanically Ventilated Patients

CASE STUDY 1

LM, a previously healthy 33-year-old woman, was admitted to the medical intensive care unit (MICU) with a 7-day history of a viral upper respiratory illness and new signs and symptoms of acute respiratory failure. The patient exhibited fever (39.3°C), tachypnea (respiratory rate 30), hypotension (blood pressure [BP] 90/60 mm Hg), impaired gas exchange (partial pressure of oxygen, arterial [PaO_2], 60 mm Hg; partial pressure of carbon dioxide, arterial [$PaCO_2$], 36 mm Hg on face mask; fraction of inspired oxygen [FIO_2], 0.40), use of accessory respiratory muscles, and declining mental status. Pertinent laboratory values included blood urea nitrogen, 14.3 mmol/L; serum creatinine, 132.6 μmol/L; hemoglobin, 110 g/L; and hematocrit, 30%. The team decided intubation was necessary to support oxygenation and ventilation to provide airway protection. Midazolam (2 mg) and succinylcholine (50 mg) were given intravenously, and LM was intubated orally with a size 7.5 ID endotracheal (ET) tube. Mechanical ventilatory support was initiated using the assist-control mode at a rate of 22, tidal volume (V_T) of 10 mL/kg, FIO_2, 1.0; positive end-expiratory pressure (PEEP), 5 cm H_2O. Admission chest radiographs revealed diffuse, bilateral interstitial infiltrates. The patient received 1 liter of 0.9% sodium chloride infused over 10 minutes for hypotension, followed by a continuous rate of 150 mL/hr to provide circulatory support and enhance tissue perfusion. Antibiotics were initiated for empiric coverage of secondary bacterial pathogens.

Two hours following initiation of ventilator support, the patient's mental status improved slightly, and LM was able to communicate her anxiety and fear about her illness as well as discomfort associated with the ET tube. Sedative and analgesic therapies were begun using intermittent IV boluses of lorazepam 0.5–1.0 mg and fentanyl 50 to 100 μg as needed.

An 8-point sedation scale was used to assess the level of sedation and guide drug administration. Despite increasing bolus doses of sedatives, the patient's respiratory status deteriorated over the next 4 hours. Arterial blood gas measurements showed progressive worsening of gas exchange (pH, 7.28; PaO_2, 55 mm Hg; $PaCO_2$, 41 mm Hg; serum bicarbonate, 22 mmol/L), and chest radiographs showed increasing deterioration with bilateral diffuse infiltrates. The peak airway pressure was 65 cm H_2O, and the plateau pressure was 57 cm H_2O. Continued hypoxemia was believed to be related to the development of acute respiratory distress syndrome and partially affected by the patient's intermittent agitation and subsequent ventilator dysynchrony. Hemodynamic parameters were BP, 100/60 mm Hg; pulmonary capillary wedge pressure, 8 mm Hg; and cardiac output, 7.9 L/min. Intravenous fluids were increased to 200 mL/hr.

To protect the lung from injury, low V_T ventilation was initiated at 6 mL/kg and PEEP was increased to 10 cm H_2O. A pancuronium 2 mg IV bolus was provided to allow hypercapnia to ensue (ie, "permissive hypercarbia") without compensatory patient respiratory efforts. Additional bolus doses of pancuronium were administered every 2 to 4 hours as needed to suppress respiratory effort. Train-of-four (TOF) peripheral nerve stimulation was used to achieve at least 1 thumb twitch out of 4 prior to redosing (see Figure 6–1).

LM's clinical course continued to deteriorate despite multiple interventions and was also complicated by a pneumothorax requiring chest tube placement. Pancuronium was discontinued, and a continuous infusion of atracurium was initiated on day 2 due to increasing pancuronium requirements despite upward titration of both analgesics and sedatives. Each morning a trial of discontinuance was attempted to assess neurological status, sedation requirements, and continuing need for neuromuscular blockade. Once atracurium

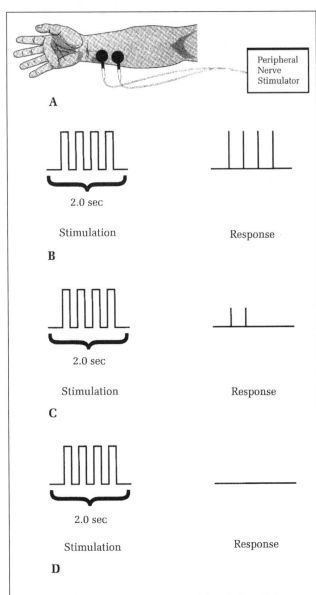

FIGURE 6–1   Peripheral Nerve Stimulation Using Train-of-Four Pattern

(A) Electrode placement for train-of-four (TOF) stimulation of the ulnar nerve; 4 stimuli are delivered over 2 seconds; response is determined by counting thumb adductions toward the palm. TOF patterns demonstrating (B) no blockade; (C) 50% blockade; and (D) 100% blockade.

Adapted from Chulay M, Guzzetta C, Dossey B. *AACN Pocket Handbook of Critical Care Nursing.* Stamford, Conn: Appleton & Lange; 1997.

degree of neuromyopathy in the upper extremities was identified by physical examination and documented by electromylogram. Physical therapy was initiated, and the patient was discharged on hospital day 32.

CASE STUDY 2

LJ is a 65-year-old, 90-kg man with a history of chronic obstructive pulmonary disease , diabetes mellitus, hyperlipidemia, hypertension, and chronic headaches of unknown etiology. He presented to the emergency department after 2 episodes of hematemesis, saying he felt lethargic and lightheaded. He reported compliance with his medications, which include albuterol and ipratropium inhalers, ultralente insulin; lovastatin, aspirin, and lisinopril. His wife told the emergency department staff that he consumed a 24-count bottle of ibuprofen 200 mg over 2 to 3 days in an attempt to relieve a particularly bad headache. She also said that the patient experiences occasional anxiety and sleepless nights for which he takes triazolam 3 to 4 nights per week.

The patient was transferred to the MICU for supportive care and management of upper gastrointestinal bleeding. Fluid resuscitation with crystalloids and blood products, as well as intravenous proton pump inhibitor therapy, was initiated. Vital signs were stable (BP, 110/60; heart rate, 80). Premedication for diagnostic esophagogastroduodenoscopy included midazolam 2 mg and fentanyl 50 µg, each administered IV over 1 minute. Ten minutes into the procedure, the patient vomited 500 mL of dark red blood.

Within 12 hours, LJ became hypoxic, febrile, and tachycardic with fluctuating mental status. An ET tube was placed for airway protection. A size 7.5 mm inner diameter oral ET tube was inserted, and the patient was placed on intermittent mandatory ventilation of 15 breaths per minute, FIO_2 of 1.0, VT of 500 mL, and PEEP of 5 cm H_2O. The patient woke 20 minutes following intubation and attempted to remove his ET tube, nasogastric tube, and IV lines. Intravenous boluses of lorazepam 2 mg were administered every 4 hours to relieve anxiety and promote rest. This regimen produced a calm, cooperative state, but LJ did not sleep at night, so the late evening (10 PM) dose was increased to 4 mg.

The next morning's physical examination revealed new crackles and diminished breath sounds in both lung apices. Chest radiographs indicated the presence of a new infiltrate in the right lower lobe. Antibiotic therapy was initiated. The patient's anxiety level increased due to fear of his worsening illness, discomfort associated with the ET tube, and sleep deprivation. Fentanyl 25 µg/h by continuous IV infusion was initiated to control pain, with intermittent boluses of lorazepam 2 mg to relieve anxiety and ensure patient safety. Despite multiple bolus doses of both agents and further increases in infusion rates, the patient showed no significant improvement.

Over the next 6 hours, the patient became increasingly agitated. The patient's nurse observed LJ occasionally "picking" invisible objects out of the air and reported that he

was discontinued, the lorazepam infusion was interrupted once each morning to assess LM's mental status and continued sedative requirements.

LM required ventilatory support for a total of three weeks. The sedative and analgesic infusions were weaned over the second week. Following discontinuation of neuromuscular blockade and sedative infusions, a moderate attempted to hit her once during routine care. Fearing that LJ would be difficult to wean from the ventilator given his history of chronic obstructive pulmonary disease and requirement for large doses of sedatives, the MICU team decided to try IV haloperidol for suspected delirium. A 5-mg dose was administered, but produced little effect, as evidenced by continued thrashing movements. After a 15-minute observation period, haloperidol 10 mg was administered. LJ remained in bed but continued to be disoriented and agitated. After an additional 15 minutes, a 20-mg IV dose of haloperidol was administered, and within 20 minutes the patient was resting comfortably. Haloperidol was administered every 1 to 4 hours to control symptoms of delirium. QTc intervals were monitored hourly with the initiation of haloperidol and increased from .34 to .39 seconds over a 24-hour period. Ultimately, LJ received 20 mg IV every hour for 6 hours with additional boluses of lorazepam and haloperidol as needed. Over the next 24 hours, haloperidol was increased to 20 mg IV every 4 hours, with additional 20 mg doses every hour as needed to control delirium. The patient remained on this haloperidol regimen while lorazepam, and then fentanyl, infusions were tapered over 2 days. As the patient's pneumonia resolved, ventilator support was decreased without incident and the haloperidol dose was decreased to 10 mg every 4 hours. The patient was successfully extubated from the ventilator following a 1-hour trial of 5 cm H_2O continuous positive airway pressure trial. Haloperidol was tapered and discontinued over the next 24 hours, and the patient was transferred out of the MICU the following day. No adverse effects associated with haloperidol were observed, including excessive QT prolongation (and associated cardiac arrhythmias) or extrapyramidal signs.

GENERAL DESCRIPTION

Technological advances in critical care offer health professionals new challenges and successes in treating patients with increasingly complicated illness. Many innovative diagnostic and therapeutic modalities are available that ultimately prolong and enhance the quality of life, yet may be associated with extended periods of immobility and discomfort.

Patients may experience pain related to surgical procedures, underlying disease, and invasive life-supporting and monitoring devices, among many other causes. They are also often anxious and agitated due to the presence of pain, fear of the unknown, inability to communicate, sleep deprivation, as well as disease- and drug-related factors. In addition, severe illness combined with sensory overload related to the ICU environment may precipitate symptoms of delirium, such as disorientation, hallucinations, and altered sleep-wake cycles.

Although it is most desirable to address and resolve the underlying cause for pain, anxiety, and/or delirium, it is not practical to assume that resolution will be rapid. Therefore, pharmacologic intervention with sedatives, analgesics, and neuroleptics is an important component of care in the criti-

cally ill patient, particularly in those requiring long-term mechanical ventilatory support. Selection of the appropriate agent(s) is based on patient-specific treatment goals, the presence of underlying disease, history of allergy or other adverse events, and cost considerations. Patients receiving sedative therapy must be carefully and continuously monitored to achieve predetermined goals of therapy, ensure stable neurologic function, and avoid oversedation or other complications. It must be emphasized that these agents may be associated with potentially dangerous side effects (see Appendix 6A) and require close monitoring (Appendix 6B). Daily interruption of sedative infusions may assist neurologic assessment and prevent complications related to oversedation, but may not be practical in all patients. The development of goal-directed sedation protocols has further advanced care by reducing the duration of mechanical ventilation, ICU and hospital stay, and neuromuscular blocker use.

The administration of neuromuscular blocking (NMB) agents (Appendix 6C) is generally reserved for patients who exhibit muscular movements or breathing patterns that interfere with the delivery of mechanical ventilation, oxygenation, and care. For example, NMB use is frequently required when inverse inspiratory-expiratory ratio or high-frequency oscillatory ventilation modes are used due to discomfort and difficulty related to synchronizing patient-initiated respiratory efforts with those of the ventilator. NMBs may also be useful in patients experiencing severe asthma by decreasing the work of breathing, preventing barotrauma secondary to elevated airway pressures, and reducing oxygen consumption.

Information about pharmacokinetic and adverse effect profiles of available NMBs is useful in selecting the best agent and method of administration for a specific patient. For example, pancuronium is associated with vagolytic effects that may not be tolerated in patients with cardiovascular disease, and is eliminated by renal and hepatic mechanisms, which may promote drug accumulation and reduced clearance in patients with impairment of these organs. Patients requiring sustained neuromuscular blockade must be frequently monitored as acute changes in the clinical course may be easily masked in the presence of pharmacologic paralysis. It is critical that a patient-specific clinical end point be identified to avoid under- or overdosing. For many patients, suppression of patient-initiated respirations is indicative of adequate paralysis; this can be easily assessed visually during routine care. However, excessive neuromuscular blockade cannot be ruled out using this method, and thus peripheral nerve stimulation using the train of four (TOF) method is commonly used to assess the depth of paralysis and prevent drug accumulation. The ideal TOF response should be that which achieves patient-specific goals for NMB therapy without producing total NMB. Another method used to assess adequacy of NMB therapy is airway pressure waveform monitoring. The reader is referred to "Respiratory Waveforms Monitoring" (Chapter 2) in *AACN Protocols for Practice: Nonivasive Monitoring* for a detailed description. And finally, the use of bispectral electroencephalograph (EEG) monitoring may be helpful to assure that patients are adequately sedated when paralytic agents are used.

Infusion rates should be periodically titrated downward to produce the lowest level of blockade and still achieve the desired goal. In addition, daily discontinuation of NMB therapy is recommended to allow reevaluation of the patient's clinical status and the adequacy of sedation. It cannot be overemphasized that paralysis without sedation can be terrifying therefore, assurance of patient comfort is crucial and must not be overlooked. Continued interest in improving patient outcomes and reducing total healthcare costs dictates that practitioners be knowledgeable about these issues and actively participate in the development and maintenance of practice protocols to achieve these goals.

Concerns regarding NMB-induced prolonged paralysis and weakness and its complications heighten the importance of specific guidelines for selecting, administering, and monitoring these agents. Residual paralysis or weakness associated with NMB administration is now a well-known phenomenon and should stimulate careful risk-benefit consideration in all patients prior to initiation.

COMPETENCY

Competency in providing appropriate sedative or NMB therapy to critically ill patients requires the clinician to do the following:

1. Assess and identify treatable causes of agitation and delirium, including hypoxia, intubation, infection, substance withdrawal, drug therapy, as well as discomfort due to confinement, injury, or surgical intervention.
2. Identify presenting signs and symptoms of pain, agitation, and delirium that indicate the need for pharmacologic intervention in patients receiving mechanical ventilation.
3. Describe the various nonpharmacologic and pharmacologic methods to provide anxiolysis, comfort, or respiratory control, and apply these to specific patient situations (eg, indication, underlying diseases, costs).
4. Identify patient-oriented end points for sedation therapy.
5. Understand currently used methods to monitor and adjust sedative and NMB therapy based on predetermined goals of therapy.
6. Recognize the complications associated with sedative and NMB agents, and use practice methods to avoid or reduce their incidence.

ETHICAL CONSIDERATIONS

The most critical ethical issue in the use of sedative and NMB agents is ensuring adequate sedation and analgesia before initiating neuromuscular blockade. It is important to remember that critically ill patients experience increased stress due to their illness, invasive procedures, and the ICU environment. Clinicians must not hesitate to provide neces-

sary relief via pharmacologic intervention. In addition, it must be emphasized that NMBs do not provide analgesic or sedative effects.

Methods to routinely assess adequacy of sedation, such as sedation scales, are recommended to avoid oversedation and prolonged awakening as well as undersedation in the presence of paralysis. Finally, frequent communication and reassurance by caregivers may provide necessary psychological support to the patient and family members during therapy with these agents.

FUTURE RESEARCH

Careful drug selection and individualization of therapy remain key issues in the provision of sedative and NMB therapy. Prospective studies assessing the impact of protocols and critical pathways on patient outcomes and total costs of care should continue to determine the safest, most effective, and least costly methods for administering and monitoring these agents. In addition, establishment and refinement of population-specific, goal-oriented sedation scales are required to enhance the consistency of caregiver observations and allow comparison of drug effects. Work in the area of EEG monitoring using the bispectral index suggests that this method may be useful in assessing the level of sedation. However, more work is needed to determine the definitive use of this technology in paralyzed and sedated patients. For example, it will be important to compare the efficacy of existing methods using selected protocols and processes of care with that of the EEG monitoring techniques. This is especially important given the cost and labor intensity of bispectral technologies.

SUGGESTED READINGS

Arbour R. Sedation and pain management in critically ill adults. *Crit Care Nurse.* 2000;20:39–58.

Brook AD, Ahrens TS, Schaiff R, et al. Effect of a nursing-implemented sedation protocol on the duration of mechanical ventilation. *Crit Care Med.* 1999;27:2609–2615.

Kress JP, Pohlman AS, O'Connor MF, et al. Daily interruption of sedative infusions in critically ill patients undergoing mechanical ventilation. *N Eng J Med.* 2004;342:1471–1477.

Ely EW, Shintani A, Truman B, et al. Delirium as a predictor of mortality in mechanically ventilated patients in the intensive care unit. *JAMA.* 2004;291:1753–1762.

Mascia MF, Koch M, Medicis JJ. Pharmacoeconomic impact of rational use guidelines on the provision of analgesia, sedation, and neuromuscular blockade in critical care. *Crit Care Med.* 2000;28:2300–2306.

Riker RR, Fraser GL. Adverse events associated with sedatives, analgesics, and other drugs that provide patient comfort in the intensive care unit. *Pharmacother.* 2005;25:8S–18S.

CLINICAL RECOMMENDATIONS

Sedation

The rating scales for the Level of Recommendation range from I to IV, with levels indicated as follows: I, manufactuer's recommendations only; II, theory based, no research data to support recommendations; recommendations from expert consensus group may exist; III, laboratory data only, no clinical data to support recommendations; IV, limited clinical studies to support recommendations; V, clinical studies in more than 1 or 2 different populations and situations to support recommendations; VI, clinical studies in a variety of patient populations and situations to support recommendations.

Period of Use	Recommendation	Rationale for Recommendation	Level of Recommendation	Supporting References	Comments
Selection of patients	Sedative or analgesic therapy should be considered during mechanical ventilation (MV) for:				
	• Patients exhibiting, or expected to exhibit, signs and symptoms of anxiety, discomfort, pain or delirium associated with critical illness, injury, or therapeutic interventions	Patients with inadequately controlled pain, agitation, or delirium face a higher risk of morbidity, mortality, and increased length of stay (LOS).	VI: Clinical studies in a variety of patient populations and situations to support recommendations	See Annotated Bibliography; 2, 3, 4 See Other References: 39, 44, 48	
	• Patients with preexisting anxiety, psychiatric, or pain disorders requiring pharmacologic intervention	Drug therapy must be continued to prevent potential withdrawal symptoms specific to the drug class(es) utilized by the patient.			
	• Patients in whom respiratory effort must be depressed or controlled, or patients with discomfort or pain associated with controlled ventilation	Diaphragmatic and chest wall movements may interfere with MV and prohibit adequate oxygenation. Also, complex ventilatory modes (eg, inverse-ratio ventilation, high frequency oscillation, or those that result in permissive hypercapnia) are nonphysiologic and may create significant patient discomfort. Pulmonary instability (high auto-PEEP and dynamic hyperinflation) may also result in hemodynamic instability such as hypotension.			Comprehensive assessment of factors affecting patient-ventilator synchrony is necessary prior to any interventions. For example, titration of flow rates and settings may improve interface with ventilation, and pharmacologic agents may not be required. Refer to Chapter 2, Invasive and Noninvasive Modes and Methods of Mechanical Ventilation.
	• Patients with history of alcohol or substance abuse	Abrupt discontinuance or decreased intake may result in drug withdrawal syndromes involving symptoms of anxiety, agitation, tachycardia, and insomnia, and progress to hallucinations, sympathetic storm, cardiopulmonary instability, and seizures if untreated.	VI: Clinical studies in a variety of patient populations and situations to support recommendations	See Other References: 20, 21	Benzodiazepines are the drugs of choice to prevent and treat symptoms of alcohol withdrawal. Benzodiazepines are also the agent of choice for prevention of anxiety and withdrawal symptoms in patients with prolonged exposure. Opioids are the agent(s) of choice to treat or prevent withdrawal in patients with prolonged exposure to opioids (eg, heroin, morphinelike agents, methadone).

Period of Use	Recommendation	Rationale for Recommendation	Level of Recommendation	Supporting References	Comments
Initial use	Recommendations for the appropriate sedative or analgesic depend on several patient-specific factors:				
	Expected duration of sedation: • Short-term (< 24 hours) Sedation: midazolam or propofol • Long-term (> 24 hours) Sedation: lorazepam Short-term analgesia infusion: fentanyl Long-term analgesia infusion: morphine	Midazolam and propofol have rapid onset. Diazepam is also recommended for rapid sedation in acute agitation. The potential for accumulation of midazolam or its active metabolite prohibits its routine use for long-term sedation.	V: Clinical studies in more than 1 or 2 different patient populations and situations to support recommendations	See Annotated Bibliography: 4, 6 See Other References: 1, 7	Small incremental doses are more appropriate in the neurologically impaired patient due to need for serial neurological assessments. Rapid bolus dosing may decrease mean arterial pressure and risk compromising cerebral perfusion. Propofol may be preferred, however, given its more rapid onset/offset of action, which facilitates serial neurologic assessments. Prolonged sedative effects may be observed with midazolam-active metabolite accumulation in renal failure, obesity, hypoalbuminemic states, and diazepam (long half-lived active metabolite).
	Presenting signs and symptoms and indication: • Anxiety, fear, insomnia or to decrease patient recall: benzodiazepines • Pain: opioids • Delirium, agitation unrelieved by other agents: haloperidol	Desired clinical goals or end points of therapy should be determined on initial evaluation. Drug therapy should be individualized to achieve the best possible patient outcomes. Drugs should be selected on the basis on proven safety and efficacy for the indication studied.	VI: Clinical studies in a variety of patient populations and situations to support recommendations	See Annotated Bibliography: 2, 4, 6, 8 See Other References: 9, 17, 23–26, 36	Combined/concurrent use of opioids and benzodiazepines will result in a significant dose-sparing effect due to synergistic effects between both drug classes. Haloperidol may be given based on a clinical determination of delirium.
	Hemodynamic status: • For critically ill patients with actual or potential hemodynamic instability, fentanyl is the preferred analgesic.	Fentanyl is not associated with histamine release or venodilating effects, resulting in a lower incidence of hypotension compared to morphine. Although with volume depletion or dependence on high sympathetic outflow to maintain cardiac output it may still cause hypotension.	V: Clinical studies in more than 1 or 2 different patient populations and situations to support recommendations	See Annotated Bibliography: 4, 6 See Other References: 35, 45	Hydromorphone may be an alternative but is much longer acting, has active metabolites, and potential for increased risk of delirium.
	• Avoid administration of morphine, propofol, or dexmedetomidine in patients with unstable hemodynamics.	Propofol-induced hypotension in ICU patients is likely related to the magnitude of the dose and rate of administration. Other risk factors include advanced age, hypovolemia, and concomitant opioid administration.		See Other References: 1, 14, 35	Revised product information for propofol recommends avoiding bolus doses in elderly, debilitated, or critically ill patients.

Period of Use	Recommendation	Rationale for Recommendation	Level of Recommendation	Supporting References	Comments
Initial use *(cont.)*	**Renal or hepatic status:** • Fentanyl is recommended for analgesia in patients with renal dysfunction.	Fentanyl is primarily cleared by hepatic metabolism. Morphine-6-glucuronide accumulation may produce prolonged sedative effects during renal impairment.	V: Clinical studies in more than 1 or 2 different patient populations and situations to support recommendations	See Other References: 11	
	• Lorazepam and propofol are recommended sedatives for patients exhibiting hepatic dysfunction.	Both are conjugated by the liver, a pathway generally spared until significant hepatic insufficiency occurs.	V: Clinical studies in more than 1 or 2 different patient populations and situations to support recommendations	See Annotated Bibliography: 4 See Other References: 1, 40, 50	
	Anticipated need for neuromuscular blockade (NMB): Concomitant sedative and analgesic infusions are indicated.	NMB agents provide no sedative or analgesic effects. Assessment of pain and anxiety is not possible with any reliability in the paralyzed patient based on the clinical examination. Aggressive dosing of an opioid-benzodiazepine combination may allow reduction or avoidance of NMB drugs. Dosing of concurrent sedative/opioid infusions should be dictated by clinical goals or end points of therapy such as deep sedation, and then reevaluating need for NMB therapy as indicated. Even during NMB, aggressive dosing with sedative/analgesic agents is appropriate to minimize risk of awareness and pain while paralyzed.	V: Clinical studies in more than 1 or 2 different patient populations and situations to support recommendations	See Annotated Bibliography: 4, 6, 7, 12 See Other References: 32	
	The method of sedative/analgesic administration should be based on the following considerations:				
	Pharmacokinetic properties of the sedative: Continuous infusions should be administered with caution in critically ill patients.	Even for short-acting agents, accumulation of parent drug or metabolites may have adverse effects such as hypotension, and oversedation leading to prolonged recovery/LOS in patients with impaired liver or renal disease associated with critical illness.	V: Clinical studies in more than 1 or 2 different patient populations and situations to support recommendations	See Annotated Bibliography: 4, 6	

Period of Use	Recommendation	Rationale for Recommendation	Level of Recommendation	Supporting References	Comments
Initial use *(cont.)*	**Dosage/duration requirement:**				
	• Intermittent bolus administration may safely achieve the goals of sedation in patients requiring low dose, as-needed, or short-term sedation.	Continuous infusions may be impractical and result in oversedation if not closely titrated according to frequent assessment of level of sedation. Intermittent administration allows reassessment before each dose.	IV: Limited clinical studies to support recommendations	See Annotated Bibliography: 4, 9, 12	
	• Continuous infusion of intermediate-acting sedatives such as lorazepam may be required when frequent intermittent doses are required to maintain goals of sedation	Lower dosage requirements and greater consistency in sedation level may be achieved. Concerns about missed doses would be eliminated. Drug tolerance may become an issue where increased doses are required to achieve the same clinical effect.			
	Concomitant neuromuscular blockade: Sedatives and analgesics should be administered by continuous infusion in paralyzed patients.	Caregiver assessment of patient awareness or pain during paralysis is not possible to do reliably based on clinical assessment.	V: Clinical studies in more than 1or 2 different patient populations and situations to support recommendations	See Other References: 32, 42	
	Patient's fluid status: Intermittent infusion or continuous infusion of undiluted lorazepam, or via syringe pump is recommended for patients at risk for fluid overload.	Problems associated with continuous lorazepam infusion include drug crystallization, large fluid volumes required from poor solubility, drug adsorption (binding) to polyvinyl chloride infusion bags, and propylene glycol toxicity, characterized by lactic acidosis, acute tubular necrosis, and hyperosmolar states.	IV: Limited clinical studies to support recommendations	See Annotated Bibliography: 4 See Other References: 2, 3, 5, 10, 31, 46, 49	Osmol gap correlates with propylene glycol concentration and can be used as a marker to identify toxicity. Hemodialysis may be required for propylene glycol removal and correction of osmolar gap.
Ongoing monitoring	Identify goal(s) for sedative/analgesic therapy (eg, obliterate respiratory effort, prevent symptoms of alcohol withdrawal).	Monitoring the level of sedation alone is meaningless without a predetermined, patient-specific end point. Multidisciplinary awareness of patient goals improves efficiency and enhances the quality of care.	IV: Limited clinical studies to support recommendations	See Annotated Bibliography: 4, 6 See Other References: 45	
	Assess and document the patient's baseline mental and neurologic status.	Identifying the patient's return to baseline mental status is facilitated if it is clearly defined before initiating therapy.			

Period of Use	Recommendation	Rationale for Recommendation	Level of Recommendation	Supporting References	Comments
Ongoing monitoring *(cont.)*	Assess the patient's level of sedation, agitation, pain, and delirium (SAPD) using a validated scoring systems in accordance with goals for therapy.	Drug therapy can be individualized and adjusted on the basis of desired patient outcomes. Detailed descriptions of patient behaviors related to scores promote consistency among caregivers.	IV: Limited clinical studies to support recommendations	See Annotated Bibliography: 4 See Other References: 15, 16, 19, 27, 33, 38, 45	See Appendix 6B.
	Document SAPD levels as often as vital signs are measured.	Complications associated with over- or undersedation may have a significant impact on patient morbidity and use of healthcare resources. Prevention demands frequent assessment to document patient-specific trends.	IV: Limited clinical studies to support recommendations	See Annotated Bibliography: 4	
	Maintain the lowest possible dose to achieve the stated goal of therapy.	Dosage adjustment directed at a defined outcome should minimize complications attributed to over- or undersedation. Periodic dosage reduction allows for continual assessment of need and mental status evaluation.	II: Theory based, no research data to support recommendations; recommendations from expert consensus group	See Annotated Bibliography: 4, 5, 6 Other References: 2, 3, 49	If propofol is selected as the primary sedative, adjustments in nutritional lipid administration must be considered.
		Prolonged (> 2–3 weeks), high-dose lorazepam infusions (> 18 mg/hr) may be associated with development of hyperosmolar state, lactic acidosis, and renal dysfunction. If signs and symptoms develop, lorazepam should be tapered and replaced with other benzodiazepines, propofol, and/or opioid analgesics.		Other References: 13, 41	
		Prolonged (> 48 hr), high-dose propofol infusion (> 66 µg/kg/min) may produce cardiac arrhythmia, rhabdomyolysis, and metabolic acidosis.			
Prevention of complications	Avoid abrupt discontinuation of sedatives and analgesics, particularly in patients with a history of anxiety.	Gradual tapering is especially recommended for patients receiving large doses or for prolonged periods (> 7 days) to prevent the development of withdrawal symptoms. For example, taper by 10%-20%/day, and if withdrawal symptoms develop, then increase dose to relieve symptoms. Reinstitute taper at a slower rate or	VI: Clinical studies in a variety of patient populations and situations to support recommendations	See Annotated Bibliography: 4 See Other References: 20, 21	

Period of Use	Recommendation	Rationale for Recommendation	Level of Recommendation	Supporting References	Comments
Prevention of complications (*cont.*)		add oral agents. If intermittent therapy is used, consider switching to a longer-acting agent.			
	Avoid rapid bolus doses of propofol, morphine, or dexmedetomidine in critically ill patients.	Hypotension may occur by peripheral vasodilation (arterial and venous) or decreases in ventricular preload/afterload. Cautious administration of these agents is recommended in patients who are elderly or hypovolemic or who demonstrate unstable hemodynamic parameters.	VI: Clinical studies in a variety of patient populations and situations to support recommendations	See Other References: 1, 14, 39, 45	Propofol must be avoided in patients with known sensitivity to eggs or egg components because of the presence of egg lecithin (extracted from egg yolk) in its vehicle. Most patients with egg allergy react to the egg white, so this phenomenon is rare (Other References: 12).
	Maintain adequate ventilatory support during sedative/analgesic administration. Monitor respiratory rate and oxygen saturation continuously, and adjust the ventilator settings as necessary.	Respiratory depression is a well-known adverse effect of virtually all sedatives and opioid analgesics and may be enhanced when agents are used in combination.	VI: Clinical studies in a variety of patient populations and situations to support recommendations	See Annotated Bibliography: 4	Modes and methods of ventilation may need to be adjusted to assure adequate minute ventilation. For example, patients on spontaneous breathing modes such as pressure support or continuous positive airway pressure may significantly decrease both rate and volume with sedative and analgesic administration. In these cases, a control mode of ventilation may be needed to assure adequate ventilation.
	Convert sedative and analgesic therapy to the oral route when enteral feedings are tolerated, hemodynamic parameters are stable, and sedative requirements are decreasing.	Oral administration eliminates issues surrounding IV access (eg, infection, drug compatibilities) and reduces drug costs.	V: Clinical studies in more than 1 or 2 different patient populations and situations to support recommendations	See Annotated Bibliography: 12	
	Develop detailed dosing guidelines and protocols for initiating, titrating and withdrawing commonly used sedative and analgesic agents. Implement drug holidays each day as the clinical situation permits.	Protocols and dosing guidelines decrease confusion for house staff unfamiliar with drugs used in critical care. They also promote consistency in patient management, which may result in improved outcomes, such as decreased mechanical ventilatory support and LOS.	V: Clinical studies in more than 1 or 2 different patient populations and situations to support recommendations	See Annotated Bibliography: 2, 4, 5, 6 See Other References: 18, 27	See Appendix 6A.

Period of Use	Recommendation	Rationale for Recommendation	Level of Recommendation	Supporting References	Comments
Prevention of complications *(cont.)*	Strict adherence to aseptic technique and administration guidelines is recommended when propofol is used. • Continuous infusion: Tubing and drug product must be replaced every 12 hours. • Intermittent injection: Prepare drug immediately prior to use and discard unused portion after 6 hours.	Outbreaks of postoperative infectious complications associated with propofol are attributed to a lack of product preservative, poor aseptic technique, and lack of compliance with manufacturer's recommendations for use.	VI: Clinical studies in a variety of patient populations and situations to support recommendations	See Other References: 51	Propofol (Diprivan, AstraZeneca) contains disodium edetate 0.005% to retard the rate of microbial growth in the event of accidental contamination. However, it remains a single-use, preservative-free product. Other products (Baxter, Gesnia Sicor) contain sulfite preservatives, which may be associated with allergic reactions in sensitive patients, particularly those with asthma.

CLINICAL RECOMMENDATIONS

Neuromuscular Blockade

The rating scales for the Level of Recommendation range from I to IV, with levels indicated as follows: I, manufactuer's recommendations only; II, theory based, no research data to support recommendations; recommendations from expert consensus group may exist; III, laboratory data only, no clinical data to support recommendations; IV, limited clinical studies to support recommendations; V, clinical studies in more than 1 or 2 different populations and situations to support recommendations; VI, clinical studies in a variety of patient populations and situations to support recommendations.

Period of Use	Recommendation	Rationale for Recommendation	Level of Recommendation	Supporting References	Comments
Selection of patients	Neuromuscular blockade is indicated for the following situations when sedation, analgesia, and other modalities have been maximized without achieving the desired goal:				
	• Patients who require obliteration of respiratory effort	Elimination of asynchronous breathing patterns may facilitate ventilation and oxygenation and hemodynamic stability. Also, compliance with complex ventilator modes (eg, PC-IRV or those resulting in permissive hypercapnia) may be improved and the risk of barotraumas/volutrauma and hemodynamic instability potentially reduced.	VI: Clinical studies in a variety of patient populations and situations to support recommendations	See Annotated Bibliography: 6, 7 See Other References: 39, 42, 45, 47	
	• Patients exhibiting severe agitation or combativeness uncontrolled by any other modality and interfering with the provision of mechanical ventilation	Uncontrolled movements may interfere with the provision of care and increase the risk for complications from self-inflicted harm or medical device removal. They also risk injury to caregivers from combative behavior.			
	• Patients with persistent, severe hypoxemia (eg, ARDS, status asthmaticus) uncontrolled by other modalities	Paralysis decreases work of breathing and reduces oxygen consumption in patients with acute respiratory failure and sepsis. It may also facilitate oxygenation/ventilation and hemodynamic stability by reducing the respiratory workload. In patients with high minute ventilation requirements, the potential for barotrauma and volutrauma secondary to auto-PEEP and high plateau and peak airway pressures is high. NMB in these cases may be life saving.			Refer to Chapter 2, Invasive and Non-invasive Modes and Methods of Mechanical Ventilation for more on this.

Period of Use	Recommendation	Rationale for Recommendation	Level of Recommendation	Supporting References	Comments
Initial use	Identify a clinical end point for NMB therapy.	Predetermination of goals for therapy guides dosage titration and enhances consistency of care among providers.		See Annotated Bibliography: 6, 7, 9 See Other References: 42, 52	
	Select NMB therapy on the basis of organ function, adverse effects, and cost considerations:				
	• Pancuronium is the NMB of first choice for patients with adequate renal function and stable hemodynamic parameters.	Pancuronium is primarily eliminated renally; prolonged paralysis has been reported with various degrees of renal impairment. Transient hypertension and tachycardia (that may be noted after bolus doses due to cardiac vagolytic effects and also possible histamine release) are clinically insignificant in most patients. Pancuronium is the least costly agent.	V: Clinical studies in more than 1 or 2 different patient populations and situations to support recommendations	See Annotated Bibliography: 6, 7	
	• Atracurium or cisatracurium are recommended in patients with renal or hepatic failure.	These agents are cleared by organ-independent Hofmann elimination and ester hydrolysis and do not accumulate in the presence of organ dysfunction.	V: Clinical studies in more than 1 or 2 different patient populations and situations to support recommendations	See Annotated Bibliography: 6, 7	
Ongoing monitoring	Clinical monitoring by direct observation of diaphragmatic or body movement is recommended.	Prolonged recovery of muscle activity may signal the need for downward dosage adjustment.	II: Theory based, no research data to support recommendations; recommendations from expert consensus group may exist	See Annotated Bibliography: 7	
	Using the train-of-four (TOF) method of peripheral nerve stimulation (PNS), determine and record the supramaximal stimulus before administration of NMB agents (the current beyond which no further tactile response can be elicited).	Baseline evaluation of the neuromuscular junction identifies the level of stimulation required for therapeutic paralysis. Omission of this step may result in underestimation of depth of blockade as all nerve fibers may not be stimulated.	V: Clinical studies in more than 1 or 2 different patient populations and situations to support recommendations	See Annotated Bibliography: 6, 7 See Other References: 37	Sedate prior to assessment. Supramaximal stimulation is controversial because of the difficulty in discerning maximal response.
	Using PNS, determine the depth of blockade (the number of twitches observed) required to achieve the goal of NMB therapy.	Patients' responses vary according to concomitant disease states and other drugs received. Outcome-directed NMB titration may reduce dosage requirements, drug accumulation, and prolonged paralysis. Patient responses also depend on factors such as	V: Clinical studies in more than 1 or 2 different patient populations and situations to support recommendations	See Annotated Bibliography: 6, 10, 13	

Period of Use	Recommendation	Rationale for Recommendation	Level of Recommendation	Supporting References	Comments
Ongoing monitoring *(cont.)*		anasarca, fluid and electrolyte balance, concurrent drug therapy, as well as technical issues with device (eg, electrical conductivity).			
	TOF assessment should be performed at least every 2 to 3 hours until the goal of therapy is achieved. Once the patient is stable, TOF may be performed every 8 hours. In a rapidly changing clinical situation, TOF assessment should be completed prior to each NMB dose or every 2 to 3 hours.	Frequent assessment during NMB initiation or periods of instability is critical in defining patient requirements. Patient-specific dosage adjustment may improve outcome.	IV: Limited clinical studies to support recommendations	See Annotated Bibliography: 7	Patients with anasarca may not have an adequate TOF response yet have diaphragmatic movement. In these patients TOF is not an adequate measure of neuromuscular blockade. Consider using airway pressure monitoring (refer to "Respiratory Waveforms Monitoring" in *AACN Protocols for Practice: Noninvasive Monitoring*) combined with daily discontinuance of the drug to prevent drug oversaturation.
	The ulnar nerve is the preferred site for PNS monitoring. Monitor response using tactile versus visual observation.	Facial nerve monitoring may be disturbing to family members. It is more likely to give false positive responses due to artifact, which may promote unnecessary increases in NMB dosage.	V: Clinical studies in more than 1 or 2 different patient populations and situations to support recommendations	See Annotated Bibliography: 10	If the ulnar nerve is not available due to edema or trauma, the facial, peroneal, or posterior tibial nerves may be used.
	The use of continuous airway pressure monitoring may be helpful to assess adequacy of NMB. It is a noninvasive, real-time measure of respiratory effort.	Refer to "Respiratory Waveforms Monitoring" in *AACN Protocols for Practice: Noninvasive Monitoring* for more on the application and interpretation of the technique with NMB.			
Prevention of complications	Ensure the provision of adequate sedation and analgesia by continuous infusion methods.	NMBs do not possess analgesic, sedative, anxiolytic, or amnesic properties. Appropriate sedative and analgesic therapies may reduce NMB requirements.	V: Clinical studies in more than 1 or 2 different patient populations or situations to support recommendations	See Annotated Bibliography: 6, 7 See Other References: 32, 39	
	Document proper functioning of ventilator alarms; provide manual ventilator bag at bedside at all times.	Paralysis caused by NMB therapy prevents patients from signaling accidental ventilator disconnections.	II: Theory based, no research data to support recommendations; recommendations from expert consensus group may exist	See Annotated Bibliography: 10 See Other References: 51	

Period of Use	Recommendation	Rationale for Recommendation	Level of Recommendation	Supporting References	Comments
Prevention of complications *(cont.)*	Schedule an NMB-free period daily as clinically appropriate.	Periodic recovery from paralysis allows assessment of neurologic and mental status, sedation adequacy, and continued need for NMB therapy.	II: Theory based, no research data to support recommendations; recommendations from expert consensus group may exist	See Annotated Bibliography: 7	
	Consider discontinuation of NMB therapy if a 0 in 4 twitch response is observed with TOF; reduce dose by 20% and restart once a 1 in 4 response is achieved.	Complete NMB is not indicated in any patient situation and may be associated with prolonged effect. TOF monitoring should be combined with clinical assessment.	II: Theory based, no research data to support recommendations; recommendations from expert consensus group may exist	See Annotated Bibliography: 10	
	In patients receiving corticosteroid therapy, discontinue NMB therapy as soon as possible.	Prolonged muscle weakness may occur after any NMB but may be enhanced when steroids are administered concomitantly. Steroid myopathy may be compounded by the use of NMBs.	VI: Clinical studies in a variety of patient populations and situations to support recommendations	See Annotated Bibliography: 1, 7 See Other References: 22, 30	
	Communicate frequently with patients while providing care.	Regardless of the lack of apparent wakefulness, explanations for procedures and regular reorientation to time and place may reduce patient anxiety and discomfort during periods of prolonged paralysis.	II: Theory based, no research data to support recommendations; recommendations from expert consensus group may exist	See Annotated Bibliography: 7	
	Initiate therapy to reduce the complications of immobility.	Range-of-motion exercises and frequent repositioning may prevent patient developing muscle atrophy, skin breakdown, nerve compression syndromes, atelectasis, and pneumonia.	V: Clinical studies in more than 1 or 2 different patient populations and situations to support recommendations	See Annotated Bibliography: 7, 11 See Other References: 52	Heavy bandages on the eye may cause pressure damage and should be avoided.
	Initiate scheduled use of ophthalmic lubricant; close lids and secure lightly as necessary.	Loss of blink reflex decreases secretion distribution and may promote corneal ulceration.	V: Clinical studies in more than 1 or 2 different patient populations and situations to support recommendations	See Annotated Bibliography:7 See Other References: 52	

ANNOTATED BIBLIOGRAPHY

1. **Behbehani NA, Al-Mane F, D'yachkova Y, et al. Myopathy following mechanical ventilation for acute severe asthma. Chest. 1999;115: 1627–1631.**

Study Sample

The sample included patients with severe acute asthma requiring hospital admission and mechanical ventilation at two institutions between 1985 and 1995.

Comparison Studied

The objective of this retrospective cohort study was to determine the incidence of acute myopathy and identify factors associated with its development.

Study Procedures

All eligible patients were evaluated by thorough chart review to determine the incidence of significant muscle weakness as defined by the presence of the following: (1) a strength rating less than 4 on a 0–5 scale in 1 or more major muscle groups, (2) inability to perform activities of daily living, or (3) the need for physical rehabilitation prior to hospital discharge. Other causes of muscle weakness associated with critical illness were documented, including sepsis, liver or renal failure, and administration of vancomycin or aminoglycoside antibiotics.

Key Results

Among 86 eligible patients, 30 received NMB treatment (pancuronium, vecuronium, or atracurium alone or in combination) for a mean duration of 3.1 ($\pm$ 2.3) days. Nine (30%) of these patients developed significant muscle weakness; 6 of these 9 patients demonstrated the presence of all 3 criteria for muscle weakness. All patients received intravenous corticosteroids; no difference was observed between patients with and without muscle weakness in terms of daily methylprednisolone-equivalent doses. No other causes for muscle weakness were documented. Patients who had muscle weakness and received NMB required a longer duration of mechanical ventilatory support (12.4 $\pm$ 7.1 vs 2.4 $\pm$ 3.0; $P < .001$) and had a longer length of hospital stay (32 $\pm$ 10 vs 9.2 $\pm$ 7.2 days; $P < .001$) Multiple logistic regression analysis showed that the duration of NMB treatment was the only independent predictor for the development of muscle weakness; each day of NMB-induced paralysis was associated with a 2.1 increase in the odds ratio (95% CI, 1.4–3.2).

Strengths and Weaknesses

Limitations include the retrospective nature of the study and the fact that only clinical assessment was used to determine the depth of neuromuscular blockade. Peripheral nerve stimulation (PNS) was not routinely used.

Clinical Implications

Close monitoring of NMB therapy in critically ill patients is necessary to reduce the incidence of muscle weakness. The routine use of a monitoring tool, such as peripheral nerve stimulation, may be useful in reducing the duration of NMB and allowing faster recovery of neuromuscular function. In addition, the use of intermittent bolus dosing may facilitate monitoring by allowing partial recovery of muscle function and ease assessment of the need for further NMB therapy.

2. **Brook AD, Ahrens TS, Schaiff R, et al. Effect of a nursing-implemented sedation protocol on the duration of mechanical ventilation. Crit Care Med. 1999;27:2609–2615.**

Study Sample

Eligible patients were adults in a medical intensive care unit (MICU) at a university-affiliated teaching hospital who required mechanical ventilation.

Comparison Studied

The objective of this study was to compare the effects on the duration of mechanical ventilation of a nurse-driven sedation protocol versus a traditional nonprotocol method of administering sedation.

Study Procedure

Patients were randomized at the time mechanical ventilation was initiated to receive sedation by nurse-driven protocol or traditional physician direction. The protocol indicated that nurses would initiate sedatives and analgesics to achieve a Ramsay score of 3 and alleviate pain, respectively, with scheduled reassessments occurring every 4 hours. The traditional method required a physician order to initiate or change any sedative or analgesic therapy, although nurses could communicate patient assessments and perceived needs to the responsible physician.

Key Results

Data from 321 patients were analyzed; 162 received protocol-driven sedation, and 159 received sedation using the conventional physician-driven method. Patient groups were similar with regard to age, APACHE II score, indication for mechanical ventilation, and underlying disease. Lorazepam and fentanyl were the primary choices for sedation and analgesia, respectively. The mean duration of mechanical ventilation was significantly shorter for patients receiving sedation by the nurse-directed protocol than for those undergoing conventional care (89.1 $\pm$ 133.6 hours vs 124.0 $\pm$ 153.6 hours; $P = .003$). Similarly, the duration of sedative infusion as well as ICU and overall hospital stay were significantly shorter in patients who received protocol-driven sedation. No differences were observed between groups regarding rates of mortality, end-organ dysfunction, or reintubation. However, the need for tracheostomy was lower in patients receiving protocol-driven versus non-protocol-driven sedation (6.2% vs 13.2%; $P = .038$). Moreover, as determined by regression analysis, the likelihood of successful weaning was significantly improved if the nurse-driven sedation protocol was used (RR 1.37; 95% CI, 1.19–1.58; $P = .026$).

Study Strengths and Weaknesses

This study provides a rational approach to the complex issue of sedation management in critically ill patients requiring mechanical ventilation and further supports the need for goal-driven therapy. This was an nonblinded study design, which may have biased physician practice. Other pertinent outcomes, such as the incidence of unplanned extubations and nosocomial pneumonia, were not addressed. Nursing compliance with the sedation protocol was also not determined.

Clinical Implications

Protocol-directed sedation may improve patient outcomes and reduce ICU costs related to complications associated with prolonged sedation and increased length of stay.

3. Ely EW, Shintani A, Truman B, et al. Delirium as a predictor of mortality in mechanically ventilated patients in the intensive care unit. *JAMA*. 2004; 291:1753–1762.

Study Sample

The sample comprised mechanically ventilated adults admitted to the medical or coronary ICU between February 2000 and May 2001.

Comparison Studied

The objective of this study was to test the hypothesis that the development of delirium in mechanically ventilated patients in the ICU is an independent predictor of 6-month mortality and hospital length of stay. Secondary outcome variables include the number of ventilator-free days and cognitive impairment at the time of discharge.

Study Procedure

Assessments of level of arousal and delirium were performed daily using the Richmond Agitation-Sedation Scale (RASS) and the Confusion Assessment Method for the ICU, respectively. Delirium was defined by a response to verbal stimulation with eye opening (RASS –3 to +4) and a positive Confusion Assessment Method for the ICU, defined by fluctuations in RASS plus the presence of inattention and either disorganized thinking or an altered level of consciousness.

Key Results

Two hundred twenty-four patients were followed for 2158 ICU days. Of these, 183 (81%) developed delirium. There were no differences between patients who developed delirium and those who did not with regard to demographics, underlying comorbidities, severity of critical illness, or admission diagnoses. Six-month mortality was significantly higher in patients who developed delirium during their ICU stay (34% vs 15%; $P = .03$). Delirious patients spent 10 more days in the hospital than nondelirious patients ($P < .001$) Multivariate analysis (adjusting for age, severity of illness, comorbidities, coma, sedative and analgesic drug use) demonstrates that delirium is independently associated with higher 6-month mortality (HR 3.2; 95% CI, 1.4–7.7; $P = .008$) and a longer hospital stay (HR 2.0; 95% CI, 1.4–3.0; $P = .001$). Similarly, delirious patients experienced significantly fewer ventilator free days and a greater risk for cognitive impairment at the time of discharge.

Clinical Implications

These outcomes data emphasize the importance of the development of protocols for routine monitoring of delirium in ICU patients. Additional studies evaluating the impact of interventions on the incidence and outcomes of delirium will be useful in promoting the importance of monitoring delirium in the ICU.

4. Jacobi J, Fraser GL, Corsin DB, et al. Clinical practice guidelines for the sustained use of sedatives and analgesics in the critically ill adult. *Crit Care Med*. 2002;30:119–141.

Description

In 1995, clinical practice guidelines were developed by a multidisciplinary task force of experts to assist critical care clinicians in the selection and appropriate use of sedatives and analgesics in the critically ill patient. Evidence-based recommendations were few at that time, due to the paucity of randomized, controlled trials, but at least provided a much-needed tool for critical care practitioners. Since that time, numerous clinical studies have evaluated new agents, methods for implementing and monitoring sedative and analgesic therapies, and validity of specific end points to improve patient outcomes. As a result, these guidelines, again supported by the Society of Critical Care Medicine, American College of Critical Care Medicine, and the American Society of Health Systems Pharmacists, have been updated. In addition to the greater availability of published science, major changes in this update include an emphasis on specific goals for sedative and analgesic therapy, monitoring, and daily discontinuation or dose adjustment to achieve specific, predefined goals. This is reflected in the substantial increase in number of recommendations, from 6 in the 1995 guidelines, to 28 in the current version. While the suggested agents have changed little, more specific, practical guidelines have been developed to facilitate safe and effective care of this complex population.

Clinical Implications

These practice guidelines encourage appropriate drug selection in critically ill patients requiring sedation and analgesic therapy; doing so will reduce the risk of drug-related adverse events and promote reductions in the use of health-care resources.

5. **Kress JP, Pohlman AS, O'Connor MF, Hall JB. Daily interruption of sedative infusions in critically ill patients undergoing mechanical ventilation.** *N Eng J Med.* **2000;342:1471–1477.**

Study Sample

Patients eligible for study included those in the MICU who required mechanical ventilatory support and continuous intravenous sedation for the management of agitation or anxiety.

Comparison Studied

The objective of this study was to determine if daily interruption of continuous intravenous sedation would reduce the duration of mechanical ventilation and ICU stay.

Study Procedure

Patients were randomized to an intervention group, in which sedation was interrupted daily, beginning 48 hours after initiation or to a control group, in which interruption of sedatives occurred only at the discretion of the ICU team. Within each group, patients were further randomized to receive midazolam or propofol, in an open-label fashion, as specified to achieve a Ramsey sedation scale score of 3 or 4. All patients received concomitant morphine infusions for analgesia. In the intervention group, a research nurse evaluated patients during the period of sedative and analgesic discontinuation, and immediately notified a study physician at the time of awakening to facilitate patient examination and determine if the sedation infusion should be resumed. When patients were also receiving a paralytic agent, the paralytic was discontinued prior to interrupting the sedation and analgesic infusions. The primary end points of the study were duration of mechanical ventilation, length of ICU stay, and length of hospital stay. Total doses of midazolam, propofol, and morphine were recorded. Additional end points included the percentage of days "awake," frequency of neurologic testing (computed tomography, magnetic resonance imaging, lumbar puncture), and adverse events.

Key Results

Data from 128 patients were available for analysis; 68 patients were randomized to the intervention group, and 60 were randomized to the control group. Groups were similar in demographics, diagnosis, severity of illness, and sedative distribution. Daily interruption was associated with a significant decrease in the duration of mechanical ventilation (median 4.9 days vs 7.3 days in the control group, *P* = .004)

and ICU stay (6.4 days vs 9.9 days; *P* = .02). Length of overall hospital stay was similar between intervention and control groups. Total doses of administered midazolam and morphine, but not propofol, were significantly lower in the intervention vs control group. Patients in the intervention group were considered to be awake a greater percentage of their ICU stay as compared to the control group (85.5% vs 9%; *P* < .001), and fewer patients required neurologic tests to assess their mental status (9% vs 27%; *P* = .02). No differences between groups were observed in the rates of self-extubation, reintubation, tracheostomy, or in-hospital mortality.

Study Strengths and Weaknesses

These findings further support the need for developing protocols for administering, titrating, and monitoring sedative therapy to improve patient outcomes and reduce ICU costs of care. A potential weakness of the study is the target Ramsay scale score chosen; one could argue that a score of 2 or 3 might have been more appropriate, allowing for a reduced risk of oversedation in the control group. In addition, the effects of daily sedative interruption on patient distress, cardiovascular parameters, or the risk for acute withdrawal during discontinuation were not discussed.

Clinical Implications

Daily interruption of sedative infusions in ICU patients may prevent complications associated with prolonged or excessive sedation and reduce costs associated with drug administration, mechanical ventilation, neurologic evaluations, and length of ICU stay.

6. **Mascia MF, Koch M, Medicis JJ. Pharmaco-economic impact of rational use guidelines on the provision of analgesia, sedation, and neuromuscular blockade in critical care.** *Crit Care Med.* **2000;28:2300–2306.**

Study Sample

Patients eligible for study were admitted to medical and surgical ICUs and required mechanical ventilation, sedatives, analgesics, and/or neuromuscular blockers during their ICU stay.

Comparison Studied

The safety and cost-effectiveness of the use of guidelines for the administration of analgesics, sedation, and neuromuscular blockers were compared with standard methods in this prospective analysis.

Study Procedure

During a 6-month baseline period (phase 1), demographic, disease severity, treatment, outcomes, and cost data were collected for 72 patients receiving scheduled intravenous doses or continuous infusions of sedative, analgesic, or NMB drugs. Simultaneously, guidelines were developed to assist drug selection, dose adjustment, determining therapeutic end points, and weaning therapies, including algorithms to facilitate decision making. In phase 2, these guidelines were instituted and enforced with educational interventions. Follow-up data were then collected in a second group of patients (n = 84), and compared with those of the baseline group.

Key Results

Patients followed in phase1 and phase 2 were similar in age gender, days of treatment and number of regimens. However, patients in the follow-up group had significantly higher APACHE II scores than patients in the baseline group. Time on the ventilator and length of stay were both shorter in phase 2 patients but mortality was not increased significantly. Maximum cost per day was decreased in phase 2 for benzodiazepines, opioid analgesics, propofol (> 24 hrs), and NMB. The largest cost reduction was associated with reduced NMB use from baseline to follow-up phases (30% vs 5%; $P < .001$). Functional status improved from baseline to follow-up, as determined by a decrease in the need for rehabilitation services following ICU discharge.

Clinical Implications

This study further supports the need for the development of goal-directed guidelines for patient, sedative, and NMB selection and monitoring to improve outcomes and reduce costs in the ICU. Specific attention to NMB use is critical in preventing associated myopathy, ventilator time, and length of stay.

7. Murray MJ, Cowen J, DeBlock H, et al. Clinical practice guidelines for sustained neuromuscular blockade in the adult critically ill patient. *Crit Care Med.* 2002;30:142–156.

Description

The use of NMB agents remains an important component of care in critically ill patients for the management of mechanical ventilatory support unresponsive to all other interventions. These clinical practice guidelines update our pharmacologic knowledge about available NMB agents as well as summarize the published literature regarding their safety and efficacy in the critically ill patient. These guidelines focus on agent selection, therapeutic end points, and methods of monitoring to achieve desired outcomes and avoid prolonged paralysis and associated complications. Similar to the guidelines for sedation and analgesia, the number of recommendations has increased significantly. The emphasis on adequate sedation and analgesia before initiating NMB therapy and the importance of daily discontinuance for patient reassessment and avoidance of drug accumulation remain integral to routine care. Assessment of neuromuscular blockade by both clinical and train-of-four monitoring is recommended, with specific goals identified as end points of therapy. The development of acute quadriplegic myopathy syndrome remains a devastating complication that may be associated with prolonged infusions

and concomitant corticosteroids, and can occur with any NMB agent.

Clinical Implications

The incidence of prolonged paralysis and its associated complications may be reduced by implementing these guidelines for practice, which promote appropriate drug selection and monitoring techniques.

8. Pohlman AS, Simpson KP, Hall JB. Continuous intravenous infusions of lorazepam versus midazolam for sedation during mechanical ventilatory support: a prospective, randomized study. *Crit Care Med.* 1994;22:1241–1247.

Study Sample

The study population consisted of 20 critically ill adult patients receiving mechanical ventilation and pharmacologic intervention for acute agitation in a MICU.

Comparison Studied

The time required to achieve adequate sedation and the dosages and number of infusion manipulations necessary to maintain adequate sedation levels were compared in patients receiving midazolam or lorazepam by continuous IV infusion. Time to recovery of baseline mental status and fluid volume administered were also measured.

Study Procedures

After a physical examination and baseline assessment of sedation and anxiety level, patients were randomized to receive either midazolam (n = 10) or lorazepam (n = 10) using an initial IV bolus, followed by a continuous IV infusion. Additional bolus doses and infusion titration was allowed to achieve a Ramsay Scale score of 2 to 3 (see Other References: 59). One hour after adequate sedation was achieved, and daily thereafter, dosages were titrated downward until the lowest dosage rate producing the goal level of sedation was reached. The use of opioid analgesics, psychotropics, and NMBs was allowed. Recovery of baseline mental status was determined using the initial assessment, degree of patient responsiveness, and ability to communicate needs.

Key Results

Although not statistically significant, patients receiving lorazepam required a longer time (124 ± 168 min) to initially achieve the goal level of sedation compared to patients receiving midazolam (105 ± 101 min). However, the number of infusion rate manipulations per day were lower in patients receiving lorazepam (1.9 ± 1.7 vs 3.6 ± 2.4). Time to recover baseline mental status was considerably, though not statistically, shorter in the lorazepam group than the midazolam group (261 ± 189 vs 1815 ± 2322 min). In both groups, daily fluid volumes greater than 1 L were necessary to deliver the maximal dosages. The ratio of lorazepam to midazolam infusion rates over the entire study period was 1:4.

Study Strengths and Weaknesses

Six of 20 patients studied received concomitant NMBs, making it impossible to assess sedation level using the Ramsay Scale. In addition, stability issues associated with lorazepam that were identified after publication (crystallization, adsorption to polyvinyl chloride infusion bags) may have contributed to difficulties in drug delivery and achievement of goal sedation levels. Finally, the small number of patients evaluated was likely not adequate to achieve statistical significance, if it did indeed exist.

Clinical Implications

Administration of lorazepam for sedation of critically ill patients requiring mechanical ventilation may be advantageous, given the reduced nursing time required to maintain adequate levels of sedation and a potentially quicker return to baseline mental status. The authors suggest reevaluation of routine administration of benzodiazepines by continuous infusion, given the difficulties encountered in rapidly achieving optimal sedation as well as the occasionally prolonged return to baseline mental status and the large volumes of fluid required.

9. Rhoney DH, Murry KR. National survey of the use of sedating drugs, neuromuscular blocking agents, and reversal agents in the intensive care unit. *J Intensive Care Med.* 2003;18:139–145.

Description

A survey was developed to characterize sedative, NMB, and reversal agent use in adults receiving care in intensive care units in the United States, assess adherence to Society of Critical Care Medicine (SCCM) guidelines, determine the use of protocols and monitoring tools for drug administration, and identify factors influencing drug selection. A total of 1934 questionnaires were mailed to SCCM physicians practicing in 780 institutions in 1998.

Results

Response rates were 50% and 24% for institutions and clinicians, respectively. Most respondents were physicians practicing in university teaching or community hospitals, with level I trauma centers and moderate to large sized ICUs. Medical and surgical ICUs were predominantly represented. Morphine, lorazepam, midazolam, haloperidol, and propofol were used most commonly to relieve agitation, anxiety, and fear. Despite SCCM recommendations that midazolam be administered only in the short term (< 48–72 hours), many respondents (~53%) used this agent for longer periods. In fact, most respondents reported using all aforementioned sedatives for longer then 72 hours. Intermittent IV bolus was the most common method of administration for morphine, lorazepam, midazolam, and haloperidol, and for propofol and fentanyl, continuous infusion was the most common method of administration. Among NMB agents, pancuronium and vecuronium were most commonly administered by continuous infusion and intermittent bolus, respectively, to facilitate mechanical ventilation. Written protocols were utilized for sedative and NMB administration in 33% and 47% of respondents, respectively. Sedation monitoring was primarily accomplished using the Glasgow Coma Scale and modified Ramsay Score. PNS was used most often to monitor NMB.

Clinical Implications

Since this questionnaire was administered in 1998, additional sedation scales have been developed and tested, so it is probable that differences in sedation assessment currently exist. However, few new agents have been introduced since that time, so it is likely that usage patterns are similar. The current SCCM guidelines recommend that monitoring of NMB be comprised of PNS combined with clinical assessment, and given the serious consequences associated with prolonged recovery following NMB administration, further study regarding monitoring approaches and outcomes will be valuable to clinical practice.

10. Rudis MI, Guslits BG, Zarowitz BJ. Technical and interpretive problems of peripheral nerve stimulation in monitoring neuromuscular blockade in the intensive care unit. *Ann Pharmacother.* 1996;30:165–172.

Description

The authors used a MEDLINE search to identify studies published from 1985 through 1994 describing the use of PNS for monitoring NMB therapy in critically ill patients. They summarize problems that may be encountered when using the TOF method to assess the depth of NMB in the ICU.

Errors in interpretation of PNS responses may be related to the device, the patient, or the technique used. Problems related to the device include weak batteries, incomplete attachment or reversal of electrodes, and inconsistent amperage delivery. The authors recommend the use of digital devices for which errors sound an alarm, and suggest using the same device consistently to reduce differences in calibration. Patient-related factors may potentially affect neuromuscular function and the depth of blockade achieved. Sepsis and multiple system organ dysfunction may diminish neuromuscular function in the absence of NMB administration. Preexisting neurologic disease (eg, stroke, myasthenia gravis) complicate the evaluation of baseline neuromuscular status. The presence of anasarca or peripheral edema requires current to flow a longer distance, which may reduce its ability to stimulate the nerve. Decreases in body temperature have been shown to enhance the depth of vecuronium blockade, possibly by increasing plasma concentrations or the sensitivity of the neuromuscular junction. In addition, concurrent drug therapies may potentiate or antagonize NMB effects. Incorrect or inconsistent PNS techniques may also influence monitoring results. Improper positioning of electrode pads, changing sites of PNS monitoring, omission of baseline testing, and failure to discern contraction of the stimulated muscle are common reasons for inconsistent results.

The authors suggest TOF monitoring using tactile quantification of the adductor pollicis muscle response as the most reliable method. They also recommend supramaximal stimulation before initiating NMB therapy to determine the level of current to use during paralysis. Further recommendations to minimize these problems are described. This article is highly recommended reading for clinicians involved in PNS monitoring.

Clinical Implications

There are currently few controlled clinical trials to support the use of PNS monitoring for NMB dosage titration or to decrease the incidence of prolonged effect (see Annotated Bibliography: 12). Given the widespread recognition of NMB-induced prolonged paralysis, many clinicians feel compelled to use PNS as the only real monitoring tool available. The problems described in this article affect the reliability of PNS devices as accurate measures of NMB. Clinical end points associated with NMB therapy must be defined and used in conjunction with PNS monitoring to achieve the optimal dose for each patient. Opponents of PNS use airway pressure waveform monitoring or end-tidal CO_2 ($ETCO_2$) monitoring to identify patient-initiated respiratory effort and ventilator asynchrony. Administration of NMB not associated with a positive response related to the clinical end point should be discontinued. Nurses must be exposed to these monitoring techniques and apply them to current practice as appropriate.

11. Watling SM, Dasta JF. Prolonged paralysis in intensive care unit patients after the use of neuromuscular blocking agents: a review of the literature. *Crit Care Med.* 1994;22: 884–893.

Description

The authors reviewed reports published from 1980 to 1993 regarding continuous infusions of vecuronium or atracurium and prolonged NMB in the ICU in order to define possible mechanisms for prolonged blockade and to suggest methods to reduce its occurrence.

The mechanisms for prolonged paralysis may be classified into two types: (1) pharmacokinetically based, attributing prolonged effects to reduced drug clearance, or (2) the result of a defect at the neuromuscular junction. Type 1 has been reported in patients with impaired renal or hepatic function who received pancuronium, vecuronium, or atracurium intermittently or by continuous infusion. Several of these studies did not use PNS to monitor NMB therapy, and the use of dosing guidelines or protocols is unclear. Type 2 has been reported in patients with normal end-organ function receiving pancuronium, vecuronium, or atracurium by either intermittent or continuous infusion. Many patients received NMB therapy at high doses, for prolonged durations, and without PNS monitoring. Concomitant use of corticos-

teroids, aminoglycoside antibiotics, and anesthetics in some patients may have contributed to a prolonged NMB effect. Further complicating the diagnosis of prolonged NMB is a syndrome of "critical illness polyneuropathy," characterized by failure to wean from mechanical ventilation, extremity weakness, and impaired deep tendon reflexes, but normal sensory function. This syndrome has occurred in patients not receiving NMBs who are recovering from multisystem organ failure or sepsis.

Methods are needed to decrease the risk of prolonged paralysis in critically ill patients. Guidelines for patient selection may reduce NMB use by offering alternative therapies for relieving anxiety and enhancing compliance with ventilator support. In addition, monitoring practices must be instituted to prevent NMB overdosage and accumulation. The authors suggest train-of-four PNS before and during NMB administration, periodic discontinuation of NMB to allow recovery of neuromuscular transmission, and consideration of intermittent administration rather than continuous infusion.

Clinical Implications

Prolonged paralysis in critically ill patients receiving NMB therapy is a serious complication that requires extended ventilator support, increasing length of stay, and excess healthcare dollars. Critical care practitioners must therefore carefully weigh the risks and benefits of instituting NMB therapy. Knowledge of NMB pharmacokinetics, concomitant drug therapies, and underlying disease states must also be used to ensure appropriate drug selection and avoid complications associated with prolonged effect. Other factors that may influence neuromuscular recovery include duration of therapy and use of neuromuscular monitoring devices. Guidelines for monitoring NMB therapy should include identification of drugs or disease states affecting NMB pharmacokinetic or pharmacodynamic properties, dosage titration based on PNS, periodic NMB discontinuation, and early institution of physical and nutritional therapies.

12. Watling SM, Johnson M, Yanos J. A method to produce sedation in critically ill patients. *Ann Pharmacother.* 1996;30:1227–1231.

Study Sample

This study sample consisted of 17 consecutive patients in a MICU diagnosed with acute respiratory failure and requiring complete respiratory rate control to facilitate mechanical ventilation.

Comparison Studied

This study evaluated the efficacy of a sedation protocol using a benzodiazepine-opioid combination to suppress respiratory drive and avoid the administration of NMB agents. Other goals of the protocol were to promote safe, effective, low-cost agents that are easily titratable by nursing and medical staffs and to avoid drugs with adverse cardiovascular effects, such as propofol and barbiturates.

Study Procedures

Patients not controlled by intermittent IV doses of lorazepam received the drug by continuous IV infusion using undiluted product administered by a patient-controlled analgesia pump. Morphine was added for synergistic respiratory depressant effects if the lorazepam infusion rate exceeded 10 mg/h or pain was anticipated. Pancuronium was administered in single bolus doses to achieve rapid control of respiratory rate. Additional sedative boluses were given when the patient triggered the ventilator or an NMB dose was administered. If respiratory control could not be achieved using large doses of both lorazepam and morphine, pentobarbital was added or substituted until the situation resolved and the combination could be resumed. Once the patient's respiratory status remained stable for 24 hours, downward titration of sedative infusions was initiated. If the expectation for sedation exceeded 5 days, the lorazepam infusion was switched to diazepam to take advantage of its lower cost and longer half-life. Lorazepam was reinstituted when the anticipated duration of sedation became less than 5 days. As patients recovered and demonstrated an ability to tolerate enteral feedings, they received both sedatives by continuous infusion through a feeding tube. Infusions were slowly tapered over 7–10 days, often with oral agents, based on the specific medical condition and indication for ventilator weaning.

Key Results

Seventeen patients required MICU care and sedation for an average of 18 days (ranges 2 to 56 and 2 to 50, respectively). Seven patients required inverse ratio mechanical ventilation to manage their respiratory failure. Twelve patients demonstrated hemodynamic instability (systolic blood pressure < 90 mm Hg), 7 had renal dysfunction (serum creatinine > 176.8 μmol/L), 9 had hepatic dysfunction (serum bilirubin > 34.2 μmol/L), and 13 were septic. Ten patients required lorazepam in dosages exceeding 30 mg/h. Ten received diazepam as the primary benzodiazepine. One patient required additional pentobarbital, and 3 patients received haloperidol for psychotic symptoms. Eight patients received feedings and sedation enterally. Fourteen patients received at least one NMB dose. NMBs were administered on 66 of 306 total days (21.6%) of sedation, with an average of 22.1 mg (pancuronium or vecuronium) administered per day. Combination therapy was well tolerated; adverse hemodynamic effects or prolonged sedation were not noted. The authors reported no delays in weaning from mechanical ventilation.

Study Strengths and Weaknesses

This study uses a goal-oriented sedation protocol in a specific population—patients with acute respiratory failure. This is important as many studies are criticized for assessing only a level of consciousness and selecting a population that is too heterogeneous to allow extrapolation of results. The successful use of diazepam, particularly in patients with end-organ dysfunction, is interesting and supports the use of a protocol-driven titration. The decreased use of NMBs in these patients is impressive, given the severity of their pulmonary illnesses. Single-dose NMB administration may be appealing given the widespread concern regarding prolonged paralysis after continuous infusions are stopped.

Clinical Implications

This observational study supports the administration of combined benzodiazepine-opioid sedation for patients receiving mechanical ventilation who require respiratory rate control. Aggressive dosing of these agents during the acute phase of illness may result in significant dosage reduction or complete avoidance of NMB therapy. In addition, establishing a protocol promotes familiarity with safe and effective agents and consistency in dosage adjustment, and may reduce the incidence of drug-related adverse events. This encourages better use of healthcare resources and reduces patient care costs.

13. Zarowitz BJ, Rudis MI, Lai K, et al. Retrospective pharmacoeconomic evaluation of dosing vecuronium by peripheral nerve stimulation versus standard clinical assessment in critically ill patients. *Pharmacotherapy.* 1997;17:327–332.

Study Sample

Seventy-seven patients admitted to a MICU and requiring vecuronium by continuous IV infusion during the period 1993 to 1995 were selected for evaluation.

Comparison Studied

This study was designed to assess the economic impact of vecuronium dosage adjustment by TOF monitoring compared to standard clinical monitoring in critically ill patients.

Study Procedures

Patients were randomized in a previous study (see Other References: 45) to receive vecuronium by continuous infusion with dosage adjustments performed by TOF monitoring (goal: 1 of 4 possible twitches or 90% blockade) or standard clinical assessment to determine the effect on respiratory and neuromuscular recovery from paralysis. Data were then evaluated retrospectively to examine the economic outcome produced by a more rapid recovery by calculating costs associated with drug administered, ICU care, and TOF monitoring. The cost of drug administered was calculated using an acquisition price of $2.09/mg. A median hourly cost of ICU care was determined from billing records for a sample of 20 patients previously studied (see Annotated Bibliography: 7). This included costs for providing mechanical ventilation, rehabilitation, ICU services, pharmacy services, neurological studies, labor, and overhead. A cost of $2.92 for each TOF assessment was ascertained via a time study of randomly selected and averaged TOF measurements performed by ICU pharmacists. These data were then extrapolated to determine the potential yearly cost savings for 198 patients receiving NMB therapy for more than 24 hours realized by dosage adjustment per routine TOF monitoring. One-way and multiway sensitivity analyses were used to assess model uncertainty.

Key Results

Patients receiving vecuronium dosage adjustments by TOF required a mean cumulative dose of 137 ± 106 mg vs 286 ± 247 mg received by controls. Mean drug costs per patient were $286 and $580, respectively. Extrapolation of these costs to 198 medical and surgical ICU patients revealed lower costs in the TOF group compared to controls ($56,693 vs $118,353). As the previous study identified prolonged recovery times in patients monitored by standard clinical methods (2198 hours) compared to those assessed by TOF (634 hours), the cost of ICU care during prolonged recovery would be increased ($118,681 vs $34,214, respectively). The average number of TOF assessments performed per patient was 7.8 ± 3.5 for a total cost of $23 per patient. The total cost of care per patient was calculated to be $1197 in the standard group and $459 in the TOF group, for a savings of $738 associated with TOF dosage adjustment. An estimated annual cost savings of $146,103 is anticipated using TOF-guided NMB dosage adjustments. A multiway sensitivity analysis demonstrated a 91% probability that dosage adjustment by TOF monitoring was less costly than standard dosing methods.

Study Strengths and Weaknesses

Monitoring NMB therapy via PNS and TOF methods has become an accepted practice in many ICUs. Despite this, many practitioners remain reluctant to incorporate it into their current practice given the lack of evidence demonstrating improved outcomes. This study is the first to identify enhanced therapeutic and economic outcomes associated with routine TOF monitoring and should stimulate development of protocols and practice guidelines involving TOF-initiated dosage adjustments.

Clinical Implications

Costs associated with critical illness, drug therapy, and potential complications are significant drains on healthcare resources. Routine TOF monitoring to individualize NMB therapy during critical illness may reduce dosage requirements and associated drug costs. Perhaps even more important is the potential therapeutic and economic impact on reducing the risk of prolonged recovery from NMB therapy. Healthcare practitioners should be knowledgeable regarding TOF technique, interpretation, and troubleshooting.

OTHER REFERENCES

1. Angelini G, Ketzler JT, Coursin DB. Use of propofol and other nonbenzodiazepine sedatives in the intensive care unit. *Crit Care Clin*. 2001;17:863–880.

2. Arbour RB. Propylene glycol toxicity related to high-dosed lorazepam infusion: case report and discussion. *Am J Crit Care*. 1999;5:499–506.

3. Arbour R. Propylene glycol toxicity occurs during low-dose infusions of lorazepam. *Crit Care Med*. 2003;31:664–665.

4. Arbour R. Continuous nervous system monitoring, EEG, the bispectral index, and neuromuscular transmission. *AACN Clin Iss*. 2003;14:185–207.

5. Arroliga AC, Shehab N, McCarthy K, et al. Relationship of continuous infusion lorazepam to serum propylene glycol concentration in critically ill. *Crit Care Med*. 2004;32:1709–1714.

6. Badr AE, Mychaskiw G, Eichhorn JH. Metabolic acidosis associated with a new formulation of propofol. *Anesthesiology*. 2001;94:536–538.

7. Bauer TM, Ritz R, Haberthur C. Prolonged sedation due to accumulation of conjugated metabolites of midazolam. *Lancet*. 1995;346:145–147.

8. Boyd AH, Eastwood NB, Parker CJR, et al. Comparison of the pharmacodynamics and pharmacokinetics of an infusion of cis-atracurium (51W89) or atracurium in critically ill patients undergoing mechanical ventilation in an intensive therapy unit. *Br J Anaesth*. 1996;76:382–388.

9. Camps AS, Rierea JASI, Vazquez DT, et al. Midazolam and 2% propofol in long-term sedation of traumatized, critically ill patients: efficacy and safety comparison. *Crit Care Med*. 2000;28:3612–3619.

10. Cawley MJ. Short-term lorazepam infusion and concern for propylene glycol toxicity: case report and review. *Pharmacother*. 2001;21:1140–1144.

11. Chan GLC, Matzke GR. Effects of renal insufficiency on the pharmacokinetics and pharmacodynamics of opioid analgesics. *Drug Intell Clin Pharm*. 1987;21:773–783.

12. Cheng EY. The cost of sedating and paralyzing the critically ill patient. *Crit Care Clin*. 1995;11:1005–1019.

13. Cremer OL, Moons KGM, Bouman EAC, et al. Long-term propofol infusion and cardiac failure in adult head-injured patients. *Lancet*. 2001;352:117–118.

14. Coursin DB, Macciolo GA. Dexmedetomidine. *Curr Opin Crit Care*. 2001;7:221–226.

15. DeJonghe B, Cook D, Griffith L., et al. Adaptation to the intensive care environment (ATICE): development and validation of a new sedation assessment instrument. *Crit Care Med*. 2003;31:2344–2354.

16. Devlin JW, Boleski G, Mlynarek M, et al. Motor activity assessment scale: a valid and reliable sedation scale for use with mechanically ventilated patients in an adult surgical intensive care unit. *Crit Care Med*. 1999;27:1271–1275.

17. Donnelly AJ, Lamb RE. Analgesic agents in critical care. *Crit Care Nurs Clin North Am.* 1993;5:281–295.

18. Earvin S, Fisher C, Merrell P, et al. The experience of four outcomes managers: an institutional approach to weaning patients from long-term mechanical ventilation. *Crit Care Nurs Clin N Am.* 2004;16:395–411.

19. Ely EW, Inouye SK, Bernard GR, et al. Delirium in mechanically ventilated patients. Validity and reliability of the confusion assessment method for the intensive care unit (CAM-ICU). *JAMA.* 2001;286:2703–2710.

20. Erstad BL, Cotugno CL. Management of alcohol withdrawal. *Am J Health Syst Pharm.* 1995;52:697–709.

21. Finley PR, Nolan PE. Precipitation of benzodiazepine withdrawal following sudden discontinuation of midazolam. *Ann Pharmacother.* 1989;23:151–152.

22. Fischer JR, Baer RK. Acute myopathy associated with combined use of corticosteroids and neuromuscular blocking agents. *Ann Pharmacother.* 1996;30:1437–1445.

23. Hall RI, Sandham D, Cardinal P, et al. Propofol vs midazolam for ICU sedation. *Chest.* 2001;119:1151–1159.

24. Higgins TL, Yared JP, Estafanous FG, et al. Propofol vs midazolam for intensive care unit sedation after coronary artery bypass grafting. *Crit Care Med.* 1994;22:1415–1423.

25. Jensen D, Justic M. An algorithm to distinguish the need for sedative, anxiolytic, and analgesic agents. *Dimens Crit Car Nurs.* 1995;14:58–65.

26. Lewis KS, Whipple JK, Michael KA, et al. Effect of analgesic treatment on the physiological consequences of acute pain. *Am J Hosp Pharm.* 1994;51:1539–1554.

27. MacLaren R, Plamondon JM, Ramsay KB, et al. A prospective evaluation of empiric versus protocol-based sedation and analgesia. *Pharmacother.* 2000;20:662–672.

28. Marik PE, Kaufman D. The effects of neuromuscular paralysis on systemic and splanchnic oxygen utilization. *Chest.* 1996;109:1038–4101.

29. Nasraway SA Jr. Use of sedative medications in the intensive care unit. *Semin Respir Crit Care Med.* 2001;22:165–174.

30. Op de Coul AAW, Lambregts PCLA, Koeman J, et al. Neuromuscular complications in patients given Pavulon (pancuronium bromide) during artificial ventilation. *Clin Neurol Neurosurg.* 1985;87:17–22.

31. Parker MG, Fraser GL, Watson DM, et al. Removal of propylene glycol and correction of increased osmolar gap by hemodialysis in a patient on high-dose lorazepam therapy. *Intensive Care Med.* 2002;28:81–84.

32. Parker MM, Schubert W, Shelhamer JH. Perceptions of a critically ill patient experiencing therapeutic paralysis in an ICU. *Crit Care Med.* 1984;12:69–71.

33. Ramsay MAE, Savage TM, Simpson BRJ, et al. Controlled sedation with alphaxolone-alphadolone. *Br Med J.* 1974;22:656–659.

34. Riker RR, Fraser GL, Cox PM. Continuous infusion of haloperidol controls agitation in critically ill patients. *Crit Care Med.* 1994;22:433–440.

35. Riker RR, Fraser GL. Adverse events associated with sedatives, analgesics and other drugs that provide patient comfort in the intensive care unit. *Pharmacother.* 2005;25:8S–18S.

36. Ronan KP, Gallagher TJ, George B, et al. Comparison of propofol and midazolam for sedation in intensive care unit patients. *Crit Care Med.* 1995;23:286–293.

37. Rudis MI, Sikora CA, Angus E, et al. A prospective, randomized, controlled evaluation of peripheral nerve stimulation vs standard clinical dosing of neuromuscular blocking agents in critically ill patients. *Crit Care Med.* 1997;225:575–583.

38. Sessler CN, Gosnell MS, Grap MJ, et al. The Richmond agitation-sedation scale. Validity and reliability in adult intensive care unit patients. *Am J Resp Crit Care.* 2002;166:1338–1344.

39. Sessler CN. Sedation, analgesia, and neuromuscular blockade for high-frequency oscillatory ventilation. *Crit Care Med.* 2005;33(Suppl):S209–216.

40. Shelly MP, Mendel L, Park GP. Failure of critically ill patients to metabolize midazolam. *Anaesthesia.* 1987;42:619–626.

41. Stelow EB, Johari VP, Smith SA, et al. Propofol-associated rhabdomyolysis with cardiac involvement in adults: chemical and anatomic findings. *Clin Chem.* 2000;46:577–581.

42. Susla GM. Neuromuscular blocking agents in critical care. *Crit Care Clin North Am.* 1993;5:297–311.

43. Tesar GE, Murray GB, Cassem NH. Use of high-dose intravenous haloperidol in the treatment of agitated cardiac patients. *J Clin Psychopharmacol.* 1985;5:344–347.

44. Tharatt R, Allen R, Albertson T. Pressure controlled, inverse ratio ventilation in severe adult respiratory failure. *Chest.* 1988;94:756–762.

45. Vender JS, Szokol JW, Murphy GS, et al. Sedation, analgesia and neuromuscular blockade in sepsis: an evidence-based review. *Crit Care Med.* 2004;32(Suppl):S554–S561.

46. Volles DF. More on usability of lorazepam admixtures for continuous infusion. *Am J Health-Syst Pharm.* 1996;53:2753–2754.

47. Wild LR. Neuromuscular blocking agents in the critically ill patient: neither sedating nor pain relieving. *AACN Clin Iss.* 1991;2(4):778–787.

48. Woods JC, Mion LC, Connor JT, et al. Severe agitation among ventilated medical intensive care patients: frequency, characteristics, and outcomes. *Intensive Care Med.* 2004;30:1066–1072.

49. Yaucher NE, Fish JT, Smith HW, et al. Propylene glycol associated renal toxicity from lorazepam infusion. *Pharmacother.* 2003;231094–1099.

50. Young CC, Prielipp RC. Benzodiazepines in the intensive care unit. *Cir Care Clin.* 2001;17:843–862.

51. Diprivan [package insert]. Wilmington, Del: AstraZeneca Pharmaceuticals, LP; 2004.

52. Tschida SJ, Hoey LL, Vance-Bryan K. The impact of practice guidelines on prescribing patterns of nondepolarizing neuromuscular blocking agents. *Pharmacother.* 1996;16:89–9904.

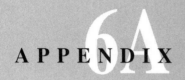

Drugs Used for Sedation and Analgesia in the ICU

Drug	Pharmacologic Properties	Route	Usual Dose[1] (minutes)	Onset (hours)	Half-life	Comments
Diazepam (Valium)	Sedative, anxiolytic, amnetic, anticonvulsant, muscle relaxant	IV	2.5 to 10 mg every 3 to 4 h	1 to 5	20 to 100	Painful IV injection; thrombophlebitis risk; active metabolite prolongs effect. Each mL contains 5 mg diazepam and 0.4 mL (400 mg) propylene glycol (PG) solvent.
Lorazepam (Ativan)	See Diazepam	IV, IM	1 to 4 mg every 2 to 4 h or 1 to 4 mg/h by continuous infusion (CI)	5 to 10	10 to 20	No active metabolite. Each mL contains 2 mg lorazepam and 0.8 mL (830 mg) PG. Accumulation of PG may be associated with hyperosmolarity (osmol gap), metabolic acidosis, due to accumulation of metabolites lactic and pyruvic acids.
Midazolam (Versed)	See Diazepam	IV	0.5 to 3 mg every 1 to 2 h or 1 to 15 mg/h by CI	1 to 5	2.5	Hepatic or renal impairment during critical illness have been associated with prolonged sedation.
Morphine	Analgesic, sedative	IV	2 to 10 mg 1 to 4 h or 2 to 20 mg/h by CI	15 to 60	2 to 4	Hypotension, respiratory depression, GI hypomotility, nausea. Duration of sedative effect may be prolonged in patients with renal impairment resulting from metabolite accumulation.
Fentanyl (Sublimaze)	Analgesic	IV	50 to 100 μg every 1 to 4 h or 50 to 300 g/h by CI	1 to 5	2 to 6	Adverse effects similar to morphine, but hypotension less prominent. Half-life increases with repeated dosing due to tissue saturation.

(Continues)

Drug	Pharmacologic Properties	Route	Usual Dose[1] (minutes)	Onset (hours)	Half-life	Comments
Propofol (Diprivan)	Sedative, hypnotic, anesthetic	IV	5 to 80 mcg/kg/min	0.5 to 1.0	0.5 to 1.0	Hypotension, bradycardia, pain can occur with peripheral IV administration; Monitor serum triglycerides and fat calories; and for increased infection risk. Propofol infusion syndrome associated with doses exceeding the upper limit recommended for > 48 hours, as well as metabolic acidosis, elevated triglycerides, rhabdomyolysis, bradycardia, hypotension, leading to asystole and death.
Haloperidol (Haldol)	Antipsychotic, mild sedative, antiemetic	IV	Rapid control: 1 to 20 mg every 15 min; Maintenance: 5 to 20 mg every 1 to 6 h *or* 10 to 40 mg/h by CI	10 to 20	12 to 36	Potential synergistic effects can occur with benzodiazepines. QTc prolongation may be associated with torsades de pointes; other adverse effects include extrapyramidal signs and neuroleptic malignant syndrome.
Dexmedetomidine (Precedex)	Sedative, anxiolytic, analgesic	IV	1.0 µg/kg over 10 minutes, then 0.2 to 0.7 µg/kg/h by CI (doses up to 2.5 µg/kg/h have been required to produce sedative effects)	18 to 24	2	Hypotension and bradycardia associated with loading dose has led to elimination of or smaller loading dose (0.4 g/kg) or slowing the infusion rate. Not recommended for > 24 hr, but studies suggest safety for up to 7 days.

[1] Loading doses recommended before continuous infusion; dosage requirements will vary among patients; titrate to desired response; increase infusion rates after additional bolus doses to maintain new steady state levels.

Note: Use of reversal agents, such as naloxone or flumazenil, are not recommended after prolonged opioid or benzodiazepine use, respectively, due to the risk of precipitating withdrawal symptoms. If needed, a single dose of flumazenil (0.15 mg) may be administered to test for oversedation after several days of benzodiazepine therapy.

Compiled from Annotated Bibliography: 4; Other References: 1, 2, 6, 7, 11, 13, 14, 17, 29, 35, 39, 40, 43, 45, 46, 50.

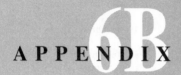
Sedation Assessment Scales With Validity and Reliability in Adult Patients

Ramsey Scale	Sedation–Agitation Scale[4]	Motor Activity Assessment Scale[2]	Richmond Agitation Sedation Scale[5,6]
6 No response	1 Unarousable (minimal or no response to noxious stimuli, does not communicate or follow commands	0 Unresponsive (does not move in response to noxious stimuli)	−5 Unresponsive (no response voice or physical stimulation)
5 Patient asleep with a sluggish response to a light glabellar tap	2 Very sedated (arouses to physical stimuli but does not communicate or follow commands, may move spontaneously	1 Responseive only to noxious stimuli (open eyes or raises eyebrows or turns head towards stimulus ormoves limb in response to noxious stimulus	−4 Deep sedation (no response to voice or physical stimulation
4 Patient asleep with a brisk response to a light glabellar tap	3 Sedated (difficult to arouse, awakens to verbal stimuli or gentle shaking but drifts off again, follows simple commands	2 Responsive to touch or name (openeyes or raises eyebrows or turnshead toward stimulus or moves limb when touched or when name is loudly spoken)	−3 Moderate sedation (any movement but no eye contact to voice)
3 Patient responds to commands only	4 Calm and cooperative (calm, awakens easily, follows commands)	3 Calm and cooperative (no external stimulus is required to elicit purposeful movement and patient follows commands)	−2 Light sedation (briefly, less than 10 seconds, awakening with eye contact to voice)
2 Patient cooperative, oriented and tranquil	5 Agitated (anxious or mildly agitated, attempting to site up, calms down to verbal instructions)	4 Restless and cooperative (no external stimulus is required to elicit movement and patient is is picking at sheets or tubes or uncovering self and follows commands	−1 Drowsy (not fully alert, but has sustained, more than 10 sec. awakening with eye contact to voice)
1 Patient anxious or agitated or both	6 Very agitated (does not calmb, despite frequent verbal reminding of limits; requires physical restraints, bites endotracheal tube)	5 Agitated (no external stimulus is required to elicit movement and patient is attempting to sit up or moves limbs out of bed and does not consistently follow commands)	0 Alert and calm
	7 Dangerous agitation (pulling at endotracheal tub, trying to remove catheter; climbing over bed rail, striking at staff, thrashing side to side	6 Dangerously agitated, uncooperative (no external stimulus is required to elicit movement and patient is pulling at tubes or catheters or thrashing side to side or striking at staff or trying to climb out of bed and does not calm down when asked)	1 Restless (anxious or apprehensive but movements not aggressive or vigorous)

(Continues)

Ramsey Scale	Sedation– Agitation Scale[4]	Motor Activity Assessment Scale[2]	Richmond Agitation Sedation Scale[5,6]
			2 Agitated (frequent non-purposeful movement or patient-ventilator dysynchronoy)
			3 Very agitated (pulls on or removes tubes or catheters or has aggressive behavior toward staff
			4 Combative (overly combative or violent, immediate danger to staff

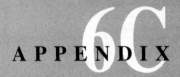
Neuromuscular Blocking Drugs Used in the ICU

Drug	Structural Class	Initial Dose	Elimination	Duration (min)	Comments
Pancuronium (**Pavulon**)	Aminosteroid	0.1 to 0.2 mg/kg every 1 to 3 h *or* 0.1 mg/kg loading dose (LD); 0.03 to 0.1 mg/kg/h by CI	Renal: 40% to 60% Biliary: 10% Hepatic: 30% to 40%	90–100	Magnitude and duration of blockade may be increased with repeated dosing; thus, lower maintenance doses may be required to achieve desired degree of blockade.
Vecuronium (**Norcuron**)	Aminosteroid	0.1 mg/kg LD, 0.05 to 0.1 mg/kg/h by CI	Hepatic: 15% to 25% Biliary: 40% Hepatic: 35% to 45%	35–45	More commonly associated with prolonged blockade following discontinuation
Atracurium (**Tracrium**)	Benzylisoquinolinium	0.3 to 0.5 mg/kg LD; 0.3 to 1.0 mg/kg/h by CI	Hoffmann elimination (produces metabolite laudanosine); plasma ester hydrolysis	25–35	Potential disadvantages: dose- and rate-related histamine release; seizures due to laudanosine accumulation with prolonged use in renal, or hepatic dysfunction.
Cisatracurium (**Nimbex**)	Benzylisoquinolinium	0.15 to 0.20 mg/kg; 0.03 to 0.2 mg/kg/h by CI	Hofmann elimination	45–60	Decreased laudanosine production due to increased drug potency; less histamine release

Note: Before initiating NMB therapy, adequate analgesia and sedation should be verified by clinical assessment; patients receiving NMB therapy should monitored by clinical, TOF, and respiratory waveform assessments.

Compiled from Annotated Bibliography: 7, 11; Other References: 22, 30, 39, 40, 42, 45.